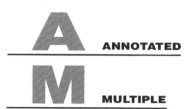 **ANNOTATED**

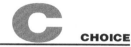 **MULTIPLE**

CHOICE

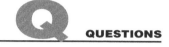 **QUESTIONS**

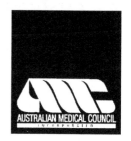

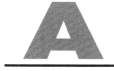 ANNOTATED

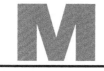 MULTIPLE

 CHOICE

 QUESTIONS

Editorial panel

Vernon C Marshall
Arthur Lindesay Clark
Anthony J Buzzard
Peter Devitt
David Gillies
Reuben Glass
Frank Hume
Barry McGrath
Roger J Pepperell
Bryan Yeo

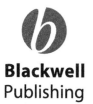

Blackwell
Publishing

© 1997 by Blackwell Publishing Ltd

First printed 1997
Reprinted 2000
Reprinted 2002
Reprinted 2004
Reprinted 2007
Reprinted 2008
Reprinted 2009
Reprinted 2010
Reprinted 2012

Blackwell Publishing, Inc., 350 Main Street, Malden, Massachusetts 02148-5020, USA
Blackwell Publishing Ltd, 9600 Garsington Road, Oxford OX4 2DQ, UK
John Wiley & Sons (Australia), 155 Cremorne Street, Richmond, Victoria 3121, Australia

The right of the Author to be identified as the Author of this Work has been asserted in accordance with the Copyright Act 1968 and all later amendments.

Cataloguing-in-Publication Data

Annotated multiple-choice questions

Includes index
ISBN 978 0 86793 377 2

Medicine – Examinations. 2. Multiple-choice Examinations. 1. Australian Medical Council.

610.76

For further information on Blackwell Publishing, visit our website:
http://www.blackwellpublishing.com

The publisher's policy is to use permanent paper from mills that operate a sustainable forestry policy, and which has been manufactured from pulp processed using acid-free and elementary chlorine-free practices. Furthermore, the publisher ensures that the text paper and cover board used have met acceptable environmental accreditation standards.

Design and typesetting by Stephanie Thompson Graphic Design

TABLE OF
CONTENTS

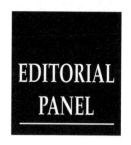

Barry McGrath

MD,FRACP

Associate Professor of Medicine, Monash University
Chairman, Board of Postgraduate Studies,
Monash Medical Centre
Senior Examiner in Medicine, Board of Examiners,
Australian Medical Council

Roger J Pepperell

MD,MGO,FRACP,
FRCOG,FRACOG

Professor of Obstetrics and Gynaecology, University of Melbourne
Consultant Obstetrician and Gynaecologist,
Royal Women's Hospital
Consultant Gynaecologist, Royal Children's Hospital
Consultant Obstetrician, Royal Melbourne Hospital
Senior Examiner in Obstetrics and Gynaecology,
Board of Examiners, Australian Medical Council

Bryan Yeo

FRACS,FRCS

Senior Lecturer in Surgery, University of New South Wales
Surgeon, Department of Surgery, Prince of Wales Hospital
Senior Examiner in Surgery, Board of Examiners,
Australian Medical Council

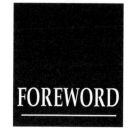

FOREWORD

The lack of familiarity with the standards and requirements of medical practice in Australia has been identified as one of the major obstacles confronting overseas-trained doctors seeking registration. The Australian Medical Council (AMC) has prepared this book to assist overseas-trained doctors who are preparing for the AMC examination. The Council believes that this book will be a valuable guide and self-assessment tool. It also illustrates best-practice principles for a wide range of medical conditions found in the Australian community.

John S Horvath
President
May 1997

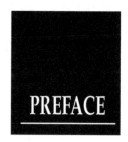

PREFACE

The Australian Medical Council (AMC) is responsible for the accreditation of Australian university medical courses and for the assessment of overseas-trained doctors applying for registration to practise within Australia. Assessment is via an initial multiple choice question (MCQ) examination and by subsequent clinical examination.

The MCQ examination for overseas-trained doctors consists of a test of medical knowledge equivalent to that attained by graduates of Australian medical schools who are about to commence intern training. The MCQ examination assessment aims to test the principles and practice of medicine in the fields of internal medicine, surgery, paediatrics, psychiatry and obstetrics and gynaecology. Most questions are designed to reflect common conditions seen in Australian clinical practice. Questions cover a range that includes prevention and pathogenesis, clinical features, laboratory findings, differential diagnosis, management and outcome. Most aim to test basic or essential knowledge; a smaller number relate to less common conditions that illustrate important principles. Questions may consist solely of written material or may incorporate radiographs or scans, colour photographs and line drawings.

This book contains a selection of multiple choice questions from the AMC Examination Bank in each of the disciplines, with accompanying commentaries. They have been chosen to give a representative overview of each of the above fields. All questions have been used previously in an AMC examination and have been subjected to computed statistical analysis to test for reliability, validity and degree of difficulty.

The Board of Examiners believes that this selection, and the accompanying discussions and commentaries, will help candidates in preparation for the AMC examinations. The AMC questions have been developed from sources which include contributions from Australian medical schools and from overseas. They are derived from a range of texts as well as from continuing review and consensus of best clinical practice. The level of difficulty of these questions has been maintained at the level attained by Australian graduates by commissioning questions from those who regularly provide questions for Australian medical school examinations and by regularly testing samples of the AMC questions in the appropriate Australian university examinations.

Their themes are thus representative of curricula of medical schools of universities within Australia.

All medical students should thus find the book of considerable value as an educational resource in preparation for their clinical assessments, as should postgraduate trainees preparing for higher degrees across the spectrum of general and specialist practice.

Arthur Lindesay Clark
Past Chairman, Board of Examiners
Australian Medical Council

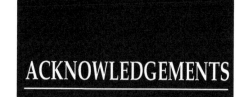

ACKNOWLEDGEMENTS

The Editorial Panel wishes to acknowledge the support of the academic and clinical staff of the Australian medical schools who provided assistance, advice and contributions to this book. We are unaware of any of the material having prior copyright and apologise for any omission in this regard.

We are also grateful to Ian Frank and the staff of the Australian Medical Council (AMC) secretariat and, in particular, to Avril Jordan and Rommy Poxleitner for their efforts in transcribing the raw material into the final form of the book.

Finally, a special note of thanks is due to Susan Buick of the AMC who has been a key part of the project since its inception. Her tireless efforts and assistance to the Editorial Panel in reviewing the MCQ banks and compiling the commentaries, as well as her role in coordinating the production of the manuscript, have ensured the successful completion of the project.

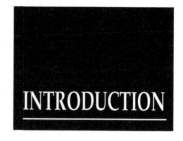

The Multiple Choice Question (MCQ) Examination

The Australian Medical Council (AMC) wishes candidates to be fully aware of the details of the examination and its assessment. Multiple choice testing methods used by the AMC aim to produce formats which validly assess a broad sample of content and of problem-solving clinical skills, efficiently and reliably. Multiple Choice Questions (MCQ) used include patient scenarios, clinical data and visual material in their stems. Many are structured to require analysis, interpretation and evaluation in their completion. Multiple choice testing comprises only one component of the total assessment system; the subsequent clinical assessment tests more fully additional clinical skills.

Classification and Mix of Questions

The mix of questions and commentaries in this book follows the pattern set for individual examinations and is broadly representative of the syllabus.

The questions are grouped into five disciplines: Medicine (ME), Surgery (SU), Paediatrics (PA), Obstetrics and Gynaecology (OG) and Psychiatry (PS). Approximately one-third of the questions are medical, approximately one-third relate to childhood and women's health, approximately one-quarter relate to surgical topics and approximately one-tenth are specific to psychiatry. Questions relating to the community and to general practice are spread over all disciplines, as are those dealing with the ethical, social and historical aspects of medicine. The proportions, in individual examinations, are approximately 35%, 25%, 15%, 15%, 10% for ME, SU, PA, OG and PS questions respectively.

Questions are classified across disciplines by the function or process involved as follows:

Function/process
A   Aetiology, epidemiology, genetics
B   Anatomy, physiology, pathology, pathogenesis
C   Clinical manifestations
D   Diagnosis and investigations
E   Treatment and prevention of disease
F   Complications and outcome
G   Ethical, legal, social, economic, humanistic, historical aspects

Questions are further grouped into principal and associated systems, regions and sub-specialties as follows:

Systems/regions/subspecialties
1   Integument/dermatology
2   Head and neck/eye/ENT
3   Nervous system/neurology
4   Musculoskeletal/orthopaedics/rheumatology
5   Circulatory system/heart/vessels
6   Respiratory system/lungs/chest wall
7   Gastrointestinal system/abdomen/abdominal wall
8   Breast/endocrine system
9   Reproductive system (male/female)
10   Haemopoietic system/haematology/blood/blood products

11   Renal system/urology
12   Mental state/intellectual function/behavioural problems
13   Major psychiatric disorders/drug and alcohol abuse
14   Developmental abnormalities
15   Nutrition/metabolism
16   Infectious diseases
17   Clinical pharmacology
18   Clinical oncology
19   Clinical immunology
20   Critical care/anaesthesia
21   Community medicine/public health

Results of investigations are usually expressed in *Système International* (SI) units. Normal values are indicated in parentheses. Abbreviations and normal values are as outlined in the publication *Manual of Use and Interpretation of Pathology Tests* (Royal College of Pathologists of Australasia, ISBN 0959 335 528).

Types of Questions and Marking

Questions are of two styles or formats (types A and J). In type A questions, one correct answer must be selected from five possible responses to the stem. Type J questions also consist of a stem and five responses, of which one or more may be correct. All type J questions will have at least one correct response.

Type A questions score either 1 or 0. The maximum mark for each type J question is again 1, as for Type A. If candidates answer all five responses without error, they score 1 mark. If there is one error the question is scored 0.6. If there are two errors the question is scored 0.2. If there are three, four or five errors, no mark is scored for the question.

Analysis and Review of Questions

The MCQ examination is marked by computer by an independent university based educational testing centre on behalf of the AMC. Questions are analysed and reviewed after each examination.

Type A ('one from five')

These comprise the great majority of questions used. The percentage of candidates answering each question correctly (degree of difficulty) is noted as is the percentage scoring distractors as correct. A statistical index is calculated to indicate the question's ability to discriminate between candidates who scored well overall and those who performed poorly. This discrimination index compares how candidates obtaining the correct answer in each individual question perform in relation to their overall mark and rank order.

Type A questions are usually considered satisfactory and are retained if analysis indicates that the range of candidates answering the question correctly was satisfactory (degree of difficulty ranging from approximately 20 to 80%), that the distractors attracted an appropriate number of responses and that the performance correlation between high and low-scoring candidates was appropriate. Questions may be retained when the proportion of correct answers is outside the range of 20–80% if other characteristics are satisfactory and if the question is considered to cover an important topic. Questions are considered for revision when they are found to have either a very high or low degree of difficulty, when they discriminate poorly across rank order, when individual distractors receive high responses and are judged too difficult or ambiguous or when a distractor is a poor one because it attracts a response from very few candidates. The analysis can also help indicate when the subject matter of the question is not well known by candidates overall or when guessing may be contributing significantly to the spread of answers.

Type J ('multiple true–false')

For type J questions each response is assessed as is the mean degree of difficulty of the question, in deciding on revision or retention of the question.

Interpretation of Questions

Candidates taking MCQ and clinical examinations can be troubled by the wording of questions, as when asked which features are *classical, characteristic* or *typical* of certain diseases, whether events are *likely, frequent, common, unusual* or *rare* and whether findings are expected in the *majority* or *minority* of cases or in *few* or *many* patients.

Many terms, such as *common* and *frequent* and other synonyms and antonyms, are not absolute in themselves. They have clearest meanings when used to compare and contrast two or more events. Frequencies are then compared by the qualifications *more* or *most*, *less* or *least*.

- 'In the Australian population, blood group O is *more common* than blood group AB.'
- 'In patients with appendicitis, vomiting is a *less common* symptom than abdominal pain.'
- 'Of the following cancers (bladder, breast, colon, lung, pancreas) cancer of the lung is the *most common* cancer in Australia per million of population.'

In everyday speech, words such as *common* are used less specifically and usage varies with context. For example 'influenza attacks are *common* this winter'; a comparison with other winters is implied but not stated. 'Influenza is a *common* illness.' 'Cancer is a *common* cause of death.' Neither of these statements implies a precise frequency; nor do they imply that influenza or cancer cause more than half of all illnesses or deaths. *Common* used as an isolated descriptor becomes clearer if additionally qualified: e*xtremely common, very common, moderately common. Moderately common* still can signify a wide range of frequencies, but a *very common* event would be expected to occur with a frequency well over 50%. An *extremely common* event would be almost invariable and an *extremely uncommon* event numerically very small, viz:

'Of the various blood groups in an Australian population, O (45%) and A (40%) are *common*, B is *uncommon* (9%) and AB is *extremely uncommon* (3%). Rhesus positivity is *very common* (85%) and Rhesus negativity is *uncommon* (15%).'

When applied to several events conjointly, *common* can signify differing percentages for each.

Question: *Common* clinical features of appendicitis include which of the following: pain, abdominal tenderness, anorexia, vomiting, fever, convulsions?

Answer: Convulsions are *rare* in appendicitis. Each of the other features is *common*; anorexia, abdominal tenderness and pain are, however, *more common* than vomiting and fever.

The gist of the question is made clearer if it is expressed as follows:

'Clinical features *characteristic* (*typical*) *of* appendicitis include which of the following?'

Convulsions would not be included within a standard description or definition deemed characteristic of appendicitis; the other features would.

For the above reasons, it is difficult to give numeric percentages (even approximate ones) to such words as *common* or *often*. We have preferred, wherever possible, to additionally qualify them or to use clear comparisons: 'A occurs *more often* than B'. However, we append a glossary of suggested definitions and, where appropriate, approximate percentages as a guide to interpretation of questions, in an attempt to minimise language problems with stems and responses.

Several terms admit of no degrees or comparatives and are NOT qualifiable by more, less, very or moderately. Examples are *unique, invariable, at all times, always, never, ideal*. If required, they can be suitably qualified by *almost*.

It is important for candidates to be aware that in clinical practice these terms, with their ranges and nuances of likelihood, often comprise steps in deductive pathways of diagnostic problem solving by probability prediction and probability analysis. Subjective probabilities and predictions need, however, to be constantly scrutinised in the light of objective data; such scrutiny helps to confirm or refute their reliability. The Board of Examiners, by continuously reviewing and revising questions, aims to minimise confusion or ambiguity in stems and responses.

GLOSSARY

Term	Definition	Approximate percentage
Characteristic of, typical of, associated with]	Significantly more frequent than in the general population; within the definition.	—
Uncharacteristic, atypical, not associated with]	Significantly less frequent than in the general population; outside the definition.	—
Invariable	At all times	100
Essential	Indispensable	100
Necessary	Indispensable	100
Requisite	Indispensable	100
Always	At all times	100
Never	Not at all	0
Nearly always	At almost all times	>90
Almost always		
The majority, many	More than half	>50
The great majority	Very much more than half	>80
The minority, few	Less than half	<50
Predominate	The main element, in the ascendancy	>50
Usual	More than half	>50
Unusual	Not usual, less than half	<50
Likely	To be expected	>50
Unlikely	Not to be expected	<50
Probable	More likely than not	>50
Improbable	Not likely	<50
More, less	Greater or smaller in amount	—
Most, least	Greatest or smallest in amount	—
Extremely common	Almost always	>90
Very common	Very much more than half	>80
Common, uncommon]	Preferably qualified and used in	Variable
Frequent, rare	comparison to other options	Variable
Often, seldom]		Variable
Can, may, possible	To be possible, not impossible	>0

Commentaries

Commentaries explanatory of correct and incorrect responses have been prepared by a multidisciplinary editorial committee of the AMC Board of Examiners, with advice from senior examiners in each discipline. The commentary sections relating to the correct response(s) are emboldened for emphasis. Historical notes of eponyms are included for their interest. They should not be taken to indicate that the AMC expects candidates for the AMC examinations to have such detailed knowledge of medical history.

Disclaimer

Reference texts are listed for further reading and as additional guides to study. The editors and publishers have made every effort to ensure that the answers and commentaries are in accord throughout with current knowledge and practice. However, clinical practice, as well as the core basic clinical sciences, is constantly evolving and today's incontrovertible facts can become tomorrow's outworn shibboleths. Furthermore, and especially in controversial areas which comprise the leavening in our daily medical bread, normal variations in emphasis will always ensure that readers, like patients, who seek multiple opinions from numerous sources, may ultimately find an opinion more in agreement with their own wishes than convention dictates.

Vernon C Marshall
Chairman, Editorial Committee

Multiple Choice Questions

Medicine
Questions

TYPE

A

Questions ME-Q1 to ME-Q125

- Type A questions consist of a stem and five responses
- **<u>One</u>** correct answer must be selected from five possible responses to the stem

ME-Q1

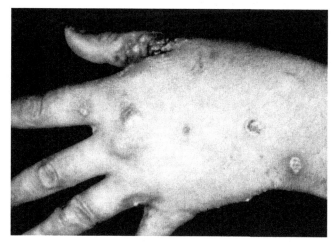

Figure 1

The skin lesions shown in the accompanying photograph (Figure 1) were found on the hands of a 73-year-old nursing home patient. She has been noted to be constantly scratching the lesions and appears poorly cared for. The MOST APPROPRIATE treatment would be

A topical steroids.
B erythromycin.
C gamma benzene hexachloride.
D miconazole cream.
E prednisone, 60 mg daily.

ME-Q2

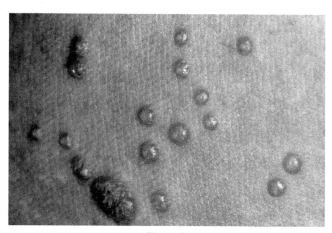

Figure 2

The lesions shown in the accompanying photograph (Figure 2) were observed on the chest wall of a 6-year-old child. The skin in other areas appears normal. The MOST LIKELY cause would be

A warts.
B herpes simplex.
C chicken pox.
D molluscum contagiosum.
E an allergic reaction.

ME-Q3

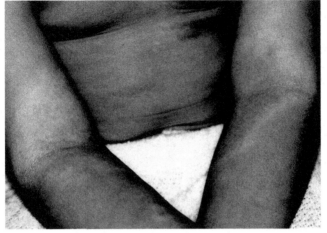

Figure 3

The skin lesions in the accompanying photograph (Figure 3) would BEST be treated by

A   moisture and wet dressing.
B   hot bathing.
C   oral steroids.
D   tar cream.
E   salicylic acid cream.

ME-Q4

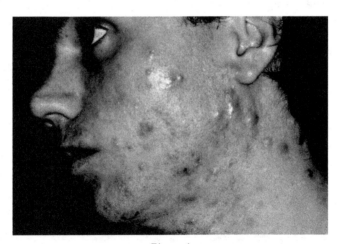

Figure 4

The MOST APPROPRIATE treatment for the lesions on the face and neck of the patient shown in the accompanying photograph (Figure 4), which have been unresponsive to conventional therapy, would be

A   benzyl peroxide.
B   isotretinoin (Roaccutane®).
C   tetracycline.
D   0.5% cortisone cream.
E   occlusive mascara.

ME-Q5

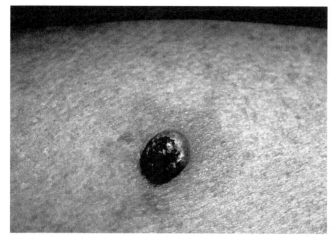

Figure 5

The lesion shown in the accompanying photograph (Figure 5) was found in a 28-year-old female patient who had a successful renal transplant 1 year ago. The MOST APPROPRIATE treatment would be

A no active treatment and await resolution.

B surgical removal.

C radiotherapy.

D removal with liquid nitrogen.

E topical podophyllin.

ME-Q6

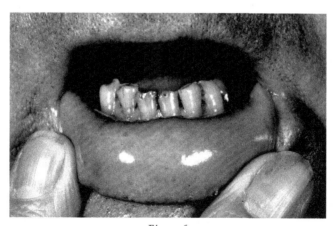

Figure 6

The lesions shown in the accompanying photograph (Figure 6) are likely to be ASSOCIATED with

A liver disease.

B small bowel tumours.

C anaemia.

D polycythaemia.

E consumption of photosensitising drugs.

ME-Q7

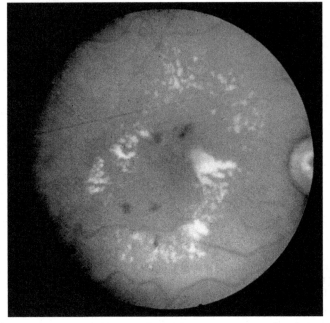

Figure 7

A 47-year-old Aborigine complains of blurring of vision. His blood pressure is normal, he smokes 40 cigarettes per day and drinks 100 grams of alcohol per day. There is no history of chest pain. On examination his blood pressure is 140/80 mmHg. The fundus is shown in the accompanying picture (Figure 7). The MOST LIKELY cause is

    A previous hypertension.

    B alcohol amblyopia.

    C a secondary cerebral tumour.

    D diabetes mellitus.

    E *Toxocara canis*.

ME-Q8

A 65-year-old overweight man complains of recent misty vision on sunny days. His vision, when tested, is 6/18 right and left. Which of the following is the MOST LIKELY basis of his complaint?

    A Chronic simple glaucoma.

    B Myopia.

    C Cataract.

    D Macular degeneration.

    E Diabetic retinopathy.

ME-Q9

Which of the following is LEAST likely to be a complication of chronic otitis media?

    A Cholesteatoma.

    B Decreased auditory acuity.

    C Meningitis.

    D Otosclerosis.

    E Thrombosis of the lateral venous sinus.

ME-Q10

A palpable and apparently solitary nodule in the thyroid is MOST COMMONLY

A a solitary cyst.
B part of a multinodular goitre.
C an adenoma of the thyroid.
D a thyroid carcinoma.
E localised Hashimoto disease.

ME-Q11

Wernicke encephalopathy is CHARACTERISED by

A neck stiffness.
B ophthalmoplegia.
C Grand mal epilepsy.
D extensor plantar responses.
E all of the above features.

ME-Q12

In a stroke, a CLEAR DISTINCTION between haemorrhage and thrombosis can be made on which of the following points?

A The degree of loss of consciousness.
B The progress of clinical features.
C The abruptness of onset.
D The presence or absence of headache.
E None of the above.

ME-Q13

Muscle tone is usually increased in lesions of all the following structures EXCEPT

A spinal cord.
B corticospinal pathways.
C cerebellum.
D basal ganglia.
E internal capsule.

ME-Q14

A 60-year-old male has had three episodes of transient left monocular blindness and right hemianaesthesia. There is a soft bruit in the neck on the left and Doppler studies show a 25% stenosis of the internal carotid artery at the bifurcation. The currently RECOMMENDED MANAGEMENT would be

A immediate carotid endarterectomy.
B carotid endarterectomy after 2 months.
C aspirin, 100 mg each day.
D warfarin (INR 3.5–4.0).
E intracarotid streptokinase infusion.

ME-Q15

A 50-year-old woman experiences an episode of shimmering lights, which spread over her left visual field during a 10 min period, leaving her with blurred vision that resolves after approximately 30 min. Which is the MOST LIKELY diagnosis?

A Migrainous aura.
B Transient carotid ischaemic attack.
C Vertebrobasilar insufficiency.
D Retrobulbar neuritis.
E Epilepsy.

ME-Q16

A 65-year-old man presents with a sudden, persisting monocular visual loss. There is a history of continual ipsilateral headache for the past 12 months. What laboratory test is MOST RELEVANT to the likely diagnosis?

A Urinalysis.

B Complete blood count.

C Erythrocyte sedimentation rate.

D Chest X-ray.

E Cerebral CT scan.

ME-Q17

When the eyes of a semiconscious accident victim are examined it is found that the right pupil is dilated and does not react to light shone into either eye. The left pupil reacts to light shone directly into the left eye but not to light shone into the right eye. This could be DUE TO injury to the

A left optic nerve and left third nerve.

B right third nerve alone.

C right third nerve and left optic nerve.

D right optic nerve and left third nerve.

E right optic nerve and right third nerve.

ME-Q18

The SUDDEN ONSET of a left third nerve palsy and a right hemiplegia involving the face, arm and leg can be explained by which one of the following?

A Left internal capsule infarct.

B Left medullary infarct.

C Right upper cervical spinal cord infarct.

D Left midbrain infarct.

E Left occipital lobe infarct.

ME-Q19

A 50-year-old man has a 12 month history of episodes of severe vertigo and vomiting; between episodes he is asymptomatic. He has noticed progressively increasing deafness in his right ear with mild tinnitus. Examination reveals that, except for a nerve deafness in one ear, there are no abnormalities in the third, fourth, fifth, sixth or seventh cranial nerves during an acute attack of vertigo. The MOST LIKELY diagnosis is

A acoustic neuroma.

B vertebrobasilar insufficiency.

C Ménière disease.

D vestibular neuronitis.

E benign positional vertigo.

ME-Q20

A 67-year-old man presents with a history of progressive dysphagia and hoarseness over the preceding 24 h. On examination there is a right Horner syndrome and the right side of the palate does not elevate on phonation. The right gag reflex is absent and the patient cannot produce an explosive cough. These signs and symptoms are MOST LIKELY due to which of the following?

A A left capsular haemorrhage.

B A meningioma at the foramen magnum.

C Thrombosis of the left posterior inferior cerebellar artery.

D A left cerebello–pontine angle tumour.

E A right-sided brain stem infarction.

ME-Q21

A 40-year-old woman presents complaining of difficulty with swallowing. Examination shows she has a nasal speech, weakness of facial and neck muscles, receding hairline and a weak and slow hand grip. The patient is MOST LIKELY to be suffering from

A   facioscapulohumeral dystrophy.

B   myasthenia gravis.

C   dystrophia myotonica.

D   bulbar palsy.

E   polyneuritis.

ME-Q22

A 38-year-old builder had acute back pain which subsided over 24 h. He now complains of increasing numbness and tingling in both legs and poor bladder and bowel control. Which of the following should be your FIRST STEP in management?

A   Physiotherapy.

B   Strict bed rest with pelvic traction.

C   Epidural local anaesthesia.

D   Spinal manipulation.

E   Urgent myelogram.

ME-Q23

A 50-year-old man presents with a 2 year history of burning pains in the feet, pins and needles in the fingers and toes and weakness and unsteadiness of the legs. There is distal wasting and weakness in all limbs, areflexia and glove and stocking sensory loss to all modalities. The MOST LIKELY diagnosis is

A   polymyositis.

B   hereditary sensorimotor neuropathy (Charcot–Marie–Tooth disease).

C   diabetic neuropathy.

D   acute postinfectious polyneuropathy (Guillain–Barré syndrome).

E   diabetic amyotrophy.

ME-Q24

A 64-year-old man complains of 6 months of increasing stiffness in his legs and difficulty with walking. On examination there is wasting of the right biceps brachii with depression of the tendon reflex, spasticity in both legs with weakness of hip flexion and bilateral brisk lower limb tendon reflexes. The MOST LIKELY cause is

A   multiple sclerosis.

B   motor neuron disease.

C   Parkinson disease.

D   cervical spondylosis.

E   vertebrobasilar ischaemia.

ME-Q25

A 35-year-old woman develops weakness of the legs over a period of 7 days. On examination the only abnormalities are generalised weakness of the legs and suppressed reflexes. The MOST LIKELY diagnosis is

A   hysterical paralysis.

B   motor neuron disease.

C   multiple sclerosis.

D   Guillain-Barré syndrome.

E   spinal cord compression.

ME-Q26

An obese 55-year-old man presents with mononeuritis multiplex. He is MOST LIKELY to have

- A infectious mononucleosis.
- B lead poisoning.
- C Guillain-Barré syndrome.
- D diabetes mellitus.
- E myxoedema.

ME-Q27

All of the following can provoke the syndrome of parkinsonism EXCEPT

- A phenytoin intoxication.
- B manganese intoxication.
- C phenothiazine intoxication.
- D methyldopa (Aldomet®) intoxication.
- E carbon monoxide intoxication.

ME-Q28

Which of the following is of PROVEN BENEFIT in the treatment of established post-herpetic neuralgia?

- A Corticosteroids.
- B Acyclovir.
- C Amitriptyline.
- D Cimetidine.
- E Phenytoin.

ME-Q29

A 60-year-old woman who has had rheumatoid arthritis for 35 years and has been managed on corticosteroids for the past 10 years, now complains of sudden onset of pain and swelling in the right knee which is warm and very tender. There is no other evidence of synovitis. The MOST LIKELY diagnosis is

- A an exacerbation of rheumatoid arthritis.
- B concurrent gout.
- C secondary osteoarthritis.
- D septic arthritis.
- E unrecognised trauma.

ME-Q30

Rheumatoid factor

- A is highly specific for rheumatoid arthritis.
- B is present in more than 95% of patients with rheumatoid nodules.
- C titres are useful to monitor disease activity in rheumatoid arthritis.
- D is positive in more than 80% of patients with rheumatoid arthritis at the onset of arthritis.
- E can be used to differentiate between rheumatoid arthritis and systemic lupus erythematosus.

ME-Q31

Ankylosing spondylitis

  A is commonly associated with a reduced lung vital capacity.

  B rarely involves the cervical spine.

  C is associated with sacroiliitis in 30–50% of patients.

  D is more common in females.

  E is characterised radiographically by a marked loss of intervertebral disc height and spinal ankylosis.

ME-Q32

Osteoarthritis

  A commonly affects the metacarpophalangeal joints.

  B is a disease of subchondral bone with cartilage abnormalities appearing later.

  C is usually associated with more than 30 min of early morning stiffness.

  D can occur secondary to rheumatoid arthritis.

  E is best treated by immobilisation of the affected joint.

ME-Q33

All of the following radiological changes are frequently found in osteoarthritis EXCEPT

  A joint space narrowing.

  B periarticular osteoporosis.

  C osteophyte formation.

  D increased density of bone ends.

  E occasional subchondral cysts.

ME-Q34

A 73-year-old woman complains of pain mainly in the limb girdles, associated with marked stiffness. Her symptoms are worse in the early hours of the morning and on waking. There is no abnormality on examination apart from mild generalised stiffness of the shoulder and hip joints. Your provisional diagnosis should MOST LIKELY be CONFIRMED by

  A X-ray of the pelvis and shoulder girdle.

  B serum calcium and phosphorus levels.

  C serum alkaline phosphatase level.

  D erythrocyte sedimentation rate of 110 mm/h.

  E latex rheumatoid factor.

ME-Q35

Which of the following statements regarding non-steroidal anti-inflammatory drugs is CORRECT?

  A They are first line drugs in the treatment of osteoarthritis.

  B Anti-ulcer therapy should be administered at the same time because of the risk of gastrointestinal haemorrhage.

  C Gastrointestinal haemorrhage is not a complication if suppositories are used.

  D They can worsen pre-existing renal impairment.

  E They are ineffective when administered with food.

ME-Q36

Finger clubbing in the adult is MOST FREQUENTLY associated with which of the following conditions?

A Pulmonary tuberculosis.

B Cor pulmonale secondary to chronic airflow limitation.

C Obstructive sleep apnoea.

D Squamous cell carcinoma of the lung.

E Recurrent pulmonary embolism.

ME-Q37

Cardiac auscultation reveals accentuation of the first heart sound at the apex, accentuation of the second pulmonary sound and a presystolic murmur at the apex. The MOST LIKELY diagnosis is

A pulmonary stenosis.

B mitral stenosis.

C aortic stenosis.

D mitral incompetence.

E functional heart murmur.

ME-Q38

Which of the following statements is NOT CORRECT? A third heart sound

A is a diastolic filling sound.

B will disappear if atrial fibrillation occurs.

C can be normal in young people.

D is often a sign of left ventricular failure.

E may occur in mitral incompetence.

ME-Q39

A 28-year-old woman presents because of lethargy, dizzy spells and occasional syncope. During a dizzy spell the heart rate is 32 beats/min and the blood pressure is 85/60 mmHg. Which of the following is the MOST LIKELY diagnosis?

A Addison disease.

B Insulinoma.

C Structural disease of the cardiac conducting system ('sick sinus syndrome').

D Sinus tachycardia with 4:1 atrioventricular block.

E Iron deficiency.

ME-Q40

A 60-year-old man who has enjoyed good health complains of increasing breathlessness, abdominal discomfort and swelling of the feet for 3 weeks. His venous pressure is elevated, the liver is enlarged and there is gross ascites. The resting respiratory rate is 25/min and there are basal crepitations. The pulse rate is 36/min and an ECG shows an atrial rate of 96/min. The blood pressure is 180/80 mmHg. The MOST EFFECTIVE IMMEDIATE treatment is

A intravenous frusemide.

B intravenous frusemide plus digoxin.

C intravenous digoxin.

D abdominal paracentesis.

E insertion of a transvenous pacemaker.

ME-Q41

In the elderly, with mild systolic hypertension (170–180 mmHg), which of the following is CORRECT?

A   Diastolic blood pressure rather than systolic blood pressure is a better predictor of cerebrovascular morbidity and mortality.

B   Effective lowering of mild systolic hypertension is associated with a decreased incidence of stroke in those aged 65–80 years.

C   A serum creatinine level of 0.15 mmol/L (<0.11) is a contraindication for anti-hypertensive therapy.

D   The lower plasma renin activity in the elderly results in a decreased efficacy of angiotensin-converting enzyme (ACE) inhibitors in this age group.

E   A history of stroke would be a contraindication to antihypertensive treatment in such patients.

ME-Q42

After a pulmonary embolus, which of the following is MOST LIKELY?

A   Low right atrial pressure and low central venous pressure.

B   Low systemic arterial blood pressure and low venous pressures.

C   High pulmonary venous pressure and pulmonary oedema.

D   High right ventricular pressure and high systemic venous pressure.

E   High left atrial pressure and functional mitral valve incompetence.

ME-Q43

The MOST COMMON site of a spontaneous rupture of an atherosclerotic aortic aneurysm is

A   ascending aorta.

B   arch of aorta.

C   descending thoracic aorta.

D   abdominal aorta above renal arteries.

E   abdominal aorta below renal arteries.

ME-Q44

Fibromuscular hyperplasia of the renal arteries as a cause of hypertension is MOST FREQUENT in

A   young adult males.

B   young adult females.

C   middle-aged males.

D   middle-aged females.

E   females of all ages.

ME-Q45

The chest is slightly larger but moves less on the right; the percussion note is less resonant on the left where breath sounds are louder. The MOST LIKELY disorder is

A   consolidation on the left.

B   pneumothorax on the right.

C   collapse on the left.

D   consolidation on the right.

E   pleural effusion on the left.

ME-Q46

Which of the following features does NOT assist in the diagnosis of severe emphysema?

- A Inspiratory indrawing of costal margins.
- B Diminished cardiac dullness.
- C Pulsus paradoxus.
- D Diffuse expiratory rhonchi.
- E Faint breath sounds.

ME-Q47

In a coal miner aged 50 years, a persistent blood-stained pleural effusion is MOST LIKELY to be due to

- A pulmonary tuberculosis.
- B coal miner's pneumoconiosis.
- C carcinoma of the lung.
- D silicosis.
- E mesothelioma.

ME-Q48

A patient with arterial blood gas analysis showing a P_aCO_2 of 55 mmHg and a P_aO_2 of 50 mmHg

- A may have hyperventilation as a cause.
- B must be cyanosed.
- C needs urgent mechanical ventilation.
- D needs controlled oxygen therapy.
- E must have a reduced diffusing capacity.

ME-Q49

Which one of the following disorders is MOST LIKELY to be associated with retention of carbon dioxide?

- A An acute asthmatic attack.
- B Lobar pneumonia.
- C Exacerbation of chronic bronchitis.
- D 'Pure' (uncomplicated) emphysema.
- E Chronic pulmonary tuberculosis.

ME-Q50

Which of the following clinical features is UNUSUAL in a patient with chronic hypercapnia?

- A Retinal venous distension.
- B Drowsiness.
- C Cold, clammy skin.
- D Headache.
- E Muscle twitching.

ME-Q51

Respiratory alkalosis is ASSOCIATED with

- A increased P_aCO_2, increased plasma bicarbonate.
- B increased P_aCO_2, decreased plasma bicarbonate.
- C decreased P_aCO_2, increased plasma bicarbonate.
- D decreased P_aCO_2, decreased plasma bicarbonate.
- E decreased P_aCO_2, decreased urinary bicarbonate.

ME-Q52

A healthy non-smoking 19-year-old man, hospitalised for an appendicectomy, is mistakenly given an overdose of his narcotic premedication. He is found unconscious and on auscultation of his chest, he has reduced breath sounds but no added sounds. Emergency chest X-ray is clear. His arterial blood gases (in mmHg), taken while breathing room air are MOST LIKELY to show

A pH 7.22, P_aO_2 70 P_aCO_2 61

B pH 7.23, P_aO_2 90 P_aCO_2 59

C pH 7.23, P_aO_2 86 P_aCO_2 30

D pH 7.39, P_aO_2 65 P_aCO_2 42

E pH 7.39, P_aO_2 75 P_aCO_2 60

ME-Q53

Which of the following is an UNLIKELY ASSOCIATION with the disease mentioned?

A Rust-coloured sputum — pneumococcal pneumonia.

B Watery consistency sputum — chronic asthma.

C Foul-smelling sputum — lung abscess.

D Pink and frothy sputum — pulmonary oedema.

E Clear mucoid sputum — chronic bronchitis.

ME-Q54

In which one of the following is the investigation result MOST CONSISTENT with the diagnosis?

A Mild asthma – arterial P_aCO_2 50 mmHg.

B Pulmonary embolism – normal chest X-ray.

C Pleural effusion due to congestive cardiac failure – pleural fluid protein concentration of 4 g/dL.

D Severe airflow limitation – forced expired volume in 1 s of 80% (FEV_1, % predicted).

E Pulmonary embolism – normal perfusion lung scan.

ME-Q55

A 24-year-old asthmatic presents to the emergency department complaining of shortness of breath. He looks unwell. His pulse is 130/min and his temperature is 38°C. The chest is hyperinflated, the breath sounds are vesicular but diminished and there is a soft, generalised expiratory wheeze. Which of the following is the MOST APPROPRIATE sequence of investigations?

A A chest X-ray.

B A chest X-ray followed by a peak expiratory flow reading.

C A chest X-ray followed by arterial blood gases and then peak expiratory flow reading.

D Peak expiratory flow reading followed by arterial blood gases and then chest X-ray.

E Sputum collected for culture followed by chest X-ray and blood cultures.

ME-Q56

In a patient with severe asthma, which of the features listed would be the MOST ominous?

A Arterial Po_2 50 mmHg.

B Arterial Pco_2 50 mmHg.

C An FEV_1 0.8 L.

D Very loud wheezes.

E A respiratory rate of 20/min.

ME-Q57

A 35-year-old woman presents with an acute onset of productive cough, pleuritic chest pain and fever. She was previously well and on no medication except for an oral contraceptive. Chest X-ray shows consolidation of the right middle lobe. What is the MOST LIKELY diagnosis?

A Staphylococcal pneumonia.

B Mycoplasma pneumonia.

C Pulmonary embolism.

D Streptococcal (pneumococcal) pneumonia.

E Viral pneumonia.

ME-Q58

Which one of the following statements concerning Pneumocystis carinii pneumonia is CORRECT?

A It is an early manifestation of HIV infection.

B Clinical examination of the chest is frequently normal.

C Chest X-ray is normal in more than 50% of cases.

D Gas exchange is usually normal.

E It is usually diagnosed by sputum culture.

ME-Q59

Infection with *Mycoplasma pneumoniae* is characterised by all of the following EXCEPT

A it affects mostly children and young adults.

B cold agglutinins are often present in the blood.

C amoxycillin is the treatment of choice.

D the chest X-ray appearance is usually more extensive than suggested by clinical signs.

E the white blood cell count is usually normal.

ME-Q60

An Asian immigrant to Australia presents with fever, weight loss and cough with haemoptysis. Physical examination is normal but chest X-ray reveals a patchy infiltrate with cavitation and fibrosis in the right upper lobe. Which of the following is CORRECT?

A The presence of a BCG scar excludes tuberculosis.

B The diagnosis of active tuberculous disease is confirmed by the chest X-ray appearance.

C Negative Mantoux test excludes active tuberculosis.

D Negative sputum smears for acid-fast bacilli exclude active tuberculosis.

E Acid-fast bacilli in sputum are highly suggestive, but not pathognomonic, for tuberculosis.

ME-Q61

You are managing a 43-year-old woman with metastatic carcinoma of the lung who has painful bone metastases and requires morphine for pain relief. Which of the following statements is CORRECT?

A   Intravenous morphine is invariably required to treat severe pain.

B   Dosing as necessary (p.r.n.) reduces the risk of addiction.

C   Morphine should be avoided in lung cancer as it could cause severe respiratory depression.

D   Anti-inflammatory drugs enhance analgesia.

E   Oral morphine is not adequately absorbed and should not be used.

ME-Q62

Acute pulmonary embolism may be associated with all of the following EXCEPT

A   increased second pulmonary heart sound.

B   syncope.

C   pleural rub.

D   dyspnoea.

E   bronchial breath sounds.

ME-Q63

A 59-year-old woman with a history of multiple previous myocardial infarctions and congestive cardiac failure presents acutely short of breath. Chest X-ray shows cardiomegaly with clear lung fields. Blood pressure is 110/80 mmHg. A ventilation–perfusion lung scan shows one unmatched segmental perfusion defect in each lung. The NEXT APPROPRIATE diagnostic or therapeutic step should be

A   obtain a Doppler ultrasound of the lower limbs.

B   bed rest and low dose subcutaneous heparin for 1 week.

C   simultaneous commencement of intravenous heparin and oral warfarin therapy.

D   pulmonary angiography to assess the extent of any pulmonary emboli.

E   intravenous thrombolytic therapy to prevent pulmonary hypertension in the long term.

ME-Q64

A 22-year-old HIV positive male with chronic cough is suspected of having pulmonary tuberculosis. A Mantoux test is performed with 10 IU human PPD (purified protein derivative) and is negative 24 h later. Which of the following statements is CORRECT regarding this patient?

A   The Mantoux result makes the diagnosis of pulmonary tuberculosis unlikely.

B   The finding of 5 mm skin induration at 72 h indicates a positive Mantoux.

C   He should receive BCG vaccination as he is at high risk of tuberculosis in the future.

D   Chemoprophylaxis should be started with isoniazid and should be continued for 18 months.

E   Microscopy of sputum for acid-fast bacilli is unnecessary following a negative Mantoux test.

ME-Q65

Dysphagia can be ASSOCIATED WITH each of the following EXCEPT

   A monilial oesophagitis.

   B myasthenia gravis.

   C iron deficiency anaemia.

   D parkinsonism.

   E oesophageal varices.

ME-Q66

The following statements concerning patients with dysphagia due to oesophageal motility disorders are correct EXCEPT

   A symptoms occur with both liquid and solid foods.

   B a history of substernal crushing chest pain can be present.

   C cold fluids can precipitate symptoms.

   D calcium channel-blocking agents can be effective.

   E symptoms are usually relentlessly progressive.

ME-Q67

A 22-year-old woman presents with painful dysphagia. There is a past history of Raynaud phenomenon. Upper gastrointestinal endoscopy reveals ulcerative oesophagitis, which proves resistant to double dose (800 mg, b.d.) cimetidine therapy. An oesophageal mano-metry study demonstrates absent peristalsis; the lower oesophageal sphincter is not identified. Which of the following is the MOST APPROPRIATE treatment?

   A Fundoplication.

   B Omeprazole.

   C Octretide.

   D Pneumatic dilatation of the lower oesophageal sphincter.

   E Ranitidine.

ME-Q68

Diagnosis of the presence of oesophageal reflux MOST USUALLY requires

   A an endoscopy plus a clinical history.

   B a barium meal.

   C a good clinical history only.

   D a nuclear scan to demonstrate reflux.

   E manometry plus a clinical history.

ME-Q69

Lactose intolerance (lactase deficiency) can frequently complicate all of the following EXCEPT

   A gluten-sensitive enteropathy.

   B viral gastroenteritis in Caucasians.

   C Crohn disease (regional ileitis).

   D viral gastroenteritis in Chinese.

   E chronic pancreatitis.

ME-Q70

In a 25-year-old woman with gluten-sensitive enteropathy, which of the following statements is CORRECT?

A The anaemia is most likely to be due to Vitamin B_{12} deficiency.

B The pretreatment biopsy will demonstrate flattened villi and an inflammatory cell infiltrate of periodic acid-Schiff positive macrophages.

C Corn contains gluten and should be excluded from the diet.

D When placed on a strict gluten-free diet, the small bowel histology will improve markedly within 2 weeks.

E There is an association with the development of lymphoma.

ME-Q71

In Wilson disease, all of the following are correct EXCEPT

A jaundice can be a presenting feature.

B there are juvenile and late onset forms, which predominantly affect different organs.

C patients can present with tic-like movements.

D there can be diagnostic changes in the eye.

E serum ceruloplasmin concentration correlates with the clinical severity of the disease.

ME-Q72

Which of the following statements about hepatitis B is CORRECT?

A Alpha-interferon is very effective in clearing surface antigen from the serum in 30–40% of patients with chronic active hepatitis B.

B Raised alanine aminotransferase (ALT) levels and jaundice precede the appearance of hepatitis B surface antigen (HBsAg) in the serum of a patient with acute icteric hepatitis B.

C The hepatitis B e antigen/e antibody (HBeAg/Anti HBe) status is a more sensitive marker of viral replication than the hepatitis B virus (HBV) DNA polymerase level.

D Hepatitis B carriers have a 90–100-fold increased risk of hepatocellular carcinoma compared with non-carriers.

E The majority of maternal–fetal hepatitis B infection occurs *in utero*.

ME-Q73

A 23-year-old Chinese woman who is known to be HBsAg–positive gives birth. The attending practitioner should

A vaccinate both mother and baby against hepatitis B.

B give anti-hepatitis B hyperimmune globulin to both mother and baby.

C give hyperimmune globulin to the baby and begin vaccination of the baby.

D do nothing, because the mother is likely to be a chronic hepatitis B carrier and the child has been infected *in utero*.

E treat the mother with alpha interferon and the baby with hyperimmune globulin.

ME-Q74

Which of the following FAVOURS organic bowel disease rather than a functional condition, such as irritable bowel syndrome?

    A Looser and more frequent stools at onset of pain.

    B Nocturnal diarrhoea with pain that wakes the patient from sleep.

    C Abdominal distension.

    D Passage of mucus in the stool.

    E Relief of abdominal pain after defaecation.

ME-Q75

The MOST COMMON cause of 'traveller's diarrhoea' is

    A enterotoxigenic *Escherichia coli.*

    B *Shigella* species.

    C *Giardia lamblia (intestinalis).*

    D *Entamoeba histolytica.*

    E *Salmonella typhimurium.*

ME-Q76

In regard to large bowel cancer, all the following statements are true EXCEPT

    A the risk of developing bowel cancer is significantly increased in first degree relatives of patients with the disease.

    B patients with large bowel cancer have approximately a three-fold increase in the risk of developing a subsequent bowel cancer.

    C patients with colonic adenomas have an increased risk of developing bowel cancer.

    D tubular adenomas are more likely to become cancers than are villous adenomas.

    E patients with Crohn colitis have an increased risk of developing cancer of the bowel than normal people.

ME-Q77

A 30-year-old woman presents with a 2 week history of bloody diarrhoea. Sigmoidoscopic examination reveals changes compatible with ulcerative colitis. A rectal biopsy is taken. The NEXT STEP should be to

    A commence salicylazosulphapyridine.

    B commence intravenous steroids.

    C order a stool culture.

    D commence rectal steroids.

    E await results of rectal biopsy.

ME-Q78

All of the following are manifestations associated with ulcerative colitis EXCEPT

    A pyoderma gangrenosum.

    B uveitis.

    C primary sclerosing cholangitis.

    D vitamin B_{12} malabsorption.

    E splenomegaly.

ME-Q79

A 19-year-old female, recently returned from Indonesia, presents with bloody diarrhoea, cramping abdominal pain, tenesmus and fever. Which of the following statements is CORRECT?

    A The patient should be isolated in view of the possibility of cholera.

    B Anti-diarrhoeal agents, such as diphenoxylate (Lomotil®) or loperamide (Imodium®) should be prescribed to control diarrhoea.

    C The finding of cysts of *Entamoeba histolytica* is diagnostic of amoebic colitis.

    D The symptoms suggest *Campylobacter jejuni* infection and antibiotics will hasten clinical recovery significantly.

    E Stool microscopy is likely to show numerous polymorph leucocytes.

ME-Q80

Most cancers of the large bowel

    A arise *de novo* in the mucosa.

    B arise from pre-existing adenomas.

    C have spread to the liver at the time of detection.

    D present first with low abdominal pain.

    E occur in the caecum.

ME-Q81

Cytological examination of the ascitic fluid from a patient with colonic cancer reveals malignant cells. The ascites is MOST LIKELY to be due to

    A malignant obstruction of the colonic lumen.

    B malignant invasion of the peritoneal tissues.

    C hepatic metastases.

    D portal venous obstruction.

    E multiple primary tumours within the intestinal wall.

ME-Q82

All of the following are common features of Cushing disease (pituitary dependent hypercortisolaemia), EXCEPT

    A diabetes mellitus.

    B failure to suppress plasma cortisol following low dose dexamethasone (0.5 mg, q.i.d.).

    C proximal myopathy.

    D bitemporal field defect.

    E hypertension.

ME-Q83

All the following are characteristic clinical features of acromegaly EXCEPT

    A thick greasy skin.

    B homonymous hemianopia.

    C hypertension.

    D cardiomyopathy.

    E glycosuria.

ME-Q84

A 38-year-old woman presents with a 2 week history of malaise, feeling hot and feverish, palpitations, sweating, tremor, pain in the neck and weight loss of 2 kg. Her pulse is 120/min and her hands are sweaty with a tremor. Her thyroid is palpable, firm, tender and enlarged. Which one of the following results CONFIRMS the MOST LIKELY diagnosis?

    A High serum thyroxine and T3 levels.

    B Low thyroid uptake of radioactive iodine.

    C Thyroid nuclear scan showing increased uptake.

    D Antithyroid antibodies present in high titre.

    E Low thyroid stimulating hormone (TSH) with flat response to thyrotropin-releasing hormone (TRH).

ME-Q85

A 47-year-old woman presents with a 3 year history of amenorrhoea and, more recently, has noted galactorrhoea. She is not troubled by headaches or visual disturbance. She has a history of hypertension for which she is taking verapamil (Isoptin). Investigations reveal a prolactin of 425 ng/mL (< 20). The MOST LIKELY cause of the elevated prolactin is

    A macroadenoma of the pituitary.

    B verapamil.

    C perimenopausal state.

    D microadenoma of the pituitary.

    E craniopharyngioma.

ME-Q86

Factors that increase the risk for osteoporosis in women include each of the following EXCEPT

    A low bodyweight.

    B smoking.

    C high alcohol intake.

    D thiazide diuretic therapy.

    E premature menopause.

ME-Q87

All of the following can occur with an ABO-incompatible blood transfusion EXCEPT

    A fever, rigors.

    B hypotension.

    C back pain.

    D bilirubinuria.

    E haemoglobinuria.

ME-Q88

A 22-year-old man presents with sudden onset of bruising, fatigue, and sore throat. The blood count shows haemoglobin 10.9 g/dL, platelets 50 x 10^9/L (150–400), leucocytes 2.2 x 10^9/L (3.5–10) and neutrophils 1.0 x 10^9/L (3.5–7.5). There are a few moderately firm, enlarged cervical lymph nodes. The MOST LIKELY diagnosis is

    A infectious mononucleosis.

    B idiopathic thrombocytopenic purpura.

    C an adverse drug reaction.

    D acute leukaemia.

    E infection with the human immunodeficiency virus (HIV).

ME-Q89

A 40-year-old woman presents with a sudden onset of bruising and nose bleeds. The blood count indicates thrombocytopenia (platelets 10 x 10^9/L) but is otherwise normal. The thrombocytopenia could have been ASSOCIATED WITH all of the following EXCEPT

A   a recent viral infection.

B   a recent blood transfusion.

C   taking quinine for nocturnal cramps.

D   the recent onset of pain and stiffness in her fingers.

E   starting to take a contraceptive pill 2 months earlier.

ME-Q90

A 60-year-old man regularly drinks the equivalent of 60 g alcohol daily. A blood count shows haemoglobin 13.0 g/dL, mean corpuscular volume (MCV) 110 fL, white blood cells (WBC) 5.8 x 10^9/L with a normal differential count and platelets 100 x 10^9/L (150–400). The gamma glutamyl transpeptidase (GGT) was 60 U/L (< 50). The liver span was 15 cm and there were no other abnormal physical signs. The MOST APPROPRIATE NEXT STEP would be

A   liver biopsy.

B   bone marrow biopsy.

C   check on serum folate and vitamin B_{12} levels.

D   check serum amylase.

E   estimation of serum iron and serum ferritin.

ME-Q91

Macrocytic anaemia is found in all of the following EXCEPT

A   hypothyroidism.

B   anti-epileptic medication.

C   regional ileitis (Crohn disease).

D   chronic alcoholism.

E   chronic uraemia.

ME-Q92

The development of a macrocytic anaemia during pregnancy is MOST LIKELY a consequence of

A   inadequate intake of folate.

B   small bowel disease.

C   inappropriate intake of vitamin B_{12}.

D   alcoholism.

E   chronic giardiasis.

ME-Q93

A 45-year-old male patient aged is found by chance to have a haemoglobin of 11.5 g/dL and an MCV of 76 fL (85–98). He is symptom free and takes no medications of any kind. The MOST APPROPRIATE INITIAL step would be

A   recommendation for follow-up blood count in 3 months.

B   test for occult blood in a series of three stools.

C   examination of the bone marrow.

D   colonoscopy.

E   estimation of serum iron, ferritin and transferrin.

ME-Q94

A 60-year-old man complains of angina. Full physical examination reveals only generalised pallor. A blood count reveals haemoglobin of 9.5 g/dL and hypochromic microcytic red cells and an ECG is normal. After confirming that the patient has an iron deficiency you would then

A prescribe oral iron and a beta-blocker and see him in 1 month's time.

B request a sigmoidoscopy and colonoscopy.

C request a barium meal.

D arrange a blood transfusion.

E request bone marrow examination.

ME-Q95

A 65-year-old woman who has been taking piroxicam (Feldene®) 20 mg daily for 3 months for 'rheumatic pains' presents complaining of epigastric discomfort. A blood count reveals a haemoglobin concentration of 9.2 g/dL, with normal white blood cells and platelets. You arrange an upper gastrointestinal endoscopy. Pending this investigation you SHOULD

A reduce the dose of piroxicam to 10 mg daily.

B continue piroxicam and add sucralfate.

C change to another oral non-steroidal anti-inflammatory agent.

D change to naproxen (Naprosyn®) suppositories.

E cease piroxicam and advise the patient to control pain with paracetamol.

ME-Q96

Which of the following SUPPORTS a diagnosis of glandular fever due to Epstein–Barr virus (EBV) infection?

A Splenic infarction.

B Eosinophilia.

C A maculopapular rash following erythromycin.

D The presence of cold agglutinins in the patient's blood.

E Abnormal liver function tests without jaundice.

ME-Q97

Which of the following effects of antidiuretic hormone leads to the PRODUCTION of a concentrated urine?

A Increase in free water clearance.

B Increase in sodium concentration in the distal tubule fluid.

C Increased active transport of water in the distal tubule.

D Increased permeability of water in the distal tubule.

E Increased reabsorption of sodium in the distal tubule.

ME-Q98

Which of the following statements about urinary tract infections is CORRECT?

A Asymptomatic bacteriuria only occurs in females.

B Asymptomatic bacteriuria does not require treatment.

C Patients with cystitis can have negative urine cultures.

D Pyuria is synonymous with a urinary tract infection.

E Most urinary tract infections arise by haematogenous spread.

ME-Q99

A 60-year-old woman is brought to the Emergency Department by her relatives who have noticed that she is 'unwell' and confused. Blood tests are requested and the initial results are: Na 139 mmol/L; K 5.4 mmol/L; Cl 113 mmol/L; HCO_3 17 mmol/L; urea 11.5 mmol/L (< 8); creatinine 0.14 mmol/L (< 0.11); arterial pH 7.28; P_aCO_2 30 mmHg; P_aO_2 90 mmHg. Which of the following statements is CORRECT?

  A The anion gap is increased.

  B The symptoms and signs are due to uraemia.

  C Metabolic acidosis has been documented.

  D The results suggest that she has been vomiting excessively.

  E An infusion of bicarbonate should be commenced.

ME-Q100

Which of the following is the MOST COMMON cause of end-stage renal failure in adults in Australia?

  A Diabetes mellitus.

  B Polycystic renal disease.

  C Analgesic nephropathy.

  D Chronic glomerulonephritis.

  E Reflux nephropathy.

ME-Q101

In patients with chronic renal failure and hypertension due to bilateral renal artery stenosis, which of the following agents is MOST LIKELY to reduce glomerular filtration?

  A Beta-blockers.

  B Calcium antagonists.

  C Angiotensin-converting enzyme (ACE) inhibitors.

  D Nitrates.

  E Corticosteroids.

ME-Q102

A 30-year-old man is awakened during the night by very severe pain in the right loin. He feels nauseated and sweaty. The pain comes and goes over intervals of about 10 min but seems better when he gets out of bed. He notices bright blood in his urine but does not see or hear a stone being passed. He is afebrile and plain X-ray of his urinary tract shows an opacity 5 mm by 3 mm in the line of the ureter just below the right sacroiliac joint. You SHOULD

  A advise him to go to bed to ease the pain.

  B send him to a urologist for urgent retrieval of the stone via cystoscopy.

  C tell him to drink lots of water, prescribe appropriate analgesia and have him return for a repeat X-ray within 2 days.

  D prescribe him allopurinol and a thiazide diuretic straight away.

  E advise him to avoid all dairy foods and foods containing calcium.

ME-Q103

A 35-year-old man has had two episodes of colicky left renal angle pain radiating to the groin. The first, 6 months ago, lasted about 4 h and had disappeared when the man woke from sleep the next day. The second, which lasted a similar time and occurred 1 week previously, was initially accompanied by red urine. No stone was seen to be passed on either occasion. Which of the following statements is CORRECT?

   A One can be certain that these symptoms are not caused by renal calculi.

   B Cystoscopy and retrograde pyelography should be the first line of investigation.

   C At the patient's age, a presumptive diagnosis of stone should be made and a low calcium diet instituted.

   D Renal ultrasound should be performed as the first investigation.

   E If the symptoms are caused by calculi, there is very little chance that a renal excretory abnormality will be found.

ME-Q104

All the following can result from hypokalaemia EXCEPT

   A cardiac arrhythmia.

   B intestinal stasis.

   C tall peaked T waves in the ECG.

   D polyuria.

   E muscular weakness.

ME-Q105

A young man, previously in good health, over 3 days develops headache, fever and becomes drowsy. Examination shows signs of meningeal irritation and a routine chest radiograph shows a well-defined rounded opacity approximately 2 cm in diameter in the right lung. The MOST LIKELY diagnosis is

   A cryptococcosis (torulosis).

   B sarcoidosis.

   C primary pulmonary neoplasm.

   D disseminated tuberculosis.

   E multiple secondaries from a melanoma.

ME-Q106

A general practitioner prescribes a course of penicillin V for a sore throat in an 11-year-old boy after diagnosing infection with a Group A haemolytic streptococcus. The boy recovers well. Ten days after the onset of the sore throat he develops malaise and mild facial and hand swelling. All of the following statements are correct EXCEPT

   A hypertension and pulmonary oedema are commonly associated with this clinical presentation.

   B urinary sediment containing red cells and hyalin casts suggests acute post-streptococcal glomerulonephritis.

   C a low antistreptolysin titre (ASOT) excludes post-streptococcal glomerulonephritis.

   D the treatment is bed rest, diuretic and antihypertensive medication.

   E the boy's family should be screened for Group A haemolytic streptococcus carriers.

ME-Q107

Which of the following micro-organisms is the MOST LIKELY causative agent of acute septic arthritis in a 4-year-old Australian boy?

A *Staphylococcus aureus.*

B Group B streptococcus.

C *Streptococcus viridans.*

D *Neisseria gonorrhoeae.*

E *Mycobacterium tuberculosis.*

ME-Q108

The MOST COMMON INITIAL manifestation of Human Immunodeficiency virus (HIV) infection is

A an opportunistic infection.

B meningitis.

C a gastrointestinal disorder.

D a mild flu-like illness.

E not a specific symptomatic pattern.

ME-Q109

An Australian-born patient with AIDS presents with meningitis. The MOST LIKELY pathogen is

A *Mycobacterium tuberculosis.*

B Human Immunodeficiency virus (HIV).

C *Neisseria meningitidis*

D *Cryptococcus neoformans.*

E *Streptococcus pneumoniae.*

ME-Q110

Coxiella burnetii infection (Q fever) is usually ACQUIRED by

A sexual transmission.

B inhalation of infective particles from animal carcasses.

C the faecal–oral route.

D eating undercooked sausages.

E drinking milk.

ME-Q111

The MAJOR lesion in tabes dorsalis is

A demyelination of posterior columns.

B isolated degeneration of dorsal nerve roots.

C isolated demyelination of ventral nerve roots.

D demyelination of the anterior spino–cerebellar tract.

E peripheral nerve demyelination.

ME-Q112

Which of the following antibiotics is MOST COMMONLY implicated in the development of pseudomembranous colitis?

A Ampicillin.
B Metronidazole.
C Vancomycin.
D Trimethoprim–sulphamethoxazole.
E Erythromycin.

ME-Q113

Metronidazole is active against all of the following organisms EXCEPT

A *Bacteroides fragilis.*
B *Giardia lamblia.*
C *Entamoeba histolytica.*
D *Toxoplasma gondii.*
E *Trichomonas vaginalis.*

ME-Q114

Ceftriaxone is effective therapy for infection CAUSED by which of the following micro-organisms?

A *Mycoplasma pneumoniae.*
B Penicillinase-producing *Neisseria gonorrhoeae.*
C *Chlamydia trachomatis.*
D *Giardia lamblia (intestinalis).*
E *Gardnerella vaginalis.*

ME-Q115

The plasma concentration of a drug declines with first order kinetics. Which of the following is CORRECT?

A There is only one metabolic pathway for the elimination of the drug.
B The elimination half-life is constant, regardless of the plasma concentration of the drug.
C The rate of elimination is independent of the plasma concentration.
D A plot of the logarithm of the plasma concentration of the drug versus time will not be a straight line.
E At therapeutic plasma concentrations, the elimination of aspirin and ethanol are typical examples.

ME-Q116

Which of the following drugs in therapeutic doses would NOT be implicated in a patient with easy bruising?

A Aspirin.
B Indomethacin.
C Prednisone.
D Paracetamol.
E Warfarin.

ME-Q117

Amoxycillin RESISTANCE in *Escherichia coli*

A can be counteracted by combining amoxycillin with cephalexin.

B does not reduce the efficacy of amoxycillin in treating urinary tract infections.

C is rarely transferred between different bacterial strains.

D can be overcome by increasing the dose of amoxycillin.

E is most commonly due to production of enzymes known as beta-lactamases.

ME-Q118

Tetracycline is the TREATMENT OF CHOICE for adults with

A acute bronchitis.

B tonsillitis in a penicillin-allergic patient.

C *Klebsiella* urinary tract infection.

D psittacosis.

E gonorrhoea.

ME-Q119

Cimetidine can reduce the hepatic metabolism of all of the following EXCEPT

A propranolol.

B phenytoin.

C warfarin.

D digoxin.

E theophylline.

ME-Q120

Which one of the following statements about anti-epileptic drugs is CORRECT?

A Sodium valproate commonly causes gingival hyperplasia.

B The incidence of birth defects in babies of epileptic mothers on treatment is about three-fold higher than in the normal community.

C The preferred treatment of status epilepticus is intravenous barbiturate.

D Phenytoin follows zero order kinetics at therapeutic doses; therefore, monitoring plasma concentrations does not help in management.

E Phenytoin is the drug of choice for Petit-mal seizures.

ME-Q121

A 75-year-old woman has taken lithium, without complication, for many years. Subsequently a non-steroidal anti-inflammatory drug (NSAID) is prescribed for osteo-arthritis. Over the ensuing weeks she develops ataxia, anorexia, nausea and tremulousness. Which of the following is CORRECT?

A These features are consistent with NSAID toxicity.

B The main therapeutic measure would be salt restriction.

C Lithium inhibits the clearance of most NSAID from the body.

D Interactions between lithium and NSAID are of little clinical significance.

E These features are consistent with lithium toxicity.

ME-Q122

Adjuvant chemotherapy has been MOST CLEARLY demonstrated to improve the survival of patients with which of the following conditions?

- A Oesophageal cancer.
- B Completely resected gastric cancer.
- C Malignant melanoma with lymph node metastases.
- D Stage 2 (node positive) breast cancer in premenopausal women.
- E Dukes A (confined to mucosa) colon cancer.

ME-Q123

In the MANAGEMENT of a patient with allergic rhinitis occurring throughout the year

- A symptoms at any time of the year, irrespective of season, exclude isolated grass pollen allergy.
- B sublingual immunotherapy with allergen extract is effective.
- C topical vasoconstrictors are effective long-term therapy.
- D desensitisation is preferred to topical steroids and antihistamines.
- E a nasal smear can show a large number of eosinophils.

ME-Q124

Smooth muscle auto-antibodies CHARACTERISTICALLY OCCUR in the sera of patients with

- A polymyositis.
- B dermatomyositis.
- C chronic active hepatitis.
- D hepatocellular carcinoma.
- E Duchenne muscular dystrophy.

ME-Q125

A 21-year-old man gives a 5 year history of recurrent purulent otitis media, bronchitis and sinusitis and two episodes of pneumonia.

- A Acquired Immune Deficiency Syndrome (AIDS) is the most likely diagnosis.
- B A normal plasma electrophoretogram excludes a diagnosis of humoral immune deficiency.
- C His history would be consistent with congenital (X-linked) agammaglobulinaemia.
- D If hypogammaglobulinaemia is found, replacement therapy with intravenous immunoglobulin would be expected to result in clinical improvement.
- E An isolated defect in cell-mediated immune function is the likely cause.

Medicine
Questions

TYPE

Questions ME-Q126 to ME-Q205

■I Type J questions consist of a stem and five responses of which **one or more** may be correct

■ All Type J questions will have at least one response correct

ME-Q126

The accompanying photograph (Figure 8) shows a young girl's skin lesion which has been present since birth. Which of the following is/are APPROPRIATE?

   A Advise the parents that it will regress with time.

   B Arrange laser therapy.

   C Recommend low dose radiotherapy.

   D CT scan of the head and skull.

   E Serum calcium, phosphate and alkaline phosphatase.

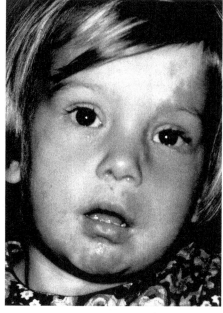

Figure 8

ME-Q127

Appropriate treatments for the lesions on the face shown in the accompanying photograph (Figure 9) INCLUDE

   A miconazole cream.

   B clotrimazole cream.

   C systemic griseofulvin.

   D hydrocortisone cream, 1%.

   E nystatin cream.

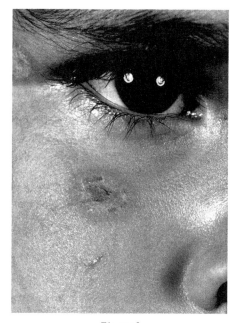

Figure 9

ME-Q136

In which of the following is a visual field disorder CORRECTLY MATCHED with a likely cause?

A Central scotoma – optic neuritis.

B Enlarged blind spot – papilloedema.

C Constricted fields – glaucoma.

D Bitemporal hemianopia – occipital infarct.

E Homonymous hemianopia – optic nerve glioma.

ME-Q137

Which of the following conditions CAUSE(S) spastic paraparesis?

A Alzheimer disease.

B Guillain–Barré syndrome.

C Lumbar canal stenosis.

D Cervical spondylosis.

E Parkinson disease.

ME-Q138

Peripheral neuropathy is FREQUENTLY observed as an unwanted effect with which of the following drugs?

A Nitrofurantoin.

B Ketoprofen.

C Sodium valproate.

D Isoniazid.

E Vincristine.

ME-Q139

Which of the following CAUSE(S) mononeuritis multiplex?

A Polyarteritis nodosa.

B Thiamine deficiency.

C Diabetes mellitus.

D Sarcoidosis.

E Vitamin B_{12} deficiency.

ME-Q140

A 60-year-old man presents with wasting and weakness of ALL the small muscles of the right hand. These symptoms and signs could be EXPLAINED by which of the following?

A Spondylitic compression of the T1 nerve root.

B Ulnar nerve lesion at the elbow.

C Cervical rib.

D Apical lung carcinoma.

E. Carpal tunnel syndrome.

ME-Q141

A herniated intervertebral disc compressing the first sacral nerve root COMMONLY results in

- A loss of bladder function.
- B loss of knee jerk.
- C loss of ankle jerk.
- D foot drop.
- E weakness of quadriceps muscle.

ME-Q142

Carbamazepine (Tegretol®) is an APPROPRIATE treatment for which of the following?

- A Absence seizures (Petit mal).
- B Complex partial seizures.
- C Trigeminal neuralgia.
- D Generalised tonic clonic seizures.
- E Cluster headache.

ME-Q143

Prochlorperazine (Stemetil®) is an APPROPRIATE treatment for which of the following?

- A Acute vertigo.
- B Unsteadiness of gait.
- C Senile tremor.
- D Parkinson disease.
- E Dizziness on standing.

ME-Q144

Osteoporosis

- A is more common in women than in men.
- B is associated with constant back pain in the majority of cases.
- C is usually associated with a normal serum calcium.
- D is a contra-indication to anti-depressant therapy.
- E may be caused by oral contraceptives.

ME-Q145

A 62-year-old man presents to you with his first attack of gout. On examination you find splenomegaly. Which of the following would you consider to be the LIKELY CAUSE(S) of the enlarged spleen?

- A Polycythaemia vera.
- B Portal hypertension.
- C Myelofibrosis.
- D Chronic lymphocytic leukaemia.
- E Systemic lupus erythematosus.

ME-Q146

Nutritional rickets is ASSOCIATED with

- A prominent costochondral junctions.
- B haemorrhagic tendency.
- C increased serum alkaline phosphatase.
- D nephrocalcinosis.
- E hypertrophy of the gums.

ME-Q147

In cardiac tamponade
    A there is sinus bradycardia.
    B the blood pressure falls with inspiration.
    C the jugular venous pressure is usually raised.
    D the chest X-ray shows pulmonary oedema.
    E a pericardial friction rub excludes an effusion.

ME-Q148

Which of the following statements about mitral valve prolapse is/are CORRECT?
    A The valve may become the site of infective endocarditis.
    B It is more common in men than in women.
    C It may cause systemic embolism.
    D It always causes a click and late systolic murmur.
    E It is usually accompanied by left ventricular hypertrophy.

ME-Q149

Which of the following statements about ventricular septal defect of the heart is/are CORRECT?
    A The condition usually produces a left to right shunt.
    B The condition can be diagnosed by cardiac ultrasound.
    C Atrial fibrillation is commonly present.
    D The condition predisposes to infective endocarditis.
    E Decreased pulmonary vascular markings are seen on chest X-ray.

ME-Q150

A hypertensive patient presents with atrial fibrillation, a ventricular rate of 120 beats/min, and chronic congestive cardiac failure (CCF). With respect to the management, which of the following statements is/are CORRECT?
    A Appropriate initial therapy could include vasodilation with captopril.
    B Digoxin would be appropriate treatment.
    C One frequently encountered side effect of therapy with captopril is hypokalaemia.
    D A cardioselective beta-blocker should be used to control the heart rate.
    E Angiotensin-converting enzyme (ACE) inhibitors can reduce sodium and water retention.

ME-Q151

A 65-year-old, previously well woman presents because of chest pain, nausea, vomiting and sweating. The respiration rate is 20 /min. The blood pressure is 90/60 mmHg and the pulse is regular at 130 /min. The venous pulse is visible 8 cm above the clavicle at 45° of recumbency and the liver is palpable 2 cm below the costal margin. The chest is clear to auscultation and there is no dependent oedema. The ECG shows sinus tachycardia and changes of acute inferior myocardial infarction. Intravenous therapy during the next 4 h should APPROPRIATELY INCLUDE
    A thrombolytic medication.
    B fluids to control blood pressure.
    C vasodilators.
    D diuretics.
    E narcotics.

ME-Q152

A 30-year-old male smoker on no medical therapy, height 170 cm, weight 100 kg, has a blood pressure of 170/96 mmHg. Silver wiring is present in the optic fundi. Twelve-lead ECG, serum electrolytes and serum creatinine are normal. You SHOULD

A   counsel him to stop smoking.

B   check his serum cholesterol and fasting blood sugar.

C   request a CT scan of the pituitary fossa.

D   advise him to moderate salt and alcohol intake.

E   have the urine microscopically examined.

ME-Q153

Which of the following statements is/are CORRECT concerning the drug treatment of hypertension?

A   The incidence of death from heart failure is reduced.

B   Thiazide diuretics have favourable effects on plasma lipids.

C   Adrenergic beta-blocking agents are relatively contraindicated in patients with symptomatic peripheral vascular disease.

D   Only the diastolic pressure is of importance in assessing progress.

E   Lowering the blood pressure below 130/80 mmHg increases the risk of myocardial infarction.

ME-Q154

A 64-year-old man with a history of well controlled hypertension has had a small thrombotic stroke. On examination he has a mild hemiparesis, an irregular pulse and blood pressure 120/80 mmHg. An ECG shows moderate left ventricular hypertrophy and atrial fibrillation with a ventricular rate of 95 /min. Which of the following long-term treatments is/are APPROPRIATE?

A   Continuation of antihypertensive treatment.

B   Cessation of antihypertensive medication and periodic reviews of blood pressure.

C   Aspirin, 100 mg, each morning.

D   Warfarin (INR range 1.8–2.2).

E   Digitalisation.

ME-Q155

Plasma cholesterol in a 51-year-old woman is found to be 6.8 mmol/L (< 5.5), triglycerides 3.2 mmol/L (< 2.0), high-density lipoprotein (HDL)–cholesterol 1.0 mmol/L (1.0–2.2). She is 160 cm tall and weighs 72 kg, giving her a body mass index (BMI) of 28. Her blood pressure is between 160/100 and 170/110 mmHg on repeated readings. Her mother died at the age of 60 from a myocardial infarction and her 55-year-old brother has had a coronary artery bypass graft. Which of the following statements is/are CORRECT?

A   Giving up her 20 cigarettes per day habit will immediately lower her blood pressure.

B   Her strong family history makes it more important than usual to lower her risk factors.

C   It is likely she will show insulin resistance.

D   Thiazide diuretics are good agents to begin her antihypertensive treatment.

E   She needs a renal angiogram to exclude renal arterial disease as a cause of her arterial hypertension.

ME-Q156

A 62-year-old man with high blood pressure has been prescribed atenolol, 100 mg daily, for the past 6 years. He believes that his high blood pressure is partly the result of heavy alcohol intake at weekends. He has increasing breathlessness and now sleeps propped on three pillows. He is conscious of his heart going faster than usual but has no chest pain. Blood pressure is 180/116 mmHg and his cardiac apex is very forceful and thrusting, but only moderately displaced in the fifth left intercostal space. The ECG shows conspicuous left ventricular hypertrophy confirmed on echocardiography. This also shows concentric wall thickening with an ejection fraction of 60%. Which of the following is/are CORRECT?

- A   In spite of a normal ejection fraction, he may have left ventricular failure.
- B   Beta-blockers are contraindicated because of the risk of precipitating or worsening cardiac failure.
- C   His left ventricular hypertrophy, by itself, places him at a significantly higher risk of heart attack, heart failure, stroke and early death.
- D   It is very unlikely his blood pressure control will be improved by doubling his atenolol dosage.
- E   His alcohol intake contributes significantly to his arterial hypertension and cardiac hypertrophy.

ME-Q157

The association of heart failure with a new systolic murmur in the setting of an acute myocardial infarction COULD BE DUE TO

- A   tricuspid regurgitation.
- B   papillary muscle dysfunction.
- C   papillary muscle rupture.
- D   ventricular septal defect.
- E   left ventricular outflow tract obstruction.

ME-Q158

The cough CAUSED BY angiotensin-converting enzyme (ACE) inhibitor therapy

- A   usually disappears if the patient is changed to another ACE inhibitor.
- B   usually occurs within 1 week of commencing medication.
- C   is usually not productive of sputum.
- D   is frequently accompanied by wheezing.
- E   is an absolute contraindication to future ACE inhibitor therapy.

ME-Q159

A 65-year-old woman is commenced on digoxin 0.125 mg/day to control the ventricular response rate to atrial fibrillation. The elimination half-life of digoxin is approximately 24 hours. Which of the following is/are CORRECT?

- A   It will take 3–5 days before steady state plasma concentrations of digoxin are achieved.
- B   The control of her ventricular response rate could be achieved more rapidly if she were given an initial loading dose of 0.5 mg digoxin.
- C   The addition of verapamil to her therapy would be expected to increase her plasma digoxin levels.
- D   If the cause of her atrial fibrillation is thyrotoxicosis, a lower dose should be used.
- E   Cholestyramine therapy may reduce the absorption of digoxin.

ME-Q160

A 65-year-old man with a 20 year history of hypertension presents with severe central chest pain radiating through to the back. The blood pressure is 190/110 mm Hg. An ECG shows ST segment depression and left ventricular hypertrophy. Which of the following is/are APPROPRIATE?

A Control blood pressure with a beta-blocking drug.

B Await cardiac enzymes before commencing tissue plasminogen activator (tPA).

C Arrange urgent CT scan of the chest.

D Commence on heparin.

E Commence on aspirin.

ME-Q161

Appropriate early management of unstable angina would INCLUDE

A admission to a coronary care unit for monitoring.

B aspirin.

C thrombolytic therapy.

D intravenous heparin.

E exercise test.

ME-Q162

A 68-year-old heavy smoker with chronic airway obstruction presents with increasing dyspnoea and confusion. His arterial blood gases reveal: P_aO_2 40 mmHg, P_aCO_2 34 mmHg, pH 7.22. Which of the following is/are CORRECT?

A Supplemental oxygen is dangerous in this man.

B These features could be due to superimposed acute left ventricular failure.

C These features could be due to acute bacteraemic shock.

D The deterioration is likely to be due to the administration of a sedative drug.

E Lactic acidosis is a likely associated finding.

ME-Q163

OCCUPATIONAL ASTHMA occurs after EXPOSURE TO

A silica.

B toluene di-isocyanate.

C asbestos.

D western red cedar dust.

E flour.

ME-Q164

In respiratory disease or heart disease, dyspnoea USUALLY reflects

A arterial hypoxaemia.

B hypercapnia.

C a decreased diffusing capacity of the lungs.

D an awareness of increased effort with breathing.

E lowered arterial pH.

ME-Q165

In auscultation of the chest

  A the presence or absence of rhonchi (wheezes) gives a reliable indication of the presence or absence of airway obstruction.

  B bronchial breathing can be heard above a pleural effusion.

  C inspiratory stridor suggests severe asthma.

  D crepitations (crackles) are commonly heard throughout inspiration in the presence of airways obstruction.

  E bronchial breathing tends to be heard over consolidated lung.

ME-Q166

Bronchogenic carcinoma

  A is surgically resectable in approximately 50% of patients.

  B can be excluded if the chest X-ray is normal.

  C has a 5 year survival of 50% after surgical resection.

  D can only be diagnosed reliably by bronchoscopy.

  E can present with hypokalaemia.

ME-Q167

Which of the following statements is/are CORRECT concerning small cell carcinoma of the lung?

  A It is the only histological type of lung carcinoma that produces ectopic hormone.

  B Its occurrence is poorly correlated with a history of cigarette smoking.

  C Chemotherapy with cyclophosphamide as the sole agent is the appropriate treatment.

  D At diagnosis, most patients have metastases beyond the hilar lymph nodes.

  E It may be associated with cerebellar degeneration.

ME-Q168

Concerning pulmonary sarcoidosis

  A pulmonary lesions characteristically cavitate.

  B the tuberculin skin test is usually positive.

  C erythema nodosum is a typical skin manifestation.

  D spontaneous resolution is usual.

  E hypercalcaemia suggests skeletal involvement.

ME-Q169

Idiopathic pulmonary fibrosis (cryptogenic fibrosing alveolitis) is COMMONLY ASSOCIATED with

  A hypercapnic respiratory failure.

  B positive antinuclear and rheumatoid factors.

  C finger clubbing.

  D inspiratory crepitations.

  E increased neutrophil and eosinophil count in alveolar washings.

ME-Q170

In cigarette smokers with chronic bronchitis, long-term worsening of airflow obstruction can be PREVENTED BY

- A continuous prophylactic antibiotic treatment.
- B regular oral theophylline compounds.
- C treatment with cortisone-like compounds.
- D ceasing to smoke cigarettes.
- E regular inhalation of bronchodilators.

ME-Q171

Barrett oesophagus

- A is lined by columnar epithelium.
- B is a congenital condition.
- C is caused by gastro-oesophageal reflux.
- D predisposes to oesophageal cancer.
- E is reversible.

ME-Q172

Concerning hepatitis A infection

- A fulminant hepatitis can occur.
- B faecal shedding of the virus usually diminishes with onset of clinical disease.
- C pooled gamma-globulin, if given within 2 weeks of exposure, will reduce the attack rate markedly.
- D parenteral transmission is uncommon.
- E the infection does not become chronic.

ME-Q173

Which of the following statements about viral hepatitis is/are CORRECT?

- A Delta hepatitis (hepatitis D) is caused by a defective virus dependent upon the presence of hepatitis B-DNA for its infectivity.
- B Hepatitis C is usually a self-limiting disease.
- C Plasma-derived vaccines for hepatitis B are more efficacious than recombinant vaccines.
- D With hepatitis A infection, jaundice is more common in adults than in children.
- E Acute hepatitis A infection is diagnosed by the presence of anti-hepatitis A virus IgG antibodies.

ME-Q174

Concerning hepatitis B immunisation

- A babies born to hepatitis B-infected mothers should receive both hepatitis B hyper-immune serum and vaccine.
- B administration of hepatitis B vaccine to chronic hepatitis B carriers is not harmful.
- C the vaccine is given orally.
- D recombinant vaccines elicit higher seroconversion rates than the plasma-derived vaccine.
- E recombinant vaccines can be used to boost immunity after primary immunisation with plasma-derived vaccine.

ME-Q175

In chronic pancreatitis
  A   serum amylase is markedly raised.
  B   the diagnosis can be excluded by the absence of calcification.
  C   associated diabetes requires low doses of insulin.
  D   the most usual association is with cholelithiasis.
  E   an abdominal mass is usually present.

ME-Q176

Which of the following is/are chemosensitive malignancies?
  A   Small cell lung cancer.
  B   Lymphoma.
  C   Chondrosarcoma.
  D   Testicular cancer.
  E   Breast cancer.

ME-Q177

Concerning pseudomembranous enterocolitis
  A   it is only associated with prolonged antibiotic therapy.
  B   the condition generally responds to treatment with vancomycin.
  C   the condition generally responds to treatment with tetracycline.
  D   stools of affected patients contain a toxin produced by *Clostridium difficile*.
  E   it is not associated with the use of ampicillin.

ME-Q178

Gynaecomastia in the male
  A   is usually due to excessive prolactin secretion.
  B   can result from treatment with histamine H_2 receptor antagonist drugs.
  C   occurs in liver cirrhosis.
  D   is best treated with testosterone.
  E   can occur during long-term spironolactone therapy.

ME-Q179

A RAISED serum prolactin level
  A   occurs in patients with severe primary hypothyroidism.
  B   can be a reversible cause of hypogonadism in acromegaly.
  C   is usually suppressed by bromocriptine.
  D   is responsible for gynaecomastia in the majority of males with this finding.
  E   is usually associated with a normal skull X-ray.

ME-Q180

Adrenal cortical failure can RESULT from
  A   tuberculosis.
  B   autoimmune adrenalitis.
  C   metastatic carcinoma.
  D   amyloidosis.
  E   meningococcal septicaemia.

ME-Q181

Concerning phaeochromocytomas

A sweating, nervousness and flushing are due to the secretion of catecholamines.

B urinary catecholamine excretion is markedly increased in more than 95% of cases.

C fasting blood sugar may be increased.

D blood pressure may be normal.

E blood pressure may be continually raised.

ME-Q182

A 25-year-old woman complains of 2 weeks of dysphagia and soreness in her neck, especially when swallowing. She has earache and her two children have had 'colds'. She is anxious and tremulous and her heart rate is 95 /min. Her thyroid gland is enlarged and tender. Thyroid hormone levels are as follows: T4 225 nmol/L (85–160); T3 3.6 nmol/L (1.5–2.6); TSH < 0.1 mU/L (0.4–-4.0). Which of the following is/are likely to be CORRECT?

A She does not have Graves disease.

B Antithyroid antibody titres will be high.

C A thyroid scan will show low iodine uptake.

D She has been taking thyroxine surreptitiously.

E Radioiodine would be the treatment of choice.

ME-Q183

Which of the following is/are SIDE EFFECTS of high dose oestrogen oral contraceptives?

A Increased incidence of thrombosis.

B Frigidity and depression.

C Migraine.

D Dysmenorrhoea.

E Hypertension.

ME-Q184

Changes in male sexual responses that occur with ageing INCLUDE

A a decreased ability to enjoy sexual activity.

B a need for more direct stimulation of the penis to achieve an erection.

C an increased tendency to premature ejaculation.

D a decreased volume of semen.

E a lengthened refractory period between erections.

ME-Q185

The erythrocyte sedimentation rate (ESR) is LIKELY to be elevated in which of the following?

A Acute gouty arthritis.

B IgG myeloma.

C Congestive cardiac failure.

D Polycythaemia rubra vera.

E Subacute bacterial endocarditis.

ME-Q186

Kidney stones

- A require extracorporeal lithotripsy in the majority of cases.
- B can be associated with hypercalciuria (urine calcium in excess of 7.5 mmol daily).
- C usually occur without demonstrable abnormalities of calcium metabolism.
- D can occur as a complication of excessive ascorbic acid consumption.
- E can be symptomless.

ME-Q187

Which of the following is/are TRANSMITTED PREDOMINANTLY in an autosomal dominant manner?

- A Alpha$_1$ antitrypsin deficiency.
- B Neurofibromatosis type II (von Recklinghausen disease).
- C Glucose-6-phosphate dehydrogenase deficiency.
- D Congenital spherocytosis.
- E Polycystic disease of kidney (adult form).

ME-Q188

Potential causes of hypercalcaemia INCLUDE

- A calcium-containing medications.
- B immobilisation.
- C oral contraceptive preparations.
- D carcinoma of the breast.
- E hyperparathyroidism.

ME-Q189

Tetracyclines can be used in the TREATMENT or PROPHYLAXIS of which of the following?

- A *Plasmodium falciparum* malaria.
- B Brucellosis.
- C Q fever.
- D Staphylococcal osteomyelitis.
- E Non-gonococcal urethritis.

ME-Q190

A 52-year-old patient with acute myeloid leukaemia and chemotherapy-induced neutropenia develops fever (39°C) and a cough. Blood count shows 0.5 x 10^9/L (2.0–7.5) neutrophils. On chest X-ray there is right lower lobe pneumonia. Which of the following organisms is/are LIKELY to be responsible?

- A *Mycoplasma pneumoniae.*
- B *Staphylococcus aureus.*
- C *Pneumocystis carinii.*
- D *Pseudomonas aeruginosa.*
- E *Klebsiella pneumoniae.*

ME-Q191

Hydatid disease can be ACQUIRED by humans by which of the following means?

- A Eating inadequately cooked lamb's liver.
- B Contact with the contents of hydatid cysts in the abattoir or on the farm.
- C Contact with hydatid cysts in a dog.
- D Ingestion of parasite ova from an infested dog.
- E Eating inadequately cooked pork.

ME-Q192

Which of the following pairings of a drug with a common adverse effect is/are CORRECT?

- A Levodopa — confusion.
- B Amantadine — choreiform movements.
- C Propranolol — nightmares.
- D Haloperidol — tardive dyskinesis.
- E Chlorpromazine — parkinsonism.

ME-Q193

Concerning digoxin therapy

- A it is effective in controlling the ventricular rate in atrial fibrillation.
- B the presence of hypokalaemia may potentiate the effects of digoxin.
- C the presence of hypercalcaemia may potentiate the effects of digoxin.
- D atrial fibrillation is a frequent toxic effect.
- E pulsus trigeminus is a sign of good digitalisation.

ME-Q194

Angiotensin-converting enzyme (ACE) inhibitors

- A are contraindicated in patients with diabetes and renal impairment.
- B should not be used with diuretics.
- C can cause an irritating cough.
- D should always be the 'first-line' therapy for heart failure.
- E reduce the rate of subsequent ischaemic events in patients with impaired left ventricular function after myocardial infarction.

ME-Q195

The SHORT-TERM effects of systemic treatment with high doses of corticosteroids INCLUDE

- A Cushing syndrome.
- B mood changes.
- C osteoporosis.
- D hypokalaemia.
- E hyperglycaemia.

ME-Q196

Patients with haematological malignant disease often receive prolonged courses of high dose corticosteroid therapy (prednisolone 100 mg, daily), as part of their treatment. Which of the following effects can RESULT from this prolonged corticosteroid therapy?

- A Insomnia.
- B Loss of appetite.
- C Fluid retention.
- D Increased muscle bulk.
- E Avascular necrosis of bone.

ME-Q197

Which of the following side effects COMMONLY occur(s) with intravenous amphotericin B administration?

A Hypokalaemia.
B Optic neuritis.
C Anaemia.
D Hypercalcaemia.
E Rise in serum creatinine.

ME-Q198

Which of the following drugs require(s) DOSE MODIFICATION in the presence of chronic renal failure?

A Digoxin.
B Aminophylline.
C Promethazine.
D Gentamicin.
E Paracetamol.

ME-Q199

Major tranquillisers (phenothiazines and butyrophenones) are LIKELY CAUSE(S) of which of the following involuntary movements?

A Dystonic attacks (oculogyric crises).
B Hand tremor at rest.
C Inability to sit still (akathisia).
D Flapping tremor (asterixis).
E Action myoclonus.

ME-Q200

Which of the following clinical conditions due to malignancy is/are USUALLY amenable to palliative irradiation?

A Superior vena caval obstruction.
B Bony pain.
C Tumour fungation.
D Established paraplegia.
E Chronic debilitating haemorrhage.

ME-Q201

With long-term treatment with immunosuppressive agents, there is an INCREASED risk of

A skin cancer.
B aseptic bone necrosis.
C lens cataract.
D renal tract calculi.
E viral infections.

ME-Q202

Common neurological manifestations of HIV infection INCLUDE which of the following?

A Guillain-Barré syndrome.

B Parkinsonism.

C Dementia.

D Peripheral neuropathy.

E Trigeminal neuralgia.

ME-Q203

Concerning the condition immune thrombocytopenic purpura (ITP)

A the platelet count is very commonly normal.

B the condition may respond to treatment with intravenous gamma-globulin.

C quinine, penicillin and heparin are all known to be associated with the development of the disease.

D splenectomy is the first line of treatment in adult patients.

E the number of megakaryocytes in the bone marrow is reduced.

ME-Q204

In the evaluation of a patient with suspected systemic lupus erythematosus, which of the following is/are CORRECT?

A A positive antinuclear antibody test is diagnostic.

B The presence of sclerodactyly or digital infarction is highly suggestive of the diagnosis.

C A normal creatinine clearance excludes renal involvement.

D Joint involvement is typically symmetric and non-deforming.

E A history of pleurisy suggests infection rather than lupus.

ME-Q205

A 16-year-old girl presents 3 h after the acute onset of increasing diffuse urticaria and facial oedema with dysphonia. Which of the following is/are CORRECT?

A A fever of 39.5°C is consistent with urticaria alone.

B The presence of dysphonia requires urgent hospitalisation.

C This disorder is usually caused by inhaled allergen.

D Hereditary angioedema is the likely cause.

E A search for a specific allergen is important.

Surgery Questions

TYPE

A

Questions SU-Q1 to SU-Q107

- Type A questions consist of a stem and five responses
- **<u>One</u>** correct answer must be selected from five possible responses to the stem

SU-Q1

Of the following factors which is MOST important in determining the overall prognosis in a patient with a malignant melanoma?

A Depth of invasion in the skin and subcutaneous tissues.

B Previous history of irradiation in the area.

C The number of mitotic figures in the microscopic specimen.

D The level of carcinoembryonic antigen.

E Previous history of depigmentation of a pigmented naevus.

SU-Q2

A patient has had a mole excised from the lower leg just above the ankle with 1 mm clearance around it. Draining lymph nodes were clinically normal. Histopathology reveals malignant melanoma (extending to a depth of 0.5 mm on microscopy). Further treatment would OPTIMALLY be

A radical excision of the draining lymph nodes.

B irradiation to the primary area.

C wider excision of the primary area.

D keeping the patient under regular observation.

E reassurance of patient that the lesion has been adequately excised.

SU-Q3

An adult patient sustains a full thickness skin burn approximately the size of a 10 cent coin on his thigh as a result of a splash from molten metal. The BEST TREATMENT of the wound would be excision and

A primary closure.

B full thickness skin graft with microvascular techniques.

C split skin graft.

D pedicle graft.

E dressing.

SU-Q4

A tumour arising in a burn scar is MOST LIKELY to be

A squamous cell carcinoma.

B basal cell carcinoma.

C malignant melanoma.

D sweat-gland adenocarcinoma.

E fibrosarcoma.

SU-Q5

The lesion depicted in the accompanying photograph (Figure 11) appeared spontaneously. The following ACTION should be undertaken

A reassurance that spontaneous resolution will occur.

B incision under local anaesthetic.

C application of liquid nitrogen.

D review in 1 month.

E plastic surgical referral.

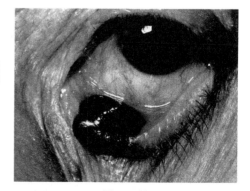

Figure 11

SU-Q6

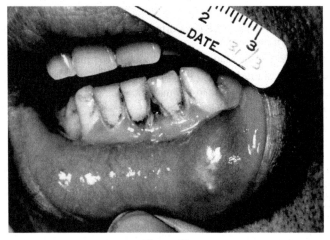

Figure 12

A 22-year-old man noticed the lesion depicted in the accompanying photograph (Figure 12) 4 weeks previously. The lesion is MOST LIKELY

    A a basal cell carcinoma.

    B a squamous cell carcinoma.

    C a sebaceous cyst.

    D an early syphilitic lip lesion.

    E a mucoid cyst.

SU-Q7

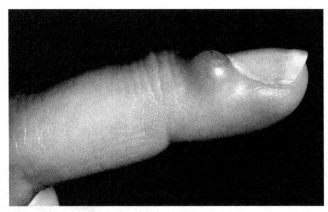

Figure 13

The lesion pictured in the accompanying photograph (Figure 13) has been present on the finger of a middle-aged woman for the past 6 months, with gradual enlargement and mild discomfort. The MOST LIKELY diagnosis is

    A osteoarthritis of distal interphalangeal joint.

    B mucous (synovial) cyst of the finger.

    C gouty tophus.

    D chronic paronychia.

    E chronic suppurative arthritis.

SU-Q8

A lipoma

    A is a premalignant condition.

    B is invariably subcutaneous.

    C often occurs in the scrotum.

    D cannot be tethered to the skin.

    E is usually lobulated.

SU-Q9

The lesion depicted in the accompanying photograph (Figure 14) was present on the back of a 43-year-old builder. You should ADVISE him the lesion

    A should be excised because it is malignant and will extend locally but NOT to the draining lymph nodes.

    B is benign but is likely to become malignant, so should be excised.

    C should be excised because it is malignant and is likely to extend to the draining lymph nodes.

    D is benign, but should be excised because it may become an abscess.

    E is benign and has no inflammatory or malignant complications and does not need to be excised.

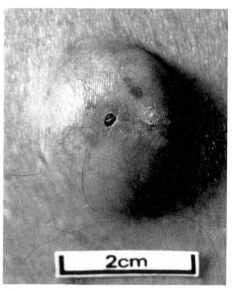

Figure 14

SU-Q10

Which of the following lesions of squamous epithelium is NOT premalignant?

    A Leucoplakia.

    B Intradermal naevus.

    C Bowen disease.

    D Chronic radiation dermatitis.

    E Solar keratosis.

SU-Q11

Which of the following is the MOST LIKELY pathological diagnosis of the lesions in the accompanying photograph (Figure 15), which were noted on the back of an elderly woman?

    A Pigmented basal cell carcinomas.

    B Seborrhoeic keratoses.

    C Mycosis fungoides.

    D Solar keratoses.

    E Hutchinson melanotic freckles.

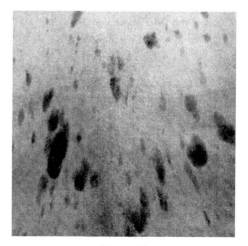

Figure 15

SU-Q12

A 63-year-old woman has the lump depicted in the accompanying photograph (Figure 16) on the left side of her face. It has been very slowly increasing in size over 10 years. The MOST LIKELY DIAGNOSIS is

A carcinoma of the parotid.
B carcinoma of the submandibular gland.
C adenolymphoma (Warthin tumour) of the parotid.
D parotid calculus.
E pleomorphic adenoma of the parotid.

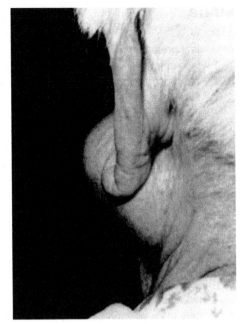

Figure 16

SU-Q13

Facial nerve palsy in association with a parotid tumour SUGGESTS which of the following diagnoses?

A Warthin tumour (adenolymphoma).
B Mixed parotid tumour of the superficial lobe.
C Adenoid cystic carcinoma.
D Mixed parotid tumour of the deep lobe.
E Associated chronic parotitis.

SU-Q14

Which of the following normal structures in the neck is MOST LIKELY to be mistaken for malignant enlargement of a lymph node?

A The Adam apple (anterior aspect of thyroid cartilage).
B The greater horn of the hyoid bone.
C The sternoclavicular joint.
D The sternomastoid tendon.
E The thyroid gland.

SU-Q15

A branchial cyst

A usually makes its first appearance in the second or third decade of life.
B is situated in the upper third of the neck.
C protrudes around the anterior border of the sternomastoid.
D is usually lined by squamous epithelium.
E exhibits all of the above characteristics.

SU-Q16

Papillary carcinoma of the thyroid gland

    A is a slow growing tumour which is influenced by thyroid stimulating hormone secretion.

    B is multifocal and spreads mainly by the blood to the bone.

    C is sometimes associated with phaeochromocytoma and skin lesions.

    D produces calcitonin and the syndrome of malignant hypocalcaemia.

    E is extremely radiosensitive and should be treated by irradiation of the thyroid gland.

SU-Q17

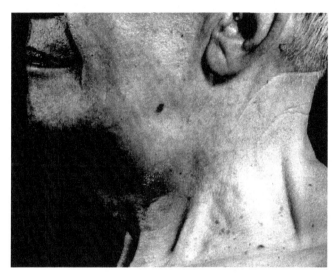

Figure 17

A previously well 59-year-old man developed sudden onset of acute pain in the left cervical region at 19.45 h. He subsequently became aware of a tender swelling which is illustrated in the accompanying photograph (Figure 17). The precise cause of the swelling would BEST be DETECTED BY

    A palpation of the cervical lymph nodes in the anterior triangle of the neck.

    B palpation of the cervical lymph nodes in the posterior triangle of the neck.

    C plain X-ray of the posterior part of the mandible.

    D examination of the tonsils after local anaesthetic spray.

    E bimanual palpation of the floor of the mouth.

SU-Q18

A ranula

    A is an inflamed sublingual salivary gland.

    B is usually situated on the lower lip.

    C results from obstruction of a minor salivary gland duct.

    D often extends down through the mylohyoid.

    E often presents as a sinus in the neck.

SU-Q19

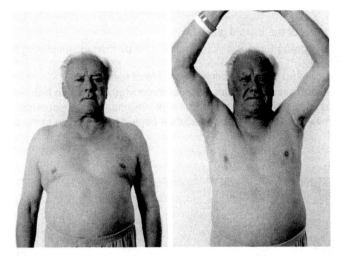

Figures 18 and 19

The patient in the accompanying photographs (Figures 18 and 19) presented with a neck swelling, and a feeling of dizziness when he reaches upwards. The photographs show the findings when he lifts his arms above his head. The change in facial appearance on arm elevation is DUE TO

A   traumatic asphyxia caused by an old fibrosing haematoma of the neck.

B   vascular steal syndrome with retrograde flow of blood from brachial to carotid arteries.

C   venous obstruction from retrosternal extension of the neck mass.

D   compression of a medullary thyroid carcinoma causing localised serotonin release.

E   compression of the sympathetic trunks crossing the first rib.

SU-Q20

An unconscious patient is on his back. Which one of the following statements is INCORRECT?

A   The tongue may be obstructing the airway.

B   Tilting the head back may open the airway.

C   The patient should be transported in the supine position.

D   If airway obstruction is remedied the patient may regain consciousness.

E   The patient should be rapidly assessed for other injuries.

SU-Q21

In assessing progress of a patient with a head injury the MOST IMPORTANT clinical observation is

A   examination of the fundi.

B   the state of the pupils.

C   the level of consciousness.

D   plantar responses.

E   blood pressure.

SU-Q22

Chronic subdural haematoma

   A is best managed in elderly patients with oral corticosteroids and diuretics.

   B is usually associated with a skull fracture.

   C commonly presents with headache and dementia.

   D is rare in alcoholics.

   E usually results from bleeding from cortical vessels.

SU-Q23

A patient lacerates the ulnar nerve just above the wrist. Which of the following physical findings is MOST LIKELY to be present? Inability to

   A extend the wrist.

   B flex the wrist.

   C flex the distal phalanges of the fourth and fifth digits.

   D oppose the thumb and index finger.

   E spread the fingers.

SU-Q24

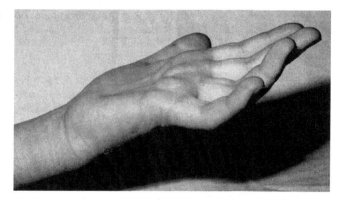

Figure 20

The deformity pictured in the accompanying photograph (Figure 20) is TYPICAL of

   A congenital finger contracture (clinodactyly).

   B ulnar nerve palsy.

   C Dupuytren contracture.

   D rheumatoid arthritis.

   E Volkmann contracture of tendons.

SU-Q25

A patient presents with a history of low back pain and right sided sciatica. Pain extends to the small toes, the ankle reflex is absent and there is eversion weakness of the foot. Which nerve root is ENTRAPPED?

   A Lumbar 3.

   B Lumbar 4.

   C Lumbar 5.

   D Sacral 1.

   E Sacral 2.

SU-Q26

Volkmann ischaemic contracture is MOST COMMONLY associated with

- A wrist fracture.
- B fracture of both bones of the forearm.
- C dislocation of the elbow.
- D supracondylar fracture of the humerus.
- E epicondylar fracture of the humerus.

SU-Q27

After successful resuscitation, which of the following is the MOST COMMON CAUSE of death in patients with multiple skeletal and soft tissue injuries?

- A Renal failure.
- B Hypovolaemic shock.
- C Septic shock.
- D Pulmonary embolism.
- E Ventilatory failure.

SU-Q28

A 55-year-old labourer feels a sharp pain in his right shoulder as he is lifting a heavy crate. On examination he has moderate pain and tenderness in the shoulder. The shoulder can be moved passively through most of its range of movement, but active abduction can only be achieved if assisted through the initial 90°. The MOST LIKELY diagnosis is

- A rupture of the long head of the biceps.
- B rupture of the subscapularis tendon.
- C rupture of the supraspinatus tendon.
- D rupture of the short head of biceps.
- E slipped upper humeral epiphysis.

SU-Q29

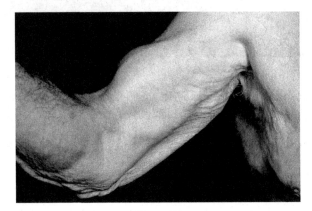

Figure 21

A 60-year-old doctor who has recommenced playing tennis, noticed one morning a swelling in his upper arm. The appearance is shown in the accompanying photograph (Figure 21). The MOST LIKELY diagnosis is

- A rupture of a valve in a brachial vein producing a large varix.
- B haematoma of the biceps/brachioradialis muscle group.
- C rupture of the short head of the biceps muscle.
- D rupture of the long head of the biceps muscle.
- E acute false aneurysm of the brachial artery.

SU-Q30

What is the preferred treatment in the management of MOST fractures of the neck of the humerus in elderly women?

    A Manipulative reduction under general anaesthetic and application of hanging cast.

    B Rest the arm in a sling for comfort and commence active shoulder movements as early as possible.

    C Open reduction and internal fixation.

    D Immobilisation in a shoulder spica.

    E Bed rest and traction using a pulley and weights.

SU-Q31

Which one of the following statements about scaphoid fractures is INCORRECT?

    A The patient may require special X-ray views (besides lateral and anteroposterior) to demonstrate the fracture.

    B The fracture may not be seen on any X-ray film before 3 weeks.

    C The fracture is often undisplaced.

    D The fracture may result in avascular necrosis of the distal half of the bone.

    E The fracture may require treatment by internal fixation.

SU-Q32

Which of the following is the most frequent LATE complication of a Colles fracture in an elderly woman?

    A Median nerve weakness.

    B Stiffness of wrist and fingers.

    C Ischaemic necrosis of distal fragments.

    D Delayed union of fracture.

    E Ulnar nerve weakness.

SU-Q33

A 13-year-old boy presents to his general practitioner complaining of poorly localised pain in his knee for the past 6 weeks. His mother has observed a limp for the same period of time and he walks with his foot externally rotated. Examination of the knee is normal. The MOST LIKELY diagnosis is

    A osteochondritis dissecans of the knee.

    B Perthes disease of the hip.

    C old undiagnosed congenital dislocation of the hip.

    D slipped upper femoral epiphysis.

    E Osgood–Schlatter osteochondritis of the knee.

SU-Q34

The LEAST likely fracture to occur in a 7-year-old child who falls on an outstretched arm is

    A fracture of both bones of the forearm.

    B dislocation of the distal radial epiphysis.

    C Colles fracture.

    D supracondylar fracture.

    E greenstick fracture of the ulna.

SU-Q35

A 23-year-old man has suffered for 6 years from a recurrent ulcer on the medial aspect of his left lower leg. Eight years ago he suffered a fractured femur. The cause of this ulcer is MOST LIKELY to be

  A diabetes.
  B syphilis.
  C perforator vein incompetence.
  D arterial injury.
  E osteomyelitis.

SU-Q36

The signs evident in the patient depicted in the accompanying photograph (Figure 22) SUPPORT a diagnosis of

  A vena caval obstruction.
  B aorto–vena caval fistula.
  C recent right axillo–femoral arterial bypass.
  D portal vein obstruction.
  E right external iliac vein thrombosis.

SU-Q37

Which one of the following is NOT consistent with a diagnosis of superficial femoral artery occlusion?

  A Claudication in the thigh.
  B Gangrene of the great toe.
  C Rest pain.
  D Calf claudication at 50 metres.
  E Improvement in claudication distance during period of observation.

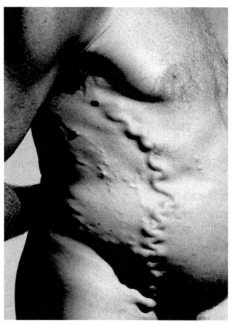

Figure 22

SU-Q38

Which one of the following clinical features is NOT consistent with the diagnosis of ACUTE arterial occlusion in a limb?

  A Pain.
  B Paralysis.
  C Pallor.
  D Oedema.
  E Coldness of the limb.

SU-Q39

A 57-year-old patient is admitted to hospital with sudden pain in the left leg 2 weeks after an acute myocardial infarction. Examination reveals a cold and white left leg with absent arterial pulses and a normal right leg. Which of the following is the MOST APPROPRIATE immediate management?

  A Arteriography followed by observation.
  B Heparin therapy and observation.
  C Heparin therapy followed by urgent embolectomy.
  D Embolectomy without anticoagulant therapy.
  E Elevation of the head of the bed with cooling of the affected limb.

SU-Q40

Nine days after anterior resection of the rectum in an obese 57-year-old man, his left leg becomes swollen with tenderness of the calf. He has a slight fever and tachycardia. The MOST IMPORTANT aspect of his treatment WOULD be

A   elevation of the foot of the bed.
B   an elastic stocking.
C   anticoagulant therapy with heparin.
D   insertion of an inferior vena caval filter.
E   ligation of the left femoral vein.

SU-Q41

A 45-year-old woman presents with a 2 day history of a painful left leg. Examination reveals bilateral varicose veins and an elongated area of tender induration in the subcutaneous tissue with surrounding erythema on the medial aspect of the left lower thigh. Which of the following is the MOST APPROPRIATE treatment?

A   Therapy with a non-steroidal anti-inflammatory agent (NSAID), supportive bandages and bed rest.
B   Antibiotic therapy and bed rest with elevation of the foot of the bed.
C   Anticoagulant therapy, supportive bandages and ambulation.
D   Analgesia as required, supportive bandages and ambulation.
E   Analgesia as required and bed rest with elevation of the foot of the bed.

SU-Q42

Which of the following is NOT a feature of vasovagal syncope (faint)?

A   Reduction in cardiac output.
B   Increase in heart rate.
C   Cold, pale skin.
D   Hypotension.
E   Poorly palpable pulse.

SU-Q43

A 25-year-old man with haemorrhagic shock is alert and anxious, has a blood pressure of 70/30 mmHg and a pulse rate of 130 beats/min. The patient was previously healthy. What percentage of total blood volume is MOST LIKELY to approximate the blood loss?

A   5%.
B   10%.
C   20%.
D   40%.
E   80%.

SU-Q44

You are performing external cardiac massage on a patient who has just suffered a cardiac arrest. Which of the following provides BEST indication that resuscitation is proving effective?

A   Electrocardiography.
B   Palpation of the femoral pulse.
C   Colour of skin and mucous membranes.
D   Size and reaction of the pupils.
E   Response to stimuli.

SU-Q45

A 65-year-old man develops sudden excruciating interscapular pain radiating into the right lower limb. On physical examination, the right femoral pulse is not felt and the left femoral pulse is weak. There is an aortic diastolic murmur. The blood pressure is 160/90 mmHg, and the pulse rate is 100 /min. The MOST LIKELY diagnosis is

A myocardial infarction.
B embolus of the abdominal aorta.
C dissecting aortic aneurysm.
D pulmonary embolus.
E spontaneous pneumothorax.

SU-Q46

Which of the following is the MOST SPECIFIC DIAGNOSTIC test in the patient described in the previous question (SU-Q45)?

A Electrocardiogram.
B Chest X-ray.
C Serum transaminase determination.
D Haematocrit determination.
E Aortography.

SU-Q47

Which of the following features is NOT a contraindication for attempted curative surgical resection of bronchogenic carcinoma?

A Superior vena cava obstruction.
B Hoarseness of voice.
C Blood-stained pleural effusion.
D Pulmonary osteoarthropathy.
E Very poor exercise tolerance.

SU-Q48

Seven days after an elective right hemicolectomy a 65-year-old man collapses complaining of sudden onset of chest pain and shortness of breath. Which one of the following is likely to be the MOST HELPFUL in establishing the cause of his chest pain?

A Electrocardiography.
B Ventilation–perfusion lung scan.
C Chest X-ray.
D Calf and thigh venography.
E Duplex scan of thigh veins.

SU-Q49

During the first 24 h after a gastrectomy your patient develops a fever of 38.5°C. The MOST LIKELY cause is

A atelectasis.
B urinary tract infection.
C wound infection.
D deep venous thrombosis.
E superficial thrombophlebitis.

SU-Q50

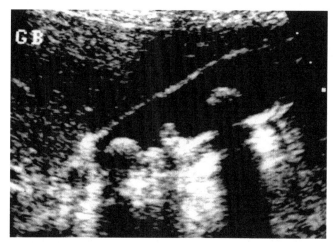

Figure 23

A 43-year-old woman with recurrent severe lower retrosternal pain and a normal electro-cardiogram has the investigation depicted in the accompanying photograph (Figure 23). No other abnormality is demonstrated on scanning the upper abdomen. The NEXT STEP in management should be

  A cholecystectomy.

  B endoscopic retrograde papillotomy of the sphincter of Oddi.

  C bile salt dissolution therapy alone.

  D lithotripsy and bile salt dissolution.

  E non-surgical management and strict fat-free dieting.

SU-Q51

A patient with a known duodenal ulcer presents with haematemesis and melaena requiring admission to hospital. Which of the following is the MOST IMPORTANT consideration favouring early surgical intervention?

  A The ulcer is over 1 cm in diameter.

  B The patient is female.

  C The patient is 65 years old.

  D The patient's blood group is O negative.

  E Previous acid secretory studies indicated a high acid output.

SU-Q52

An alcoholic man is admitted with a 10 day history of epigastric pain and vomiting. He has minimal epigastric tenderness and muscle guarding. The white blood cell count is 13 000 with 90% neutrophils and the serum amylase is 750 units/L (70–400). Two weeks after admission a non-tender mass in the epigastrium is palpable. Which one of the following investigations would you recommend to BEST EVALUATE the mass?

  A Repeat serum amylase.

  B A plain X-ray examination of the abdomen.

  C An oral cholecystogram.

  D An ERCP (endoscopic retrograde cholangiopancreatogram).

  E A computed tomography (CT) scan of the abdomen.

SU-Q53

The diagnosis of chronic fissure-in-ano is BEST made as a result of
A careful inspection of the anal verge.
B sigmoidoscopy.
C colonoscopy.
D barium enema.
E digital rectal examination.

SU-Q54

The MOST COMMON outcome after surgical drainage of a perianal abscess is
A development of a perianal fistula.
B subsequent identification of regional ileitis (Crohn disease).
C recurrence of the abscess.
D healing of the sinus.
E prolapsed anal mucosa.

SU-Q55

Seven days after a moderate myocardial infarction, a 65-year-old man develops abdominal pain and diarrhoea with passage of blood. The abdomen is slightly tender and a plain X-ray examination shows a distended small intestine but no fluid levels. Serum amylase is slightly elevated and the temperature is 38°C. The MOST LIKELY diagnosis is
A mesenteric ischaemia.
B stress ulceration of the duodenum.
C diverticulitis.
D disseminated intravascular coagulopathy (DIC).
E heparin-induced bleeding.

SU-Q56

A 32-year-old man complains that he has recently noticed the presence of small amounts of bright blood on the toilet paper after defaecation. His bowel habit is normal and regular. On proctoscopy second degree haemorrhoids are seen. His FURTHER MANAGEMENT should be
A treatment of his haemorrhoids.
B sigmoidoscopy, then treatment of his haemorrhoids if sigmoidoscopy is normal to 25 cm.
C sigmoidoscopy, colonoscopy, then treatment of his haemorrhoids if both investigations are normal.
D sigmoidoscopy, colonoscopy, air-contrast barium enema, then treatment of his haemorrhoids if all three investigations are normal.
E sigmoidoscopy, air-contrast barium enema, then treatment of his haemorrhoids if both investigations are normal.

SU-Q57

Which of the following is MOST LIKELY to be the initial symptom in acute pancreatitis?
A Vomiting.
B Sweating.
C Faintness.
D Pain.
E Constipation.

SU-Q58

The MOST USUAL type of operation performed for benign GASTRIC ulceration is

- A highly selective vagotomy.
- B bilateral truncal vagotomy and drainage.
- C gastrojejunostomy.
- D partial gastrectomy.
- E pyloroplasty.

SU-Q59

Which of the following MOST SUGGESTS the presence of strangulated bowel in intestinal obstruction?

- A Absolute constipation.
- B Generalised abdominal pain which has become constant.
- C Multiple fluid levels on abdominal X-ray examination.
- D Profuse vomiting.
- E Onset of mucous diarrhoea.

SU-Q60

A 50-year-old woman presents to the emergency department with a 36 h history of upper abdominal pain, initially epigastric, but now in the right upper quadrant. On examination she has a temperature of 38.5°C and a tachycardia. There is marked tenderness under the right costal margin. The MOST HELPFUL diagnostic investigation at this stage is

- A cholecystogram.
- B abdominal ultrasound.
- C liver function tests.
- D X-ray examination of the abdomen.
- E serum amylase.

SU-Q61

All of the following features occur in both Crohn disease and in ulcerative colitis EXCEPT

- A diarrhoea.
- B granulomatous inflammation.
- C response to steroids.
- D extra-intestinal disease.
- E a chronic course.

SU-Q62

A 36-year-old accountant presents with abdominal pain, nausea and vomiting of bright red blood. For several days his stools have been black and malodorous. He has had no previous similar episodes, but for some time he has been taking antacids for indigestion. On examination he is pale with a cool, moist skin, pulse rate 110 /min, and blood pressure 90/60 mmHg. No abdominal masses can be felt, but he is tender in the epigastrium. His haemoglobin is 10 g/dL. The MOST LIKELY diagnosis is

- A bleeding duodenal ulcer.
- B diffuse gastritis.
- C carcinoma of the papilla of Vater.
- D carcinoma of the stomach.
- E bleeding oesophageal varices.

SU-Q63

A 14-year-old boy presents with a swelling in the right groin which has been present for only 1 month. On palpatation, the swelling is felt over the external inguinal ring accompanied by an impulse on coughing, but disappears when lying down. Scrotal examination is normal in the supine and erect positions. You should ADVISE

A   an operation for an inguinal hernia.

B   a cystoscopy to exclude a diverticulum of the urinary bladder.

C   a barium enema.

D   an ultrasound examination of the testes.

E   an intravenous pyelogram with bladder examination.

SU-Q64

A 23-year-old woman consults you with a history of rectal bleeding with defaecation over the past 4 weeks. Defaecation is associated with severe acute pain which persists afterwards. She also has difficulty initiating micturition. The blood is bright and of small amount and is seen on the surface of the stool, and on the paper. The discomfort has worsened progressively and is now incapacitating her in normal activities and interfering with sleep. At the INITIAL consultation you should undertake

A   proctoscopy.

B   rigid sigmoidoscopy.

C   flexible sigmoidoscopy.

D   anal dilation with copious paraffin lubricant.

E   inspection of the anal verge with a view to establishing the diagnosis.

SU-Q65

A 65-year-old woman has a 2 year history of mucous diarrhoea due to a large villous adenoma of the rectum. She is also taking digoxin and diuretics for chronic congestive failure. Which of the following investigations would be the MOST HELPFUL prior to surgery?

A   Serum chloride.

B   Serum digoxin.

C   Serum calcium.

D   Serum potassium.

E   Haemoglobin.

SU-Q66

Calcification seen on a plain abdominal X-ray of a 63-year-old East European woman is MOST LIKELY to be due to

A   tuberculous lymph nodes.

B   calcified gallstones.

C   chronic pancreatitis.

D   uterine fibroids.

E   an abdominal aortic aneurysm.

SU-Q67

A 65-year-old patient presents with left iliac fossa pain, nausea, vomiting and distended loops of small bowel on abdominal X-ray. He is MOST LIKELY to be suffering from

A   a calculus impacted in the left ureter.

B   diverticulitis and paracolic abscess.

C   perforated appendicitis.

D   psoas abscess.

E   pseudomembranous colitis of the descending colon.

SU-Q68

The most COMMON complication seen after splenectomy is

- A left lower lobe atelectasis.
- B left subphrenic abscess.
- C deep venous thrombosis secondary to thrombocytosis.
- D pancreatic fistula.
- E prolonged paralytic ileus.

SU-Q69

Which one of the following operations is MOST LIKELY to be followed by prolonged paralytic ileus?

- A Gastrectomy.
- B Repair of right inguinal hernia.
- C Resection of ruptured abdominal aortic aneurysm.
- D Repair of a hiatus hernia.
- E Removal of an inflamed appendix.

SU-Q70

A 26-year-old man presents with a 3 week history of pain and a swelling in the left side of his scrotum. Which of the following is CORRECT?

- A If the swelling is within the scrotum and separate from the testis, it is probably a hydrocele.
- B If the swelling transilluminates then malignancy can be excluded.
- C If the examiner cannot get his hand above the swelling then the patient probably has an inguinoscrotal hernia.
- D The patient may have a twisted hydatid of Morgagni (appendix of the testis) which is a swelling at the lower pole of the testis.
- E Tuberculous epididymo-orchitis is a common cause of such a swelling.

SU-Q71

A 53-year-old farmer presents with a 2 month history of a painless swelling in the right groin. On examination he has a firm 3 cm NON-TENDER swelling immediately below and lateral to the pubic tubercle. Which of the following statements is CORRECT?

- A If there is no cough impulse he may well have a strangulated hernia.
- B The lump could well represent a secondary deposit from a testicular neoplasm.
- C The lump is probably a saphena varix.
- D The next investigation should be a computed tomography (CT) scan.
- E Anal canal tumours can metastasise to groin lymph nodes.

SU-Q72

In a patient with an appendix abscess, which of the following organisms is LEAST likely to be found in the abscess?

- A *Bacteroides fragilis.*
- B *Bacteroides melanococcus.*
- C *Streptococcus faecalis.*
- D *Escherichia coli.*
- E *Staphylococcus aureus.*

SU-Q73

The MOST COMMON factor causing an abdominal wound dehiscence is

A premature suture material breakdown.
B deficient surgical technique.
C vitamin C deficiency.
D anaemia.
E hyponatraemia.

SU-Q74

Which of the following investigations should FIRST be performed in a 65-year-old man with a history of altered bowel habit?

A Barium meal and follow through.
B Barium enema.
C Sigmoidoscopy.
D Computed tomography (CT) scan of the abdomen.
E Chest X-ray.

SU-Q75

A patient has cancer of the rectum. Which of the following clinical features is MOST LIKELY to be present?

A Rectal bleeding.
B Anaemia.
C Intestinal obstruction.
D Constipation.
E Diarrhoea.

SU-Q76

The MOST COMMON cause of a fistula between the sigmoid colon and vagina is which of the following?

A Carcinoma of the colon.
B Foreign body.
C Carcinoma of the uterus.
D Radiation therapy.
E Diverticulitis of the colon.

SU-Q77

All of the following statements concerning Paget disease of the nipple are correct EXCEPT

A the basic lesion is an intraductal carcinoma.
B the nipple epithelium is infiltrated with cancer cells.
C the tumour can usually be detected on careful palpation.
D the first symptom is often itching or burning of the nipple.
E the diagnosis is readily established by biopsy of the erosion.

SU-Q78

Which of the following statements about the use of adjuvant chemotherapy in patients with carcinoma of the breast is CORRECT?

    A There is no evidence that it causes second tumours of the breast.
    B It is now established as standard therapy in all patients with breast cancer.
    C It does not prolong survival.
    D It is more effective in postmenopausal patients than in premenopausal patients.
    E One drug alone is as effective as two or three combined.

SU-Q79

A discrete mobile mass in the breast of a 25-year-old woman is MOST LIKELY to be

    A carcinoma.
    B fibroadenoma.
    C intraduct papilloma.
    D fibroadenosis.
    E fat necrosis.

SU-Q80

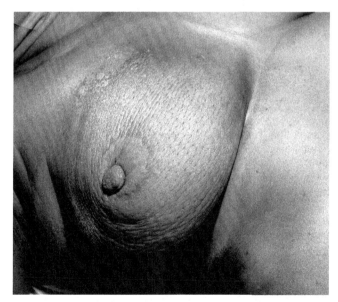

Figure 24

A 67-year-old woman recently noticed a non-painful lump in the right breast. The accompanying photograph (Figure 24) shows the appearance of the breast on inspection. The MOST LIKELY diagnosis is

    A subacute mastitis with early abscess formation.
    B advanced adenocarcinoma of the breast.
    C early intraduct carcinoma with obstruction of ductal ampullae.
    D severe fibrocystic disease of the breast (fibroadenosis with multiple cysts).
    E extensive fat necrosis of the breast.

SU-Q81

Which of the following is NOT correct? A varicocele is

- A usually associated with an inguinal hernia.
- B more common on the left.
- C often asymptomatic.
- D sometimes associated with infertility.
- E sometimes associated with a renal carcinoma.

SU-Q82

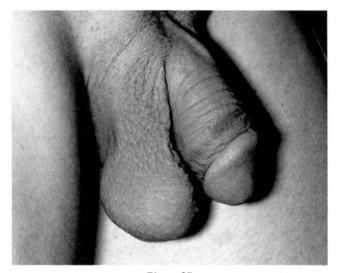

Figure 25

A 15-year-old boy has experienced, over the past month, two episodes of pain in the right lower abdomen, groin and scrotum. The last attack occurred 1 week previously. The pain lasted 2 h but since then he has had no pain. The appearance of his right groin and scrotum while standing is illustrated in the accompanying photograph (Figure 25). No tenderness can be elicited and he has no urinary or gastrointestinal symptoms. He has no fever and is eating normally. RECOMMENDED MANAGEMENT should be to ARRANGE

- A reassurance of him and his mother and ask him to return if the pain recurs.
- B three microscopic examinations of his urine and cultures and then start antibiotic therapy.
- C mumps serology.
- D cystoscopy.
- E operation.

SU-Q83

A 7-year-old boy is seen in the emergency room with a history of acute painful swelling in the right scrotum, which prevents him from sleeping. The right side of the scrotum is found to be swollen, firm, and extremely tender. The overlying skin is reddened and oedematous. The MOST LIKELY diagnosis is

- A acute hydrocele.
- B acute epididymitis.
- C traumatic orchitis.
- D torsion of the testis.
- E testicular tumour.

SU-Q84

A 64-year-old man presenting with lassitude is found to have iron deficiency anaemia. He gives no history of blood loss. Sigmoidoscopy and barium enema reveal no abnormality. The NEXT STEP in management should be

A   colonoscopy.

B   angiography.

C   oral iron supplements.

D   replacement of iron stores and repeat full blood count in 1 month.

E   cystoscopy.

SU-Q85

A symptomatic pulmonary embolus USUALLY arises from

A   deep calf veins.

B   arm veins.

C   iliofemoral veins.

D   superficial calf veins.

E   superficial thigh veins.

SU-Q86

In the pre-operative evaluation of a person for a possible bleeding tendency the MOST IMPORTANT of the following is

A   clotting time.

B   bleeding time.

C   clinical history.

D   prothrombin time or International Normalised Ratio (INR).

E   partial thromboplastin time.

SU-Q87

The CONDITION of overwhelming post-splenectomy sepsis

A   is seen twice as often in the splenectomised population as in the general population.

B   is most likely to occur several years after splenectomy.

C   occurs with nausea, vomiting, headache, confusion, shock and coma.

D   carries the highest risk for elderly patients.

E   is usually due to staphylococcus infection.

SU-Q88

A 74-year-old man falls astride an obstruction receiving injury to the perineum. Subsequently his temperature is elevated and there is gradually increased swelling of the perineum and genitalia. The MOST LIKELY injury is

A   contusion and haemorrhage of the perineal muscles.

B   haematoma of the scrotum.

C   fractured pelvis.

D   rupture of the bladder.

E   rupture of the urethra.

SU-Q89

The symptom of pneumaturia is MOST LIKELY to be an indication of

A ruptured bladder.

B urachal cyst.

C carcinoma of the colon.

D diverticular disease of the colon.

E pneumatosis cystoides intestinalis.

SU-Q90

Oliguria following a major surgical operation is probably NOT due to primary renal failure if urine examination shows

A high osmolality and low sodium concentration.

B high osmolality and high sodium concentration.

C low osmolality and high sodium concentration.

D low osmolality and high creatinine concentration.

E low osmolality and low creatinine concentration.

SU-Q91

A patient is admitted with a crush injury to his lower abdomen and pelvis. He has a severely fractured pelvis on X-ray and has fresh blood at the external urethral meatus. You should FIRST

A pass a soft urethral catheter into the bladder.

B arrange an excretion urogram.

C arrange urethroscopy.

D arrange urethrography.

E encourage him to attempt to void urine.

SU-Q92

Which one of the following statements concerning ureteric colic is CORRECT?

A Intravenous pyelography is contraindicated.

B A calcified opacity in line with the transverse processes will confirm the diagnosis.

C Delayed urographic films will often show the level of obstruction in the ureter.

D Red cells in the urine are a sign of infection occurring as well as a stone being present.

E Medullary sponge kidney is only rarely associated with renal stones.

SU-Q93

Which of the following BEST describes the daily intake of potassium required by a normal adult?

A 5 mmol.

B 25 mmol.

C 55 mmol.

D 155 mmol.

E 30 g.

SU-Q94

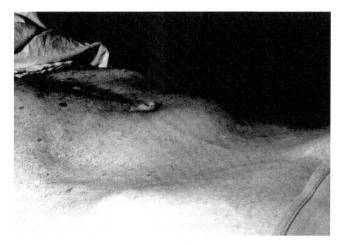

Figure 26

A 55-year-old man with a 20-year history of episodic epigastric pain which radiated through to the back, developed upper abdominal fullness and vomiting of non-bile stained material which had included some vegetables eaten 3 days before. Viewed from the right side, his abdomen appeared as illustrated in the accompanying photograph (Figure 26). He was clinically markedly 'dehydrated' and was passing only a small amount of urine of specific gravity 1038. Which of the following is the MOST APPROPRIATE IN THE FIRST HOURS of intravenous resuscitation for replacement of his deficit?

  A Dextrose 5% in water.

  B Dextrose 4% in N/5 (¹/₅ normal) saline.

  C Normal (isotonic) saline.

  D Hypertonic saline.

  E Hartmann solution.

SU-Q95

The APPROXIMATE composition in each litre of normal (0.9%) saline solution for intravenous administration is

  A sodium 141 mmol, potassium 5 mmol, calcium 2 mmol.

  B sodium 155 mmol, chloride 155 mmol.

  C sodium 31 mmol, chloride 31 mmol.

  D sodium 31 mmol, chloride 31 mmol, dextrose 220 mmol.

  E sodium 31 mmol, potassium 27 mmol, chloride 58 mmol, dextrose 166 mmol.

SU-Q96

All of the following significantly influence wound healing EXCEPT

  A diabetes mellitus.

  B vitamin C deficiency.

  C vitamin B group deficiency.

  D renal failure.

  E liver failure.

SU-Q97

The MOST IMPORTANT step in treating 'gas gangrene' is

- A adequate antitoxin.
- B adequate surgical removal of devitalised tissue.
- C a high initial dose of parenteral antibiotic.
- D a prolonged course of parenteral antibiotic treatment.
- E hyperbaric oxygen treatment prior to operative treatment.

SU-Q98

A patient presents to the Emergency Department with a penetrating wound of the sole of the foot after stepping on a rusty nail. He has never been previously immunised against tetanus. There is a bleeding puncture wound on the sole. Apart from wound toilet and debridement, which one of the following should you GIVE?

- A Tetanus toxoid.
- B Tetanus toxoid and penicillin.
- C Tetanus immunoglobulin intravenously and penicillin.
- D Tetanus immunoglobulin intramuscularly and penicillin.
- E Tetanus toxoid, tetanus immunoglobulin intramuscularly and penicillin.

SU-Q99

The most serious IMMEDIATE threat to life when an echinococcal cyst ruptures intraperitoneally is

- A haemorrhage.
- B peritoneal seeding of daughter cysts.
- C sepsis.
- D anaphylaxis.
- E hepatorenal syndrome.

SU-Q100

Which of the following is LEAST LIKELY to become malignant?

- A Leucoplakia in the mouth.
- B Hutchinson melanotic freckle.
- C Blue naevus.
- D Thyroid irradiated in infancy.
- E Skin irradiated in infancy.

SU-Q101

A hamartoma is a

- A malignant liver tumour.
- B blood clot.
- C developmental malformation.
- D hamstring muscle tumour.
- E bone tumour.

SU-Q102

The MOST COMMON malignant tumour occurring in the mouth is

- A adenocarcinoma.
- B osteogenic sarcoma.
- C ameloblastoma.
- D squamous cell carcinoma.
- E muco-epidermoid carcinoma.

SU-Q103

In patients treated by radiotherapy for cancer of the cervix the MOST COMMON site of radiation injury producing clinical effects is the

A small intestine.

B bladder.

C rectum.

D sigmoid colon.

E ureter.

SU-Q104

A 42-year-old man complains of excruciating pain to the slightest pressure on the nail of his left thumb. The MOST LIKELY diagnosis is

A dermatofibroma.

B fibroadenoma of the nail.

C giant cell tumour of the terminal phalanx.

D glomus tumour of nail bed.

E liposarcoma of the finger.

SU-Q105

A 58-year-old man had a 1.0 cm nodule excised from his forearm. Histology revealed it to be a squamous cell carcinoma which microscopically extended to the lateral margin of the resected tissue suggesting that it could be incompletely excised. There was no palpable lymphadenopathy. You should ADVISE

A wider local excision.

B wider local excision plus excision of the draining lymph nodes.

C radiotherapy to the wound and the surrounding area.

D radiotherapy to the draining lymph nodes.

E wider local excision plus radiotherapy to the draining lymph nodes.

SU-Q106

Metastatic tumours to bone are SELDOM found in the

A skull.

B vertebrae.

C long bones.

D bones below the knee or elbow.

E pelvis.

SU-Q107

A young man injured in a motor vehicle crash has fractures of three ribs anteriorly on the left and a minimal left pneumothorax. Peritoneal lavage is positive for blood, and laparotomy is planned for intraperitoneal haemorrhage. The MOST IMPORTANT step prior to laparotomy is

A insertion of a nasogastric tube.

B determination of P_aO_2 and P_aCO_2.

C to delay surgery until blood pressure has been restored to normal.

D insertion of a central venous pressure line on the right side.

E insertion of an intercostal drainage tube.

Surgery
Questions

TYPE
J

Questions SU-Q108 to SU-Q187

- Type J questions consist of a stem and five responses of which **one or more** may be correct
- All Type J questions will have at least one response correct

SU-Q108

Basal cell carcinomas

   A occur more commonly on the face than on other parts of the body.

   B rarely metastasise.

   C spread by local invasion.

   D are associated with solar exposure.

   E only occur on exposed areas.

SU-Q109

Concerning pilonidal sinus

   A it usually occurs in men aged 40–50 years.

   B the cause is persistence of a congenital tract containing hair follicles.

   C the primary sinus is usually in the midline.

   D it can occur also at the umbilicus and between the fingers.

   E rupture of an abscess can cause a sinus lateral to the midline.

SU-Q110

The lesion pictured in the accompanying photograph (Figure 27) has been present for several years. The clinical features and appearance SUGGEST

   A a lesion with negligible risk of malignant transformation.

   B Hutchinson melanotic freckle.

   C an intradermal naevus.

   D a pigmented basal cell carcinoma.

   E a seborrhoeic keratosis.

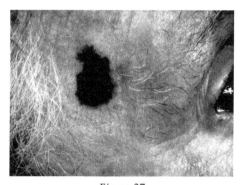

Figure 27

SU-Q111

The accompanying photograph (Figure 28) shows the perineum and scrotum of an elderly man. Concerning his MANAGEMENT

   A intravenous antibiotic treatment is the most important aspect of his management.

   B metronidazole is the preferred antibiotic.

   C surgery should be delayed until local abscess formation is evident.

   D prolonged hyperbaric oxygen treatment should be undertaken before surgery.

   E associated diabetes mellitus is likely.

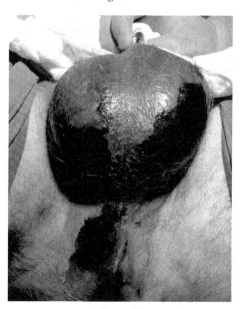

Figure 28

SU-Q112

A thyroglossal cyst

- A   is usually midline.
- B   moves with protrusion of the tongue.
- C   almost always presents before the age of 10 years.
- D   is attached to the upper pole of a lateral lobe of the thyroid gland.
- E   often undergoes malignant change.

SU-Q113

Benign nodular goitre

- A   can cause oesophageal obstruction.
- B   can cause tracheal obstruction.
- C   usually causes recurrent laryngeal palsy.
- D   can cause Horner syndrome.
- E   when malignancy of the thyroid supervenes, is usually associated with thyrotoxicosis.

SU-Q114

Concerning cancer of the lip

- A   cervical lymph node metastases are best treated with radiotherapy.
- B   the lesion usually occurs on the upper lip.
- C   pathology is nearly always squamous cell carcinoma.
- D   90% occur in males.
- E   the 5 year survival rate is better than for cancer of the tongue.

SU-Q115

In the accompanying photograph (Figure 29)

- A   P is the glabella.
- B   Q is the site of the lacrimal gland orifice.
- C   R is the columella.
- D   S is the philtrum.
- E   T is the vermilion border.

SU-Q116

Submandibular duct calculus

- A   is almost always radio-opaque.
- B   can cause swelling of the sub-mandibular gland.
- C   is best investigated by an immedi-ate submandibular sialogram.
- D   can be palpated in the floor of the mouth.
- E   can pass spontaneously.

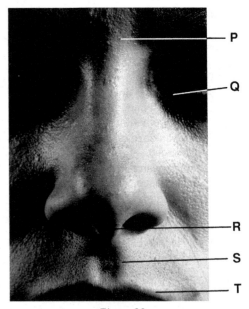

Figure 29

SU-Q117

Concerning the aetiology, diagnosis and treatment of pharyngo-oesophageal diverticulum

  A these are true diverticula consisting of all layers of the wall of the oesophagus.

  B they usually occur in elderly patients.

  C dysphagia is the main symptom and oesophageal carcinoma is the main differential diagnosis.

  D a two-stage resection is always preferred because it is safer.

  E the diverticulum is usually located on the right side of the neck.

SU-Q118

In left sided Horner syndrome there is

  A weakness of the left orbicularis oculi muscle.

  B dilatation of the left pupil.

  C sweating of the left side of the face.

  D weakness of the left levator palpebrae superioris muscle.

  E weakness of lateral eye movement.

SU-Q119

A plate-glass worker is seen in the emergency room with a deep laceration to the back of his right medial epicondyle, which exposes the underlying bone at the right elbow. Examination is LIKELY to reveal

  A anaesthesia of the thumb and index finger.

  B reduced power on flexion of the wrist.

  C an inability to oppose thumb and index finger.

  D an inability to abduct the fingers.

  E anaesthesia of the little finger.

SU-Q120

Neuropathic joints can OCCUR in

  A diabetes mellitus.

  B syringomyelia.

  C progressive muscular dystrophy.

  D syphilis.

  E motor neuron disease.

SU-Q121

The patient in the accompanying photograph (Figure 30) has been asked to look to her left (towards the right of the picture) following the movement of a pin. The pupils are of equal size. Which of the following is/are CORRECT?

  A Appearances suggest a lesion of her left oculomotor nerve.

  B She is likely to be suffering from diplopia.

  C The corneal reflex of the affected eye will be lost.

  D Appearances suggest a lesion of her left abducens nerve.

  E The consensual light response of the affected eye will be lost but the direct response will be maintained.

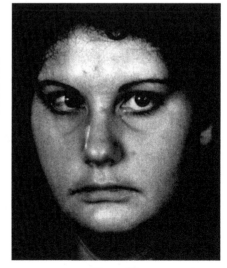

Figure 30

SU-Q122

The patient in the accompanying photograph (Figure 31) has been asked to close both eyes. Which of the following is/are CORRECT?

A Appearances suggest a lesion of the patient's right facial nerve.

B Involvement of the upper facial musculature in the paralysis suggests a lesion of the upper motor neuron.

C Preservation of taste sensation to the anterior part of the tongue on the side of the lesion is compatible with a lesion within the parotid gland.

D The corneal reflex will be preserved unless an associated trigeminal nerve lesion is present.

E Collapse of the cheek on the affected side due to buccinator paralysis would suggest an associated trigeminal nerve lesion.

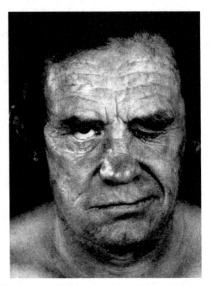

Figure 31

SU-Q123

'Stress' fractures occur TYPICALLY in the

A upper tibia.

B lower femur.

C second metatarsal.

D horizontal ramus of the mandible.

E first rib.

SU-Q124

Dupuytren disease

A is due to fibrosis of the palmar flexor tendons.

B is usually painless.

C commonly involves all fingers and the thumb.

D rarely affects females.

E can also affect the feet.

SU-Q125

Concerning fractures of the wrist and hand

A Colles fracture involves dorsal displacement of the distal fracture segment.

B Smith fracture involves volar displacement of the distal fracture segment.

C scaphoid fracture usually involves no displacement.

D Bennett fracture involves the first carpo–metacarpal articulation.

E Monteggia fracture involves dislocation of the wrist.

SU-Q126

Varicose veins are ASSOCIATED with

A arterio–venous fistulae.

B previous deep venous thrombosis in the calf.

C sapheno–femoral incompetence.

D previous fractured tibia.

E a familial predisposition.

SU-Q127

Five days after laparotomy and drainage of a pancreatic abscess, a 63-year-old woman develops a painless swelling of her right lower leg and thigh. Appropriate action INCLUDES

A ask for a compression stocking to be applied.

B order a Duplex–Doppler study or venogram.

C commence heparin; 1000 units/h, intravenously.

D commence heparin; 5000 units, twice daily, subcutaneously.

E arrange a ventilation–perfusion scan.

SU-Q128

A lumbar sympathectomy is SOMETIMES performed in peripheral vascular disease because it

A greatly improves claudication distance.

B encourages the recanalisation of major arteries.

C interrupts afferent pain fibres.

D often improves skin circulation in the foot.

E reduces the risk of venous thrombosis.

SU-Q129

A 68-year-old man collapses in the toilet one night. He rouses himself and returns to bed. He is unaffected subsequently and feels well again in the morning. Which of the following might REASONABLY EXPLAIN his syncope?

A Gastrointestinal haemorrhage.

B Bladder neck outflow obstruction.

C Myocardial infarction.

D Cerebral transient ischaemic attack.

E Aortic stenosis.

SU-Q130

Concerning the varicose veins illustrated in the accompanying photograph (Figure 32)

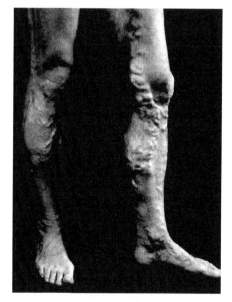

A Trendelenburg test on the patient's left leg would be expected to confirm sapheno–femoral valvular incompetence at the groin.

B a doubly positive Trendelenburg test means that both the long and short saphenous venous systems are involved.

C the lower part of the thigh over the subsartorial canal is a frequent site for a perforating vein joining the superficial and deep venous systems.

D as well as superficial venous varicosities, the patient's left leg shows obvious and gross evidence of severe long-standing deep venous insufficiency.

E emergency treatment for haemorrhage from an eroded superficial varicose vein involves elevation of the leg and compression at the bleeding point.

Figure 32

SU-Q131

A healthy young man fractures his femur in a motor cycle accident and develops adult respiratory distress syndrome ('shock lung'). Clinical features after 48 h are likely to INCLUDE

A tachycardia.

B tachypnoea.

C increased arterial $P_a CO_2$.

D hypertension.

E decreased arterial $P_a O_2$.

SU-Q132

A 49-year-old man with a 6 year history of abdominal pain and diarrhoea had a 10 cm narrowed segment demonstrated in the terminal ileum on a barium contrast study. No other obvious lesion is demonstrated.

A Both Crohn disease and 'backwash' ulcerative colitis are likely causes.

B Surgical treatment should only be recommended if a fistula develops.

C There would be an 80% risk of recurrence of his disease after surgery.

D Renal calculi can develop as an associated finding.

E Biliary calculi can develop as an associated finding.

SU-Q133

Factors known to be ASSOCIATED with an increased incidence of carcinoma of the colon are

A high roughage ingestion.

B familial adenomatous polyposis.

C a first degree relative with colonic cancer.

D ulcerative colitis.

E amoebic colitis.

SU-Q134

Concerning gall-bladder disease

A almost all people with gallstones eventually develop symptoms.

B an abnormal DIDA scan (technetium-labelled di-ethyl-iminodiacetic acid) supports a clinical diagnosis of acute cholecystitis.

C carcinoma of the gall-bladder in 'Western' countries is usually associated with long-standing gallstone disease.

D 50% of patients with gall-bladder calculi also have stones within the bile duct.

E calcified gallstones are suitably treated by oral bile salt therapy after shock wave lithotripsy.

SU-Q135

While recovering from an attack of acute pancreatitis, a 50-year-old man develops a clearly defined pancreatic pseudocyst. On ultrasound examination, the cyst is in the body of the pancreas and measures 15 cm.

A Such a cyst is likely to have developed over some weeks.

B The cyst can present clinically as an epigastric mass which moves with respiration.

C The amylase concentration of the pseudocyst fluid is likely to be elevated, but will be less than the serum amylase concentration.

D Pancreatic pseudocysts are due to obstruction of the pancreatic duct by gallstones.

E Such a pseudocyst will almost always resolve spontaneously without any intervention.

SU-Q136

A 48-year-old man is admitted to hospital 48 h after drinking 15 large glasses of beer (225 g alcohol). Abdominal examination reveals generalised tenderness with rebound tenderness. He is tachycardic and hypotensive and has passed no urine for 16 h. The accompanying photograph (Figure 33) shows the appearance of his abdomen around the umbilicus. Likely sequelae INCLUDE

    A acute renal failure.
    B blood loss requiring blood replacement.
    C tetany due to hypocalcaemia.
    D pancreatic abscess.
    E a mortality risk of over 20%.

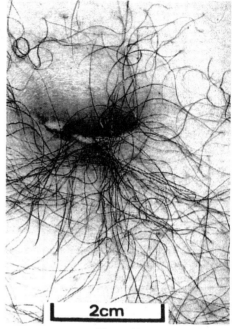

Figure 33

SU-Q137

Abdominal wound dehiscence or rupture ('burst abdomen')

    A usually occurs in the first 10 days after operation.
    B is more common with transverse incisions than with vertical incisions.
    C is usually associated with a serosanguineous discharge.
    D does not predispose to later incisional hernia.
    E is often associated with distension of the abdomen.

SU-Q138

Plain X-rays of the abdomen reveal severe dilatation of the colon and fluid levels within the colon. Likely causes INCLUDE

    A carcinoma of the sigmoid colon.
    B carcinoma of the lower half of the rectum.
    C severe ulcerative colitis.
    D faecal impaction.
    E retroperitoneal inflammation or haemorrhage.

SU-Q139

Surgical resection of the terminal ileum will SIGNIFICANTLY reduce the absorption of which of the following?

    A Bile salts.
    B Iron.
    C Folic acid.
    D Vitamin C.
    E Calcium.

SU-Q140

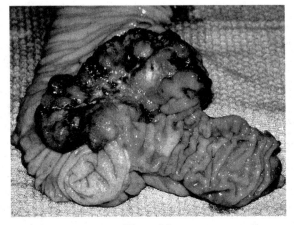

Figure 34

The accompanying photograph (Figure 34) shows the ileocaecal segment of a length of intestine surgically removed from a 68-year-old man. Histological examination of the resected lymph glands revealed no tumour. Clinical features likely to be ASSOCIATED WITH this lesion INCLUDE

A a clinically palpable mass.
B bright rectal bleeding.
C back pain.
D tiredness.
E a 5 year survival prospect of approximately 10%.

SU-Q141

Oesophageal achalasia

A is associated with failure of relaxation of the lower oesophageal sphincter.
B if long-standing, is characterised by absence of the gastric air bubble.
C is associated with Hirschsprung disease.
D can show an air–fluid level in the oesophagus.
E can be associated with late malignancy.

SU-Q142

A non-visualised gall bladder on oral cholecystography can be DUE TO

A obstructive jaundice.
B patient non-compliance.
C gastroenteritis.
D hepatocellular failure.
E acute cholecystitis.

SU-Q143

Which of the following ASSOCIATIONS are well recognised?

A Villous adenoma of the rectum and hypocalcaemia.
B Marfan syndrome and aortic incompetence.
C Coeliac disease and lymphoma.
D Immunosuppressive drugs and skin neoplasms.
E Oesophageal atresia and maternal hydramnios.

SU-Q144

Concerning ultrasound of the biliary tract
- A obesity improves resolution and diagnostic accuracy.
- B the (common) bile duct lies anterior to the portal vein.
- C a bile duct measuring 13 mm in diameter is within normal limits.
- D gallstones which do not contain calcium cannot be seen.
- E pregnancy contraindicates its use.

SU-Q145

Intussusception in children
- A is usually ileocolic.
- B usually has no focal lesion identified as lead point.
- C can be successfully treated without open operation.
- D rarely causes gastrointestinal bleeding.
- E may be associated with Henoch–Schönlein purpura.

SU-Q146

In patients with liver disease, hepatic encephalopathy may be INDUCED by
- A hypokalaemic alkalosis secondary to vomiting.
- B gastrointestinal bleeding.
- C portosystemic shunt.
- D neomycin treatment.
- E acute pneumonia.

SU-Q147

INCREASED incidence of gastrointestinal cancer is FOUND in
- A pernicious anaemia.
- B cathartic colon.
- C coeliac disease.
- D melanosis coli.
- E *Helicobacter pylori*-associated gastritis.

SU-Q148

In familial adenomatous polyposis
- A inheritance is sex linked.
- B the rectum is spared.
- C malignancy is an inevitable complication if untreated.
- D clinical presentation is usually in the fifth decade.
- E polyps rarely appear before the age of 10 years.

SU-Q149

Clinical features likely in a 23-year-old man with an acutely inflamed retrocaecal appendix INCLUDE
- A right iliac fossa tenderness.
- B temperature 37.5°C.
- C anorexia.
- D back pain.
- E macroscopic haematuria.

SU-Q150

Which of the following is/are CONSISTENT with the diagnosis of a perforated anterior wall duodenal ulcer of 3 h duration?

A   The patient complains of severe back pain.
B   The patient lies supine with knees drawn up and is afraid to move.
C   There is pallor, sweating and shallow respirations.
D   The abdomen is lax and tender in the epigastrium.
E   Liver dullness to percussion is decreased.

SU-Q151

With regard to eliciting tenderness on examination of a patient with ACUTE abdominal pain

A   rebound tenderness can be assessed by finger percussion.
B   tenderness associated with colonic disease is usually present in the midline suprapubically.
C   if tenderness is present without guarding, then peritonitis will not be present.
D   tenderness on rectal examination is highly suggestive of a pelvic abscess.
E   localised tenderness in the right iliac fossa is the most important single clinical sign of acute appendicitis.

SU-Q152

Carcinoma of the caecum in its clinical features can TYPICALLY

A   mimic appendicitis.
B   present as anaemia.
C   cause a 'small bowel obstruction'.
D   present as a palpable mass.
E   present as dyspepsia.

SU-Q153

Chronic perianal fistula is TYPICALLY associated with

A   recurring perianal abscesses.
B   faecal perianal discharge.
C   persistent pain.
D   diarrhoea.
E   purulent perianal discharge.

SU-Q154

Anal fissure is TYPICALLY associated with

A   an anal skin tag.
B   colicky abdominal pain.
C   anal pain on defaecation.
D   bleeding on defaecation.
E   faecal soiling.

SU-Q155

The accompanying photograph (Figure 35) shows the abdomen of a patient presenting with abdominal swelling. Which of the following statements is/are CORRECT?

A A small central area of resonance with dullness to percussion laterally suggests ascites.

B The minimum volume of ascitic fluid which can be detected on physical examination is 2.5 L.

C With gross ascites due to cirrhosis, the mid-clavicular liver span is always greater than 20 cm.

D The appearances could be due to an ovarian cyst.

E If distension is due to pseudo-cyesis, generalised dullness to percussion will be present.

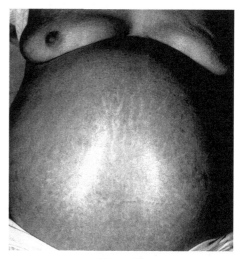

Figure 35

SU-Q156

Clinical features LIKELY to be RELATED TO the abnormality illustrated in the accompanying photograph (Figure 36) INCLUDE

A central abdominal pain.

B abdominal hysterectomy 10 years previously.

C an irreducible tender swelling below and lateral to the pubic tubercle.

D back pain.

E an irreducible tender swelling above and medial to the pubic tubercle.

SU-Q157

Primary hyperparathyroidism

A is most commonly due to a solitary parathyroid adenoma.

B is associated with high serum calcium and phosphate levels.

C can present as a psychiatric disorder.

D is predominantly a disease of adults.

E is rarely asymptomatic.

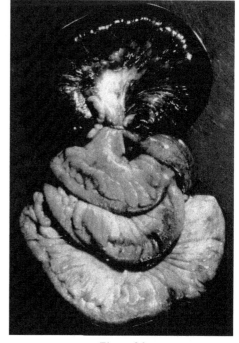

Figure 36

SU-Q158

Concerning the Zollinger–Ellison syndrome
- A there can be multiple tumours.
- B the tumour can be malignant.
- C there is associated gastric hypersecretion.
- D there is often hypoglycaemia.
- E total vagotomy prevents recurrence.

SU-Q159

Concerning simple colloid goitre
- A dietary deficiency of iodine is a cause.
- B increased uptake of iodine-131 is seen on scanning.
- C nodules can occur later if untreated.
- D antithyroid antibodies occur.
- E it is more common in females.

SU-Q160

A fine needle aspiration cytology report of your 60-year-old patient confirms that the lump in the upper outer quadrant of the right breast is a ductal carcinoma. You have performed a mammogram. After discussing the diagnosis with the patient she requests you to consider conservative surgery and not mastectomy. Which of the following FEATURES would cause you to argue in favour of mastectomy?
- A The lesion is 7 cm in diameter.
- B The mammogram shows three separate foci of suspicious calcification.
- C Peau d'orange of the overlying skin extends into another quadrant.
- D She is postmenopausal.
- E She has palpable axillary nodes on the right.

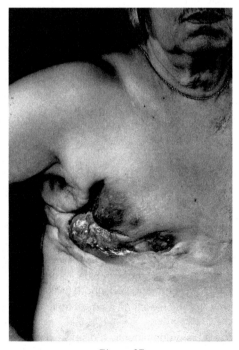

SU-Q161

Two years after a modified radical mastectomy for breast cancer, a 65-year-old woman presents with the clinical features illustrated in the accompanying photograph (Figure 37). Which of the following treatments should you RECOMMEND at this stage?
- A Tamoxifen.
- B Testosterone.
- C Local conservative excisional surgery.
- D Chest wall radiotherapy.
- E Excision of part of the chest wall and skin graft.

Figure 37

SU-Q162

Concerning carcinoma of the prostate

A multifocal carcinoma *in situ* is rarely associated with metastases to regional lymph nodes.
B the majority of patients present with early stage disease.
C the serum prostatic acid phosphatase is always elevated in the presence of bony metastases.
D pedal lymphangiography reliably detects lymphatic spread.
E Paget disease may confound the interpretation of a positive bone scan.

SU-Q163

Testicular seminoma is ASSOCIATED with

A spread to para-aortic lymph nodes.
B spread to inguinal lymph nodes.
C pulmonary metastases.
D increased serum beta human chorionic gonadotrophin (HCG).
E increased serum alpha-fetoprotein.

SU-Q164

There is a PREDISPOSITION to deep venous thrombosis in

A carcinoma of the stomach.
B peptic ulceration treated non-operatively.
C pelvic surgery.
D surgery for uncomplicated varicose veins.
E polycythaemia rubra vera.

SU-Q165

A bleeding problem after massive blood transfusion can be DUE TO

A deficiencies of factors V, VIII and XI.
B fibrinolysis.
C platelet deficiency.
D prostaglandin deficiency.
E calcium deficiency.

SU-Q166

Continued bleeding after operation for a ruptured abdominal aortic aneurysm is LIKELY to be DUE TO a general haemostatic disorder if

A bleeding occurs from venipuncture sites.
B fresh blood continues from the abdominal drain.
C the platelet count is found to be less than 30×10^9/L (less than 30 000 /µL).
D the serum fibrinogen level is found to be elevated.
E the international normalised ratio (INR) is three-fold normal.

SU-Q167

The finding of massive splenomegaly extending across the midline WOULD SUGGEST

A chronic malaria.
B Hodgkin disease.
C chronic myeloid leukaemia.
D portal hypertension.
E chronic lymphatic leukaemia.

SU-Q168

Macrocytic anaemia can be ASSOCIATED with

  A   stagnant blind small intestinal loop.
  B   gastric resection.
  C   hiatus hernia.
  D   tropical sprue.
  E   Crohn disease.

SU-Q169

Regarding classic haemophilia

  A   the incidence in the general population is 1:10 000.
  B   it is inherited as an autosomal dominant with variable penetrance.
  C   muscle compartment bleeds are the most common orthopaedic problem.
  D   factor VIII component therapy is required before any elective surgery.
  E   therapy with cryoprecipitate is free of risk for hepatitis.

SU-Q170

In a normal sized adult, the right ureter

  A   commences at the 11th thoracic vertebral level.
  B   is approximately 25 cm long.
  C   receives blood supply from the right renal artery.
  D   receives blood supply from the inferior vesical artery.
  E   receives blood supply from the inferior mesenteric artery.

SU-Q171

Dehydration prior to intravenous urography is CONTRAINDICATED in

  A   leukaemia.
  B   myelomatosis.
  C   raised intracranial pressure.
  D   chronic renal failure.
  E   renovascular hypertension.

SU-Q172

Which of the following types of urinary calculi are radiolucent?

  A   Cystine.
  B   Uric acid.
  C   Xanthine.
  D   Oxalate.
  E   Phosphate.

SU-Q173

Polycystic kidney disease in adults

  A   can present with haematuria.
  B   can be associated with liver cysts.
  C   can be associated with pancreatic cysts.
  D   is usually unilateral.
  E   can be associated with berry aneurysms of the cerebral circulation.

SU-Q174

Concerning renal papillary necrosis DUE TO analgesic ingestion

- A the incidence of urinary tract infection is increased.
- B dislodged papillae can cause ureteric obstruction.
- C it is associated with enlarged kidneys during the chronic phase.
- D papillae can calcify.
- E the incidence of transitional cell carcinoma is increased.

SU-Q175

Haematuria is a COMMON symptom of

- A benign prostatomegaly.
- B urinary tract calculus.
- C transitional cell tumour of the renal tract.
- D hypernephroma (renal cell carcinoma).
- E benign pelviureteric hydronephrosis.

SU-Q176

Pre-operative assessment of nutritional status and subsequent risk of postoperative complications can be helped by ASSESSMENT of

- A delayed cutaneous hypersensitivity.
- B serum albumin concentration.
- C mid-arm muscle circumference.
- D haemoglobin concentration.
- E strength of hand grip.

SU-Q177

Wound breakdown can be CAUSED by

- A inappropriate suture material.
- B infection.
- C uraemia.
- D jaundice.
- E previous radiotherapy to the area.

SU-Q178

Regarding respiratory acid–base abnormalities

- A respiratory acidosis is caused by decreased alveolar ventilation.
- B respiratory alkalosis is caused by increased alveolar ventilation.
- C respiratory alkalosis is characterised by a fall in P_a CO_2 and a rise in pH.
- D hyperkalaemia is a frequent complication of respiratory alkalosis.
- E potassium restriction is an important adjunct in the treatment of respiratory alkalosis.

SU-Q179

Pre-operative factors associated with an increased risk of wound infection INCLUDE

- A alcoholism.
- B diabetes mellitus.
- C concomitant urinary tract infection.
- D longer pre-operative hospitalisation.
- E shock.

SU-Q180

Pre-operative antibiotic administration would be APPROPRIATE in a patient undergoing

A   appendicectomy for acute appendicitis.
B   highly selective vagotomy.
C   aortic graft replacement for aortic aneurysm.
D   haemorrhoidectomy.
E   elective repair of a femoral hernia.

SU-Q181

Echinococcus granulosa (hydatid parasite)

A   has the human as its definitive host.
B   has the dog as its intermediate host.
C   is usually spread to humans by contamination from dog faeces.
D   most commonly affects the lung in human infestation.
E   can cause pathological fracture.

SU-Q182

Concerning *Echinococcus granulosa* and hydatid disease

A   the disease can develop after eating infected sheep meat.
B   calcification of the hydatid cyst implies inactivity of the parasite.
C   pulmonary cysts respond to an 8 week course of metronidazole.
D   if the cyst is multiloculated, ultrasound can be virtually diagnostic.
E   operation for liver cysts involves removal of germinal epithelium, hydatid fluid, daughter cysts and laminated membrane.

SU-Q183

Antibiotic treatment would be INDICATED for which of the following staphylococcal infections?

A   A 25-year-old man with a furuncle in the beard area.
B   A wound infection 5 days after an antireflux procedure in a fit 35-year-old woman.
C   A 40-year-old man with a perianal abscess.
D   A 25-year-old diabetic man with a carbuncle of the back of the neck.
E   A wound infection 5 days after mitral valve replacement in a fit 63-year-old man.

SU-Q184

Medications which have peptic ulceration as a side effect INCLUDE

A   aspirin.
B   paracetamol.
C   prednisolone.
D   penicillin V.
E   erythromycin.

SU-Q185

Testicular malignancy

A   metastasises first to the inguinal lymph nodes.
B   usually manifests as testicular pain.
C   is usually associated with haematuria.
D   can manifest as a hydrocele.
E   can sometimes be cured even when metastatic.

SU-Q186

A 54-year-old woman with a well-functioning renal transplant of 12 years duration develops multiple skin carcinomas on her arms and legs. Which of the following statements is/are CORRECT?

    A Squamous carcinoma is likely to be present.

    B Basal cell carcinoma is likely to be present.

    C The carcinomas are a complication of the renal transplantation itself.

    D The carcinomas are a complication of the medications following transplantation.

    E Basal cell carcinomas are likely to outnumber squamous cell carcinomas.

SU-Q187

In day care surgery performed under general anaesthesia

    A there is no need for pre-operative starvation.

    B there is no need for postoperative starvation.

    C the patient can drive home from the day surgery centre.

    D cardiac resuscitation facilities must be available.

    E oxygen and suction facilities must be available.

Paediatrics
Questions

TYPE

A

Questions PA-Q1 to PA-Q86

■ Type A questions consist of a stem and five responses

■ **One** correct answer must be selected from five possible responses to the stem

PA-Q1

Which of the following therapies is MOST APPROPRIATE for uncomplicated seborrhoeic dermatitis in infancy?

A   Salicylic acid and sulphur cream.

B   Vitamin E cream.

C   Exclusion diet.

D   Hydrocortisone cream.

E   1% aqueous gentian violet.

PA-Q2

An infant with strabismus is found to have a white pupil. POSSIBLE CAUSES include

A   cataract.

B   retinoblastoma.

C   retrolental fibroplasia.

D   toxoplasmosis.

E   all of the above.

PA-Q3

An anxious mother consults about her 18-month-old child because 'She doesn't seem to hear properly'. The child is otherwise well. Examination of the child's ears, nose and throat appears normal, including response to the noise of a rattle. You SHOULD

A   reassure the mother and reassess the child in 6 months time.

B   arrange audiometric assessment.

C   defer investigation until the child is 3 years of age.

D   perform tuning fork tests.

E   perform tympanometry.

PA-Q4

Which one of the following statements concerning cerebral palsy is CORRECT?

A   Children with cerebral palsy have a past history of perinatal hypoxia in over 90% of cases.

B   Choreoathetosis is the most common variety of cerebral palsy in Australia.

C   Treatment with diazepam produces a marked improvement in spasticity.

D   Feeding difficulties are common.

E   Most children with spastic quadriplegia have normal intelligence.

PA-Q5

A previously healthy 3-year-old child has a single generalised convulsion lasting 5 min. She is found to have a reddened throat and a rectal temperature of 39.7°C, from which she recovers uneventfully in 5 days. Three months later she again becomes febrile with an upper respiratory tract infection. Which of the following is CORRECT?

A   She should be started on oral phenobarbitone.

B   She should be put in a bath of cold water.

C   600 mg aspirin should be administered.

D   An antibiotic should be administered promptly.

E   Most such children will not have a further seizure.

PA-Q6

In Petit-mal epilepsy (typical absence seizures)

A the onset of attacks is usually between 2 and 4 years of age.

B mental retardation is common.

C attacks are brought on by hyperventilation.

D nitrazepam is the drug of first choice.

E it is rare to have associated Grand-mal epilepsy.

PA-Q7

Cerebral palsy is

A a disorder of posture and locomotion.

B the most frequent cause of intellectual disability.

C associated with epilepsy in greater than 75% of cases.

D due to birth trauma in the majority of cases.

E usually familial.

PA-Q8

A previously healthy 10-year-old girl has developed progressive weakness, areflexia, paresis of extra-ocular muscles and respiratory insufficiency over a 2 week period. The MOST LIKELY diagnosis is

A polymyositis.

B myasthenia gravis.

C acute spinal muscular atrophy.

D Guillain-Barré syndrome.

E botulism.

PA-Q9

An infant had a head circumference on the 10th percentile at 2 weeks of age, the 25th percentile at 1 month of age, the 50th percentile at 6 weeks of age and the 90th percentile at 10 months of age. The MOST LIKELY diagnosis is

A hydrocephalus due to aqueduct stenosis.

B familial macrocephaly.

C a variant of normal.

D posterior fossa brain tumour.

E a porencephalic cyst.

PA-Q10

The MOST APPROPRIATE management of pes cavus (high-arched or vaulted feet) developing in a 12-year-old boy would be

A physiotherapy.

B metatarsal bars on the shoes.

C reassurance to the parents that this is a normal variant.

D referral for investigation of a neurological disorder.

E surgical correction of the deformity.

PA-Q11

Concerning juvenile chronic arthritis (JCA)

A   persistent hectic fever in a 2-year-old child is incompatible with the diagnosis.

B   monoarticular arthritis usually affects a small joint of the hand.

C   rheumatoid factor is usually present within 3 months of diagnosis.

D   characteristic X-ray changes are usually evident within 6 months of the onset of the symptoms.

E   iridocyclitis may be an associated feature.

PA-Q12

Which of the following is the MOST APPROPRIATE treatment for flat feet (pes planus) in a 2¹/₂-year-old boy?

A   Physiotherapy to improve the strength of the small muscles of the feet.

B   Metatarsal bars on the shoes.

C   Plates in the shoes to encourage the development of an arch.

D   Reassurance of the parents that this is a normal developmental stage.

E   Referral for investigation of a neurological disorder.

PA-Q13

'In-toeing' in children under 3 years is BEST MANAGED by

A   reassuring the parents.

B   medial wedges on shoes.

C   eversion splints worn at night.

D   plaster casts.

E   rotation osteotomies of the tibiae.

PA-Q14

Which of the following USUALLY resolves spontaneously?

A   Small ventricular septal defect in a child aged 12 months.

B   Small atrial septal defect in a child aged 3 years.

C   Patent ductus in a toddler.

D   Aortic coarctation in a premature infant.

E   Congenital heart block.

PA-Q15

Each of the following is significantly associated with ventricular septal defect in childhood EXCEPT

A   frequent lower respiratory infections.

B   spontaneous functional closure.

C   Down syndrome.

D   smoking in pregnancy.

E   oesophageal atresia.

PA-Q16

A 15-year-old girl is found on routine medical examination to have a blood pressure of 140/95 mmHg. The MOST APPROPRIATE initial action would be to

A test her urine microscopically.

B recheck the blood pressure after a period of rest.

C check the blood pressure in both parents.

D measure 24 h urinary catecholamines.

E commence therapy with a beta blocker.

PA-Q17

Which of the following would be MOST USEFUL in diagnosing congestive cardiac failure in an infant aged 6 months?

A Distended jugular veins.

B A respiratory rate greater than 40 /min.

C Oedema of the ankles.

D An enlarged liver.

E A heart rate greater than 120 /min.

PA-Q18

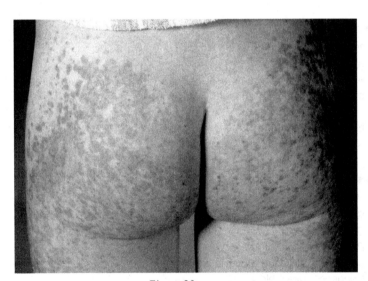

Figure 38

A 4-year-old girl pictured in the accompanying photograph (Figure 38) presents with colicky abdominal pain which has been present for 24 h. On examination, the abdomen is soft, there is localised oedema of the dorsal aspects of her feet and tenderness and swelling of the right ankle. Urticaria has been present over the buttocks and lower extremities for 4 h. The MOST APPROPRIATE investigation of this patient would be to

A test for anti-nuclear factor in serum.

B test for rheumatoid factor in serum.

C measure the levels of immunoglobulins in serum.

D arrange for a plain X-ray of the abdomen.

E perform a microscopic examination of the urine.

PA-Q19

A 6-year-old girl has had a moderately severe episode of asthma for 36–48 h. She has been treated with inhaled sympathomimetic every 3–4 h but respiratory distress recurs within 2–3 h of the inhalation. The MOST APPROPRIATE additional therapy would be

A   oral theophylline.
B   a short course of oral corticosteroids.
C   a short course of inhaled corticosteroids.
D   additional inhaled ipratropium bromide.
E   a course of oral antibiotics.

PA-Q20

In Australia the MOST LIKELY cause of a chronic unproductive cough in an otherwise healthy 10-year-old child unvaccinated for whooping cough is

A   bronchitis.
B   bronchiectasis.
C   cystic fibrosis.
D   whooping cough.
E   asthma.

PA-Q21

A 4-year-old child with asthma, associated with upper respiratory infection, walks with his mother from the bus to an Emergency Department. An hour after an inhalation of salbutamol, his shortness of breath has improved, but his mother thinks he is still too wheezy to take home. The MOST APPROPRIATE treatment would be

A   oral aminophylline elixir.
B   intramuscular antibiotic.
C   repeat inhalation of salbutamol.
D   inhalation of beclomethasone.
E   intravenous hydrocortisone.

PA-Q22

Which of the following statements is CORRECT with regard to *Bordetella pertussis* infection in children in Australia?

A   Erythromycin estolate significantly shortens the course of the disease.
B   Cough rarely lasts longer than 4–6 weeks.
C   Facial suffusion followed by vomiting during a paroxysm of coughing is highly suggestive of the diagnosis.
D   Permanent lung damage with bronchiectasis is a frequent complication.
E   It does not occur if a child has had three doses of vaccine between 2 and 6 months and a booster at 18 months of age.

PA-Q23

A previously well boy aged 18 months presents with a 24 h history of cough and wheeze and has a respiratory rate of 35 /min. There is a family history of asthma and allergy. Examination shows a boy who is generally well but he has softer breath sounds over the left hemithorax. There are bilateral wheezes, more marked on the left. The APPROPRIATE MANAGEMENT is

A   give nebulised salbutamol 4 hourly.
B   refer for physiotherapy.
C   give amoxycillin.
D   arrange inspiratory and expiratory chest X-rays.
E   admit to hospital and nurse in 30% oxygen.

PA-Q24

A 6-year-old Australian-born child presents with a 2 month history of persisting cough. Chest X-ray shows partial collapse/consolidation of the right upper lobe with associated right hilar lymph node enlargement. Which of the following is the MOST APPROPRIATE next course of action?

    A Skin prick test with dust mite antigen.

    B Needle biopsy of right upper lobe with imaging control.

    C High dose intramuscular penicillin for 5 days.

    D Therapeutic trial of oral erythromycin.

    E Intradermal injection of purified protein-derivative tuberculin.

PA-Q25

Which one of the following clinical features is MOST HELPFUL in distinguishing acute laryngotracheobronchitis ('croup') from acute epiglottitis?

    A Expiratory as well as inspiratory stridor.

    B The onset is preceded by symptoms of an upper respiratory tract infection.

    C Subcostal retraction on inspiration.

    D Barking cough.

    E Temperature greater than 38.5°C.

PA-Q26

A placid 4-week-old formula-fed baby has vomited feeds since the first week of life. Her maternal grandmother is convinced that the baby is ill. The mother is also concerned but says that the baby feeds well. You confirm that she has gained weight normally, and find no clinical abnormality. You SHOULD

    A reassure the mother and tell her to ignore anyone who says the child is ill.

    B explain that the baby probably has gastro-oesophageal reflux.

    C arrange barium swallow and meal.

    D arrange suprapubic aspiration of urine for microscopy and culture.

    E advise that the formula be diluted to make it more digestible.

PA-Q27

Which of the following statements about childhood threadworm infestation is CORRECT?

    A Recurrence after treatment is unusual.

    B It is a common and important cause of enuresis.

    C Anorexia, loss of weight and abdominal pains are frequent presenting complaints.

    D Other members of the family should receive the same treatment as the child.

    E Separation of the child from other children should occur until treatment is completed.

PA-Q28

A previously normal 3-weeks-old infant suddenly vomits a large part of his feed. Physical examination reveals no abnormality. The PROPER PROCEDURE would be to

    A thicken the feed.

    B perform a barium meal.

    C await further developments.

    D change the milk formula.

    E arrange urine microscopy.

PA-Q29

Each of the following is true of intussusception, EXCEPT

A laparotomy is indicated in more than 90% of children.
B the highest incidence is under 2 years of age.
C there is an association with Henoch–Schönlein purpura.
D there is an association with adenovirus infection.
E blood in the stools is a late feature.

PA-Q30

A boy weighing 3200 g when born at term, begins to vomit his feedings at the age of 4 weeks. When examined 1 week later, he weighs 3700 g and has a palpable pyloric tumour. He appears moderately depleted ('dehydrated') but circulation is adequate. He has had three wet nappies in the past 24 h, the last 1 h ago. Laboratory tests show

blood pH	7.50
Pa_{CO_2}	45 mmHg
base excess	+7 mmol/L
serum sodium	136 mmol/L (135–145)
serum potassium	3.5 mmol/L (3.5–4.5)
serum chloride	90 mmol/L (95–105)

APPROXIMATE REQUIREMENTS for intravenous fluid over the next 24 h would be

A 300 mL half isotonic saline with 5% dextrose and 40 mmol/L ammonium chloride.
B 300 mL half isotonic saline with 5% dextrose and 40 mmol/L potassium chloride.
C 600 mL Hartmann solution.
D 600 mL isotonic saline.
E 600 mL half isotonic saline with 5% dextrose and 40 mmol/L potassium chloride.

PA-Q31

The MOST COMMON cause of blood-stained stool in an otherwise normal infant is

A anal fissure.
B anal fistula.
C haemorrhoids.
D Meckel diverticulitis.
E intussusception.

PA-Q32

The MOST FREQUENT cause of recurrent attacks of periumbilical pain without fever in childhood is

A chronic appendicitis.
B Meckel diverticulitis.
C hydronephrosis.
D urinary tract infection.
E no recognisable organic disease.

PA-Q33

A breast-fed infant becomes jaundiced on the second day of life and is still yellow, but feeding well and thriving, after 2 weeks. Which of the following is CORRECT?

A The jaundice is probably due to conjugated bilirubin.

B The baby's urine should be checked particularly for glucose.

C Blood group incompatibility is the most likely cause.

D Weaning would probably cure the jaundice but is unnecessary.

E Thyroid function testing is not relevant.

PA-Q34

The mother of a 5-year-old boy complains that, although he was 'out of nappies' by the age of 2½ years, for the past 12 months he has been soiling his pants with faecal material several times a day. On examination there is slight abdominal distension and firm faecal masses can be felt in the lower left abdomen. The MOST LIKELY cause is

A Hirschsprung disease.

B infestation with *Giardia lamblia*.

C intermittent volvulus of the sigmoid colon.

D spina bifida occulta.

E chronic constipation.

PA-Q35

Hepatomegaly in the newborn period is a feature of each of the following EXCEPT

A galactosaemia.

B breast milk jaundice.

C neonatal hepatitis.

D Rhesus haemolytic disease.

E congestive cardiac failure.

PA-Q36

Which of the following statements about an umbilical hernia in infancy is CORRECT?

A Day surgery is indicated if the size of the defect is greater than 1 cm in a 6-month-old infant.

B Strapping of the hernia will facilitate resolution.

C Strangulation is rare.

D Hypothyroidism should always be excluded by undertaking thyroid function tests.

E It is likely to occur in subsequent siblings.

PA-Q37

A 6-month-old male infant is noted by the mother to have a swelling in the right groin for a few hours without other symptoms or signs. Examination the following day fails to reveal this swelling. Both testes are in the scrotum and the right spermatic cord is thicker than the left. You SHOULD

A arrange a surgical consultation with a view to inguinal herniotomy.

B reassure the parents that no treatment is necessary.

C re-examine at weekly intervals for reappearance of the swelling.

D arrange to review the child at 1 year of age to check if swelling has recurred.

E admit immediately to hospital for surgery because of the risk of strangulation.

PA-Q38

A 9-month-old afebrile infant presents with a 6 h history of intermittent crying, pallor and vomiting. The baby has not had a dirty nappy for 12 h. No abnormality is found on abdominal examination. Which of the following statements is CORRECT?

A The baby probably has gastroenteritis and should be commenced on an oral rehydration fluid.

B A full septic work-up should be performed.

C Intussusception should be considered as the cause of the problem.

D Babies aged 9 months often have episodes of irritability and the mother should be reassured accordingly.

E Urinary tract infection is the probable cause of the baby's illness.

PA-Q39

Which of the following statements concerning Hirschsprung disease (idiopathic megacolon) is CORRECT?

A It presents most commonly as neonatal intestinal obstruction.

B Most cases are recognised because of constipation developing at about 5 years of age.

C X-rays are diagnostic after preparation by multiple enemas.

D Biopsy of the aganglionic bowel wall is less reliable than contrast X-rays of the colon.

E Recent advances have eliminated the need for surgery in this disease.

PA-Q40

Each of the following unwanted effects has been documented with the use of topical corticosteroids EXCEPT

A thrombocytopenia.

B suppression of adrenal function.

C candidiasis.

D growth suppression in children.

E atrophy of the skin.

PA-Q41

A girl aged 5 years presents with a history of urgency of micturition, occasional enuresis and a slight, non-offensive vaginal discharge for 3 months. She has had no vaginal bleeding. Examination reveals some reddening of the labia majora. The MOST LIKELY diagnosis would be

A trichomonal infection.

B gonorrhoea.

C cystitis.

D foreign body.

E non-specific vulvovaginitis.

PA-Q42

Spontaneous petechiae on the skin are characteristic of each of the following EXCEPT

A haemophilia.

B idiopathic thrombocytopenia.

C Henoch–Schönlein syndrome.

D bone marrow aplasia.

E meningococcal septicaemia.

PA-Q43

An infant boy aged 10 months has been noticed to be tired and pale for 3 weeks. On examination he is pale but appears well nourished. There is no hepatosplenomegaly or lymphadenopathy. The peripheral blood count is as follows: haemoglobin 3.4 g/dL; haematocrit 0.16; reticulocytes 0.2%. Blood film shows hypochromic microcytic red cells, no polychromasia and no nucleated red cells; leucocytes 9.0 x 10^9 /L with 50% neutrophils, platelets 400 x 10^9 /L. The MOST LIKELY diagnosis is

A   anaemia due to blood loss.
B   iron-deficiency anaemia.
C   thalassaemia major.
D   megaloblastic anaemia.
E   anaemia of infection.

PA-Q44

An infant boy, born to parents of Greek origin, is well for the first 6 days of life, but then becomes jaundiced. On day 7 he is lethargic and his liver and spleen are palpable, 2 and 1 cm, respectively, below the costal margin. His serum bilirubin on the same day is 200 mmol/L (< 100), of which 100 mmol/L is conjugated. Which of the following blood tests is MOST LIKELY to indicate the cause of his jaundice?

A   Measurement of serum thyrotrophic hormone (TSH).
B   Blood culture.
C   Electrophoresis of haemoglobin.
D   Test for glucose-6-phosphate dehydrogenase activity in erythrocytes.
E   Test for osmotic fragility of erythrocytes.

PA-Q45

A man with haemophilia marries a non-carrier woman. The possible offspring of this marriage would be

A   all haemophilic.
B   haemophilic males, normal females.
C   female carriers, normal males.
D   male carriers, normal females.
E   all genotypically normal.

PA-Q46

Which of the following statements concerning enuresis is CORRECT?

A   Regular bed wetting is usual at the age of 4 years.
B   An intravenous pyelogram should be performed.
C   A positive family history occurs in less than 10% of cases.
D   Psychological factors predominate in the aetiology of primary enuresis.
E   The most effective treatment after the age of 8 years is a conditioning apparatus.

PA-Q47

A 3-year-old child is brought for review because of mild pallor and increasing weight over the previous 3 weeks. Examination shows generalised oedema, ascites and heavy albuminuria. You SHOULD EXPECT that

A   the serum globulin will be high.
B   the serum albumin will be low.
C   the serum cholesterol will be low.
D   there will be macroscopic haematuria.
E   the child will die within 6 months.

PA-Q48

A previously well 12-year-old boy presents with a history of pain in the scrotum for 4 h. On examination, the right hemi-scrotum is red, hot, swollen and tender; no other abnormality is found. You SHOULD

A arrange for surgical exploration of both sides of the scrotum.
B measure serum alpha-fetoprotein.
C admit him to hospital for observation.
D prescribe steroid therapy.
E prescribe penicillin and gentamicin therapy after taking blood for culture.

PA-Q49

Which of the following is CORRECT?

A Meatal ulceration is a complication of circumcision.
B The prepuce is fully retractable in 90% of uncircumcised boys aged 6 months.
C Circumcision is the first stage in the repair of hypospadias.
D Neonatal circumcision is safe in haemophilia, because of transplacental passage of factor VIII.
E Neonatal circumcision is painless.

PA-Q50

All the following statements about a normal baby are correct EXCEPT

A at 2 weeks of age the child can reach out to grasp a rattle.
B at 4–5 months the child begins to roll over.
C at 6 months the child can extend legs to stand if held upright.
D at 12 months the child can say a few words.
E at 18 months the child can put 3 or 4 words together.

PA-Q51

MOST children aged 11 months can

A walk independently.
B build a tower of four cubes.
C point to a named part of the body.
D feed themselves with a spoon.
E pick up a raisin between thumb and finger.

PA-Q52

Most children aged 48 months can do all of the following EXCEPT

A know their first and last names.
B undress themselves.
C draw a man (six parts).
D hop on one foot.
E separate easily from their mothers.

PA-Q53

Which of the following is LEAST LIKELY to cause delay in the development of speech?

A Maternal deprivation.
B Hypothyroidism.
C Tongue-tie.
D Infantile autism.
E High-tone hearing loss.

PA-Q54

Which of the following is NOT TYPICALLY DESCRIPTIVE of anorexia nervosa in adolescents?

A Marked weight loss.
B Preoccupation with food.
C Amenorrhoea.
D Decreased physical activity.
E Higher incidence among girls than boys.

PA-Q55

Each of the following conditions is a characteristic presenting feature of the child maltreatment syndrome EXCEPT

A failure to thrive.
B lacerated frenulum of the lower lip.
C burns of the feet.
D epistaxes.
E burns of the buttocks.

PA-Q56

A 3^1/2-year-old boy says only three single words, and these are poorly articulated. He uses gestures to communicate. There are no other reported problems, gross and fine motor skills are normal for age and physical examination, including tympanography, is normal. Which of the following is the MOST LIKELY explanation?

A Intellectual disability.
B Deafness.
C Manipulative behaviour.
D Dysarthria.
E Autism.

PA-Q57

Which of the following is NOT a feature of Down syndrome?

A Brachycephalic type skull.
B Prominent epicanthic folds.
C Cleft palate.
D General muscular hypotonia.
E Duodenal atresia.

PA-Q58

The parents of a newborn with Down syndrome are refusing to take the baby home. After confirming that this is their wish, which one of the following is the MOST APPROPRIATE action?

A Arrange to make the child a ward of state.
B Arrange to have the baby adopted.
C Try to persuade the parents to take the baby home.
D Arrange a temporary foster care placement.
E Keep the baby in the maternity hospital while the parents reconsider.

PA-Q59

A full-term infant is transferred to the postnatal ward when aged 1 h. On arrival, she is noticed to have cyanosed hands and feet. On examination you find the infant is responsive and cries lustily on handling. The respiratory rate is 40 /min and the lungs and heart are clinically normal. Which one of the following statements is CORRECT?

A The infant has most probably had a convulsion.

B The infant's rectal temperature should be checked.

C The infant has early signs of respiratory distress.

D Oxygen should be given.

E An immediate chest X-ray should be arranged.

PA-Q60

Which one of the following statements about obesity in children is CORRECT?

A It affects 5–10% of Australian children.

B It is defined as weight above the 97th percentile.

C 50–60% of obese 1-year-olds will be obese in adult life.

D It is readily controlled by a combination of diet and a programme of exercise.

E It is associated with an underlying metabolic or endocrine disorder in approximately 10–15% of cases.

PA-Q61

Which one of the following statements about infant feeding is CORRECT?

A Foods, other than milk, should be introduced from 2–3 months of life.

B Bottle-fed babies are more likely to be overweight than breast-fed babies.

C Test weighing is an accurate way to measure the intake for a breast-fed baby.

D Breast-fed babies should be given a multi-vitamin preparation containing iron because breast milk is low in iron.

E It is safe for a mother on lithium to breast feed.

PA-Q62

Hypernatraemic dehydration in childhood

A should be treated by rapid infusion of 4% dextrose in $^1/_5$ th isotonic saline.

B is associated with marked loss of tissue turgor.

C is most frequent under the age of 3 weeks.

D is often complicated by convulsions.

E is most commonly due to diabetes insipidus.

PA-Q63

The FINDING of glycosuria in an ill child is

A clear evidence of hyperglycaemia.

B diagnostic of diabetes mellitus.

C common in childhood and not significant in itself.

D a significant observation which demands further elucidation.

E indicative of a renal tubular disorder.

PA-Q64

A 4-year-old boy is the height of an average 2-year-old child and has a bone age equivalent to that of an 18-month-old child. Which of the following conditions is MOST LIKELY to have caused his growth retardation?

A Hypothyroidism.
B Diabetes mellitus.
C Congenital adrenal hyperplasia.
D Genetic short stature.
E Psychological deprivation.

PA-Q65

Failure to thrive in infancy is MOST COMMONLY due to

A non-organic causes.
B gastro-oesophageal reflux.
C malabsorption.
D endocrine/metabolic disorders.
E recurrent infections.

PA-Q66

Which one of the following statements is CORRECT with regard to acute viral bronchiolitis?

A Para-influenzae type 3 is the most frequent pathogen.
B The peak age group affected is infants aged 6 to 9 months.
C Inability to feed adequately is a major indication for admission to hospital.
D Beta-adrenergic agents are effective therapy.
E Approximately 25% of affected infants subsequently have asthma.

PA-Q67

An 18-month-old child is admitted with a fever of 40°C (rectal). He was well until 3 days ago when he developed malaise, fever and anorexia. One day before admission he limped and on the day of admission, he refused to walk. His entire thigh is swollen and he has limited knee movement. There is an area of point tenderness over the medial side of the distal femur. Your WORKING DIAGNOSIS SHOULD be

A cellulitis.
B undisplaced fracture.
C osteomyelitis.
D thrombophlebitis.
E osteogenic sarcoma.

PA-Q68

Which of the following MOST COMMONLY CAUSES bacterial meningitis in the first month after birth?

A *Haemophilus influenzae.*
B *Streptococcus pneumoniae.*
C *Staphylococcus aureus.*
D *Neisseria meningitidis.*
E *Escherichia coli.*

PA-Q69

A 5-year-old boy is diagnosed in the Emergency Department as having measles, the first symptoms having started 2 days previously. He has a 2-year-old sister, who has received the recommended immunisation schedule. Which of the following is APPROPRIATE MANAGEMENT?

A Treat him symptomatically and send him home.
B Refer him to the infectious diseases hospital.
C Give him gamma-globulin.
D Give gamma-globulin to the sister.
E Reassure the mother that 'he is over the worst of it'.

PA-Q70

The MOST COMMON complication of mumps in a 5-year-old boy is

A diabetes mellitus.
B orchitis.
C encephalomyelitis.
D meningo-encephalitis.
E sialectasis.

PA-Q71

A 4-year-old boy presents with a firm, mobile non-tender swelling of 3 cm diameter, high in the left anterior triangle of the neck. Three weeks earlier he had an attack of acute tonsillitis. Which one of the following is MOST LIKELY to be the cause of the swelling?

A Branchial cyst.
B Tuberculous abscess.
C Thyroglossal cyst.
D Cervical lymphadenitis.
E Lymphoma.

PA-Q72

A 2-year-old boy who has been previously well presents with foamy diarrhoea, vague upper abdominal discomfort and failure to thrive for 2 months. His weight is on the 25th percentile. Examination of the stools reveals steatorrhoea with fatty acid crystals but no other unusual feature. The MOST LIKELY diagnosis is

A *Giardia lamblia* infestation.
B coeliac disease.
C cystic fibrosis.
D *Campylobacter* infection.
E rotavirus infection.

PA-Q73

Cloxacillin is the MOST APPROPRIATE antibiotic in which one of the following infections?

A Otitis media.
B Osteomyelitis.
C 'Croup'.
D Meningococcal meningitis.
E Tonsillitis.

PA-Q74

A 14-year-old girl complains of headache and tiredness similar to her symptoms at the time of proven infectious mononucleosis, from which she had recovered 6 months previously. There are no other symptoms. On routine enquiry both the patient and her mother describe school and family life as normal. On physical examination no abnormality is found. Your ADVICE to her should be that

A these symptoms suggest a relapse of infectious mononucleosis and will resolve with time.

B she has not had adequate rest and so should have a further period of time away from school.

C her symptoms are not the result of the infection but their cause is likely to be revealed by further detailed history from the patient interviewed on her own.

D further tests, including chest X-ray and urine culture, should be undertaken.

E you now wish to discuss her ill health privately with her parents.

PA-Q75

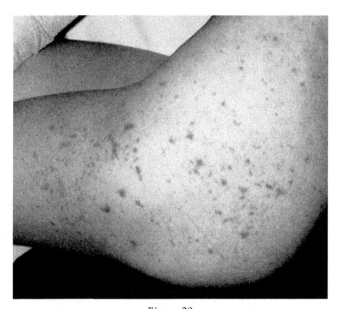

Figure 39

A 2-year-old boy presented to your surgery with the onset of the skin rash, depicted in the accompanying photograph (Figure 39), over the previous 3–4 h. He has a temperature of 38.8°C. Which one of the following responses would be the MOST APPROPRIATE?

A Send him home and tell his parents to give him paracetamol to control the fever.

B Send him to hospital immediately.

C Give him penicillin and send home.

D Give a broad spectrum antibiotic and send home.

E Give a single large dose of parenteral penicillin and send him immediately to hospital.

PA-Q76

Which of the following is the MOST COMMON organism to cause non-neonatal bacterial meningitis in children in Australia?

A   *Streptococcus pneumoniae.*
B   Beta-haemolytic streptococcus.
C   *Staphylococcus aureus.*
D   *Neisseria meningitidis.*
E   *Haemophilus influenzae* type B.

PA-Q77

Which antibiotic would be MOST APPROPRIATE for an 8-year-old with enlarged tender red tonsils covered with spots of yellow pus?

A   Cefaclor.
B   Penicillin.
C   Amoxycillin.
D   Sulphamethoxazole with trimethoprim (Cotrimoxazole®).
E   Amoxycillin with clavulanic acid (Augmentin®).

PA-Q78

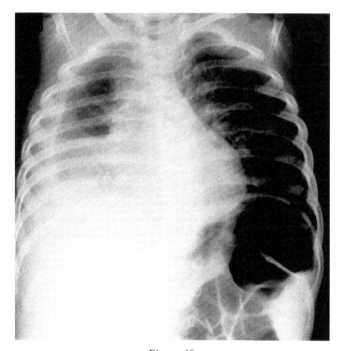

Figure 40

An X-ray of the chest of a 9-month-old infant reveals an opacity in the right lower zone and pneumatoceles. Two days later a repeat X-ray is as shown in the accompanying photograph (Figure 40). These findings are MOST LIKELY caused by

A   *Klebsiella pneumoniae.*
B   Group A streptococcus.
C   *Streptococcus pneumoniae* (pneumococcus).
D   *Haemophilus influenzae* Type B.
E   *Staphylococcus aureus.*

PA-Q79

A 4-year-old child has a 36 h history of a 'barking' cough, inspiratory stridor, and intercostal retraction. His temperature is 38.2°C and white cell count is 6.8 x 10^9/L (4.0–11.0) with a normal differential count. The MOST LIKELY diagnosis is

A   acute epiglottitis caused by *Haemophilus influenzae*.

B   'croup' caused by Group A streptococcus.

C   'croup' caused by parainfluenza virus.

D   acute bronchial asthma.

E   foreign body in the trachea.

PA-Q80

Which of the following statements about mumps is CORRECT?

A   The mumps skin test is a reliable indicator of immunity.

B   The incubation period is 7–10 days.

C   Meningoencephalitis can precede, occur simultaneously with or follow parotitis.

D   Salivary gland involvement is limited to the parotids.

E   Infertility is usual following mumps orchitis.

PA-Q81

ROUTINE treatment of a child with 'croup' should INCLUDE

A   sedatives.

B   bronchodilators.

C   observation at home or in hospital.

D   tracheostomy.

E   oxygen.

PA-Q82

A 9-month-old child has been irritable and febrile for 48 h. Today he has a generalised erythematous rash and his temperature is 37.2°C. What is the MOST LIKELY diagnosis?

A   Herpes simplex Type 1 infection.

B   Rubella.

C   Scarlet fever.

D   Roseola infantum.

E   Erythema infectiosum.

PA-Q83

A previously well 9-month-old infant has an episode of gastroenteritis with vomiting and diarrhoea. However, the diarrhoea persists after 10 days. The MOST LIKELY diagnosis would be

A   *Giardia lamblia* infestation.

B   Secondary lactase deficiency.

C   Coeliac disease.

D   Secondary bacterial enteritis.

E   Cow milk allergy.

PA-Q84

A 4-year-old girl presents with a 1 month history of loss of weight, tiredness and a protuberant abdomen. Examination reveals a large, non-tender irregularly shaped mass in the left side of the abdomen, which appears to be slightly mobile and extends just across the midline. The MOST LIKELY diagnosis would be

A   cystic dysplastic kidney.
B   left ovarian cyst.
C   retroperitoneal haematoma.
D   thalassaemia major.
E   neuroblastoma.

PA-Q85

Which one of the following is INCORRECT concerning neoplasia in children?

A   Acute lymphoblastic leukaemia is the most common neoplastic disease of childhood.
B   Appropriate treatment of Wilms tumour (nephroblastoma) results in long-term survival in over 50% of cases.
C   Most children with neuroblastoma have metastases at diagnosis.
D   Carcinoma is the most common type of solid tumour in children.
E   Intracranial tumours are most commonly infratentorial.

PA-Q86

In Australia which of the following is the MOST FREQUENT cause of death in a previously well 3-year-old?

A   Sudden Infant Death Syndrome.
B   Leukaemia.
C   Viral pneumonia.
D   Poisoning.
E   Drowning.

Obstetrics & Gynaecology Questions

TYPE

A

Questions OG-Q1 to OG-Q93

- ▮ Type A questions consist of a stem and five responses
- ▮ **One** correct answer must be selected from five possible responses to the stem

OG-Q1

The MOST ACCURATE estimation of fetal gestational age can be obtained from which of the following?

- A X-ray examination of the fetus in the second trimester.
- B Estimation of the fundal height of the uterus on abdominal palpation.
- C Pelvic examination in the first trimester.
- D The date on which fetal movements were felt by the mother for the first time.
- E Ultrasound examination of the fetus in the last trimester.

OG-Q2

The date of delivery in a primigravida is BEST predicted from which of the following?

- A The date when fetal movements were first felt.
- B The size of the uterus in late pregnancy.
- C The size of the uterus in the first trimester.
- D When the uterine fundus reaches the umbilicus.
- E The time of engagement of the fetal presenting part in the maternal pelvis.

OG-Q3

A 37-year-old female patient who has recurrent cystitis, which is clearly related to coitus, comes to you for evaluation and treatment. Which one of the following statements is MOST CORRECT regarding this condition?

- A Alteration of the coital position will usually prevent further recurrence of infection.
- B Cystoscopy is a necessary component of her evaluation.
- C An intravenous urogram is a necessary component of her evaluation.
- D The bacterial flora of her vagina plays no role in her condition.
- E The prophylactic use of postcoital antibiotics is as effective as continuous therapy.

OG-Q4

Concerning acute pyelonephritis complicating pregnancy and the puerperium, all of the following statements are correct EXCEPT

- A it affects approximately 2% of patients.
- B when unilateral it is most often right sided.
- C symptoms include anorexia, nausea and vomiting.
- D *Escherichia coli* is the predominant causative micro-organism.
- E a change in the immune mechanism in pregnancy is the major cause of this infection.

OG-Q5

The drug of choice for the TREATMENT of *Chlamydia trachomatis* infection DURING PREGNANCY is

- A metronidazole.
- B cephazolin.
- C erythromycin.
- D tetracycline.
- E clindamycin.

OG-Q6

Which of the following is CORRECT concerning GROUP B STREPTOCOCCUS infection in pregnancy?

  A The usual mode of infection is transplacental.
  B The risk of fetal infection decreases with rupture of the membranes.
  C Neonatal mortality is high once systemic infection is established.
  D The organism is usually resistant to penicillin.
  E Mature babies (those delivered after 37 weeks gestation) are able to resist infection with this agent.

OG-Q7

The MOST COMMON non-bacterial intrauterine fetal infection in Australia is

  A toxoplasmosis.
  B rubella.
  C cytomegalovirus.
  D syphilis.
  E Herpes simplex.

OG-Q8

Which one of the following bacteria produces an exotoxin causing 'toxic shock syndrome' ASSOCIATED with tampon usage?

  A *Escherichia coli.*
  B Group B streptococcus.
  C *Clostridium welchii.*
  D *Staphylococcus aureus.*
  E *Mycoplasma hominis.*

OG-Q9

If a pregnant patient has an exploratory laparotomy for possible appendicitis and the appendix and other abdominal contents appear normal for the stage of gestation, what is the TREATMENT of choice?

  A Close incision and observe.
  B Close incision and administer appropriate antibiotics and tocolytics.
  C Obtain peritoneal cytology and close incision.
  D Appendicectomy and incision closure.
  E Caesarean section if past 36 weeks gestation.

OG-Q10

Appendicitis in pregnancy is difficult to diagnose for all of the following reasons EXCEPT

  A anorexia, nausea and vomiting are common in pregnancy.
  B due to uterine enlargement the site of the vermiform appendix is changed in pregnancy.
  C leucocytosis is the rule in normal pregnancy.
  D there is immunological suppression in pregnancy, leading to the suppression of localising signs.
  E other diseases during pregnancy are readily confused with appendicitis.

OG-Q11

ACUTE appendicitis in pregnancy

    A is very often fatal.

    B is more common than in the non-pregnant state due to a reduction in cellular immunity.

    C is easier to diagnose than in the non-pregnant state.

    D occurs with the same symptoms and signs as in the non-pregnant woman.

    E occurs, but the site of maximal tenderness is higher the later the condition occurs in pregnancy.

OG-Q12

All of the following statements concerning viral hepatitis during pregnancy are correct EXCEPT

    A hepatitis A virus is usually the infecting organism.

    B it carries a worse prognosis if chronic active hepatitis is present.

    C the usual infecting organism has a proven teratogenic effect.

    D it is associated with an increased risk of premature labour.

    E the course of the disease is similar to that seen in non-pregnant individuals.

OG-Q13

A 27-year-old woman is hospitalised at 36 weeks gestation because of jaundice, haematemesis and increased confusion. For 10 days prior to admission she had nausea, vomiting, lack of appetite and fatigue. Results of laboratory studies are: urea 18 mmol/L (3–8); uric acid 0.6 mmol/L (0.15–0.40); bilirubin 60 μmol/L (2–20); alanine amino-transferase (ALT) 240 U/L (5–40), aspartate aminotransferase (AST) 210 U/L (10–45); alkaline phosphatase (ALP) 80 U/L (25–100). Serum ammonia concentration is elevated. The MOST LIKELY diagnosis is

    A acute viral hepatitis.

    B alcoholic cirrhosis.

    C pre-eclampsia.

    D acute fatty liver of pregnancy.

    E cholestasis of pregnancy.

OG-Q14

The frequency of pre-eclampsia is increased in all the following conditions EXCEPT

    A diabetes mellitus.

    B essential hypertension.

    C twin pregnancy.

    D primigravid pregnancy.

    E placenta praevia.

OG-Q15

Multiple pregnancy is associated with an increased incidence of all of the following EXCEPT

    A perinatal morbidity.

    B fetomaternal haemorrhage.

    C postpartum haemorrhage.

    D intrauterine growth retardation.

    E umbilical cord prolapse.

OG-Q16

The D antigen is present on erythrocytes of Rh-positive fetuses as EARLY as

- A 7 weeks gestation.
- B 10 weeks gestation.
- C 15 weeks gestation.
- D 20 weeks gestation.
- E 25 weeks gestation.

OG-Q17

The condition of the fetus of an Rh-negative, sensitised pregnant woman, at 28 weeks gestation, is BEST evaluated by which of the following?

- A Analysis of amniotic fluid for concentrations of bilirubin-like compounds.
- B Determination of antibody titres in the amniotic fluid.
- C A history regarding previous infants who were affected and required exchange transfusions.
- D Maternal antibody titres.
- E Ultrasound examination for fetal ascites.

OG-Q18

Recurrent glycosuria in pregnancy

- A indicates diabetes.
- B indicates prediabetes.
- C should always be investigated by a full glucose tolerance test.
- D is encountered in 10–20% of women.
- E is encountered in more than 50% of women.

OG-Q19

Pancreatitis during pregnancy is MOST OFTEN associated with

- A excessive alcohol intake.
- B hyperparathyroidism.
- C blunt abdominal trauma.
- D cholelithiasis.
- E cocaine use.

OG-Q20

Intrahepatic cholestasis of pregnancy is ASSOCIATED with

- A right upper quadrant tenderness.
- B occurrence in the first trimester.
- C high risk of recurrence in subsequent pregnancies.
- D elevation of bilirubin concentration >170 µmol/L (2–20).
- E excessive antacid use.

OG-Q21

Hypertension in pregnancy should NOT be treated with

- A methyldopa.
- B diazoxide.
- C hydralazine.
- D oxprenolol.
- E thiazide diuretics.

OG-Q22

A multigravida presents at 37 weeks gestation, not in labour, with a breech presentation and ruptured membranes. What should be done INITIALLY?

A Immediate caesarean section.

B Emergency radiological pelvimetry.

C Vaginal examination.

D Set up an oxytocin infusion.

E Urgent ultrasound scan.

OG-Q23

A young woman who is obviously pregnant is found at the side of the road at the site of an automobile accident. She is unresponsive to verbal stimuli. Assessment of her condition should give FIRST PRIORITY to

A respiratory status.

B level of consciousness.

C fetal viability.

D presence of bleeding.

E assessment of possible shock.

OG-Q24

A primigravid woman is in premature labour at 26 weeks gestation with a vertex presentation and ruptured membranes. An abdominal cardiotocograph (CTG) record is being made of the fetal heart. Which of the following patterns would be the MOST ominous?

A Baseline 170 beats/min; fair variability; no decelerations.

B Baseline 170 beats/min; fair variability; variable decelerations.

C Baseline 160 beats/min; poor variability; no decelerations.

D Baseline 150 beats/min; poor variability; late decelerations.

E Baseline 160 beats/min; fair variability; early decelerations.

OG-Q25

A 32-year-old woman, gravida (G) 5, para (P) 4, at 32 weeks gestation is admitted to hospital because of mild, bright red vaginal bleeding amounting to approximately 100 mL. Her last two children were born by lower uterine segment caesarean section. She has no pain or contractions. Vital signs are stable within the normal range. Fetal heart rate is 140 beats/min and regular and the CTG shows no deceleration and good beat to beat variation. Intravenous fluids are started, and blood is drawn for typing, cross-matching and complete blood count. In addition to bed rest, management at this time SHOULD INCLUDE

A a rectal examination.

B a vaginal examination.

C beta sympathomimetic agents.

D immediate caesarean section.

E observation and further investigation.

OG-Q26

What is the MOST LIKELY diagnosis in an antenatal patient near term with the following clinical picture: sudden onset of sharp, continuous abdominal pain, shock, a tense uterus but no vaginal bleeding?

A Placental abruption.
B Twisted ovarian cyst.
C Rupture of the uterus.
D Red degeneration of a fibroid.
E Amniotic fluid embolus.

OG-Q27

The BEST sign of PROGRESS of labour is

A position of the presenting part in relation to the maternal pelvis.
B effacement of the cervix.
C increasing frequency, strength and duration of uterine contractions.
D station of the presenting part in relation to the ischial spines.
E increasing dilatation of the cervix.

OG-Q28

Labour may be obstructed by all the following EXCEPT

A a cystocele or rectocele.
B a distended urinary bladder.
C ectopic or pelvic kidney.
D ovarian tumours.
E myomata (uterine fibroids).

OG-Q29

Conditions LIKELY to BE ASSOCIATED with shoulder dystocia INCLUDE

A prolonged gestation.
B hydrocephalus.
C non-immune hydrops.
D intrauterine growth retardation (IUGR).
E toxoplasmosis.

OG-Q30

Compared with infants delivered spontaneously, infants delivered by elective low forceps show a markedly INCREASED incidence of

A perinatal mortality and morbidity.
B speech, language or hearing abnormalities.
C cephalohaematoma.
D facial nerve damage.
E none of the above.

OG-Q31

A pudendal anaesthetic blocks which of the following nervous pathways?

A Autonomic motor pathways.
B Autonomic sensory pathways.
C T 11,12 sensory pathways.
D L 2,3,4 sensory pathways.
E S 2,3,4 sensory pathways.

OG-Q32

Which of the following maternal conditions CONTRAINDICATES epidural anaesthesia?

A   Hypertension.
B   Previous caesarean delivery.
C   Platelet count less than 40 x 10^9/L (150–400 x 10^9/L)
D   Mitral stenosis.
E   Chronic anaemia.

OG-Q33

Postpartum haemorrhage is LEAST LIKELY in which of the following situations?

A   Following birth of a 4900 g fetus of a gestational diabetic.
B   Following a 36 h labour in a 17-year-old primigravida.
C   Following a 4 h labour in a 34-year-old G5 P4.
D   Following an 8 h labour in a 21-year-old G1 P0 with mild pre-eclampsia.
E   Following a 16 h labour in a 19-year-old G2 P1 with chorioamnionitis.

OG-Q34

In evaluating fluid replacement for obstetric haemorrhage, which of the following clinical parameters is the BEST sign of adequate fluid volume?

A   Blood pressure.
B   Respiratory rate.
C   Pulse rate.
D   Urine output.
E   Pulse pressure.

OG-Q35

Each of the following situations predisposes to postpartum haemorrhage EXCEPT

A   over-distension of the uterus.
B   prolonged labour.
C   precipitate labour.
D   delivery of a growth-retarded infant.
E   sixth pregnancy over 35 years of age.

OG-Q36

In the presence of life-threatening uterine bleeding after delivery, which of the following diagnostic tests will provide the MOST USEFUL information in the SHORTEST TIME?

A   Platelet count.
B   Fibrinogen level.
C   Fibrin split products.
D   Activated partial thromboplastin time (APTT).
E   Bedside observation of clotting and bedside estimation of whole blood clotting time.

OG-Q37

The clinical presentation MOST CHARACTERISTIC of uterine inversion is

A   brisk vaginal bleeding.
B   abrupt shock with profuse vaginal bleeding.
C   vaginal bleeding with abrupt profound shock out of proportion to the bleeding.
D   sudden agonising pain.
E   no symptoms but discovery of the uterine fundus at the vaginal introitus.

OG-Q38

A 32-year-old multigravid woman has just been delivered of a 3600 g infant after successful oxytocin induction of labour at 42 weeks of gestation. With gentle traction on the umbilical cord the uterus suddenly inverted and is now approximately 10 cm outside the introitus. The MOST APPROPRIATE treatment is

A   attempt immediate replacement of the uterus.

B   remove the placenta and then attempt replacement of the uterus.

C   magnesium sulphate 4–6 g intravenously over 5–10 min, then attempt replacement of the uterus.

D   terbutaline 0.25 mg subcutaneously, then attempt replacement of the uterus.

E   ritodrine hydrochloride 350 μg intravenous bolus, then attempt replacement of the uterus.

OG-Q39

Which of the following disorders is ASSOCIATED with the HIGHEST maternal mortality?

A   Hypothyroidism.

B   Systemic lupus erythematosus.

C   Ventricular septal defect.

D   Myasthenia gravis.

E   Primary pulmonary hypertension.

OG-Q40

Which one of the following changes is a NORMAL characteristic of the puerperium?

A   Colostrum secretion for approximately 2 weeks.

B   Vascular and lymphatic engorgement of the breasts.

C   Resumption of ovulation by 2 weeks after term pregnancy.

D   Transient leucopenia.

E   Sloughing of the basal layer of the endometrium into the lochia.

OG-Q41

The organism MOST COMMONLY associated with postpartum mastitis is

A   Group B streptococcus.

B   *Escherichia coli.*

C   *Streptococcus pneumoniae.*

D   coagulase-positive *Staphylococcus aureus.*

E   coagulase-negative staphylococcal species.

OG-Q42

Admission to a psychiatric hospital for psychotic depression associated with pregnancy is MOST FREQUENT

A   in the 1st trimester.

B   in the 2nd trimester.

C   in the 3rd trimester.

D   in the puerperium.

E   after the 6 weeks postpartum check.

OG-Q43

Low Apgar scores at 1 min and 5 min in a term infant INDICATE

  A future neurological impairment.
  B the infant needs resuscitation.
  C the infant will develop seizures.
  D perinatal asphyxia.
  E significant hypoxia.

OG-Q44

Thirty minutes after receiving 50 mg pethidine intravenously for analgesia during labour, a patient delivers a 3200 g infant who remains apnoeic at 1 min following birth. There was no antecedent fetal distress. In addition to other resuscitative measures, the MOST APPROPRIATE therapy given to the fetus is

  A naloxone (Narcan®).
  B nalorphine (Nalline®).
  C theophylline.
  D caffeine sodium benzoate.
  E amphetamine sulphate.

OG-Q45

The fetus or new-born infant with intra-uterine growth retardation shows the LEAST retardation in which one of the following organs?

  A Brain.
  B Heart.
  C Liver.
  D Kidney.
  E Lymphoid organs.

OG-Q46

Abnormalities in the vessels of the umbilical cord are often associated with fetal malformation. Which of the following VESSEL PATTERNS would make you suspect an underlying cardiac abnormality may exist in the fetus?

  A One artery and two veins.
  B One artery and one vein.
  C Two arteries and a venous plexus.
  D Two arteries and two veins.
  E Two arteries and one vein.

OG-Q47

A woman has had a baby with an open neural tube defect. There is no family history of this condition. Concerning subsequent pregnancy, she should be ADVISED that if she does NOT TAKE prophylactic folate therapy

  A there is a 20% chance of recurrence.
  B there is a 10% chance of recurrence.
  C there is a 2–5% chance of recurrence.
  D there is no increased risk for recurrence.
  E no estimates can be made.

OG-Q48

Which one of the following drugs is NOT considered to have adverse effects on the human fetus?

A Diethylstilboestrol.
B Phenytoin.
C Nalidixic acid.
D Tetracycline.
E Danazol.

OG-Q49

Which one of the following statements about the circulatory transition from fetal to extrauterine life is CORRECT?

A Gaseous expansion of the lungs at birth is associated with a dramatic decline in pulmonary vascular resistance and a decrease in pulmonary blood flow.
B The foramen ovale is a flap valve and when left atrial pressure increases over the right side, the opening is functionally closed.
C With the occlusion of the umbilical cord, the large flow of blood to the placenta is interrupted causing a decrease in systemic pressure.
D Prostaglandin metabolism has been shown to play a minor role in the closure of the ductus arteriosus.
E The most dramatic increase in individual organ blood flow after delivery is to the brain.

OG-Q50

Five statements about spontaneous abortion are listed below. Choose the CORRECT statement.

A The incidence of spontaneous abortion is increased in pregnancies if the woman is over 40 years old.
B Most spontaneous abortions occur between 12–16 completed weeks of pregnancy.
C Among chromosomally abnormal spontaneous abortuses, the most common chromosomal abnormality is triploidy.
D *In utero* exposure to diethylstilboestrol (DES) increases a woman's risk of many pregnancy problems, but not spontaneous abortion.
E The karyotypic abnormalities in spontaneous abortuses are similar to those in liveborn neonates.

OG-Q51

Which one of the following options BEST fits the diagnosis of an INEVITABLE abortion?

A Vaginal bleeding.
B Vaginal bleeding with cramping.
C Vaginal bleeding with cramping and an open cervix.
D Vaginal bleeding with cramping, an open cervix and passage of tissue.
E Vaginal bleeding, cramping, an open cervix and complete uterine emptying.

OG-Q52

A patient presents for her first visit in her second pregnancy with a history of a second trimester miscarriage in her previous pregnancy. Which of the events listed below should cause you to suspect that her miscarriage had been DUE TO an incompetent cervix?

A   Onset of contractions.

B   Rupture of membranes.

C   Reduction in fetal movements.

D   Vaginal bleeding.

E   Purulent vaginal discharge.

OG-Q53

The RISK of spontaneous abortion following second trimester amniocentesis is

A   1:50.

B   1:200.

C   1:500.

D   1:1000.

E   1:2000.

OG-Q54

Which one of the following is LEAST LIKELY in a 14-year-old girl with an imperforate hymen?

A   Cyclic lower abdominal pain.

B   Cyclic chills and fever.

C   Urinary retention.

D   Diffuse lower abdominal pain.

E   Lower abdominal distension.

OG-Q55

Danazol (Danocrine®) causes each of the following EXCEPT

A   exacerbation of fibrocystic disease of the breasts.

B   clitoral hypertrophy in female fetuses when given during pregnancy.

C   labial fusion in female fetuses when given during pregnancy.

D   acne.

E   fluid retention.

OG-Q56

Which of the following statements is NOT correct concerning anorexia nervosa?

A   It is an illness of young women characterised by severe malnutrition without associated lethargy.

B   The most frequent age distribution is between 11 and 21 years.

C   90% of the patients are female.

D   There is a pathological obsession with body size resulting in a refusal, or inability, to recognise hunger.

E   Follicle-stimulating hormone (FSH) levels are pathognomonic.

OG-Q57

A 16-year-old girl has severe acne unresponsive to conventional therapy including the oral contraceptive pill and tetracyclines. Which of the following laboratory studies should be done BEFORE prescribing isotretinoin?

A Complete blood count.
B Liver function studies.
C Lipid profile.
D Measurement of blood urea.
E Pregnancy test.

OG-Q58

An inhibited sexual excitement phase in marital sex is MOST COMMONLY caused by

A fear of pregnancy.
B menopause.
C hysterectomy.
D marital discord.
E 'empty nest' syndrome.

OG-Q59

A 19-year-old girl, prescribed a triphasic oral contraceptive for the first time 1 month ago, complains of frequent spotting. The MOST APPROPRIATE management is to

A increase the dose of oestrogen.
B increase the dose of progestogen.
C advise alternative contraception.
D continue the medication and review in 2 months.
E change to a biphasic pill.

OG-Q60

All of the following are proven to be established benefits of the oestrogen/progestogen oral contraceptive pill EXCEPT

A reduction in incidence of menorrhagia.
B reduction in incidence of benign breast disease.
C reduction in incidence of pelvic inflammatory disease.
D reduction in incidence of cervical carcinoma.
E reduction in incidence of ovarian carcinoma.

OG-Q61

The Pearl Index (formula) is expressed as

A per cent of women who become pregnant using a contraceptive.
B per cent of women who do not become pregnant using a particular contraceptive.
C number of pregnancies per 100 women-years use of a particular contraceptive.
D number of pregnancies per 1000 women-years use of a particular contraceptive.
E number of pregnancies per 100 000 women-years use of a particular contraceptive.

OG-Q62

Which of the following is the MOST COMMON cause of death attributable to tubal sterilisation in developed countries of the world?

A Anaesthesia.
B Haemorrhage from the tube.
C Sepsis.
D Myocardial infarction.
E Pulmonary embolus.

OG-Q63

Primary amenorrhoea is the USUAL feature in which of the following?

A Pregnancy.

B Anorexia nervosa.

C Polycystic ovary syndrome.

D Turner syndrome (45,XO).

E Premature menopause.

OG-Q64

A 30-year-old nulliparous woman has had amenorrhoea for 2 years. She has had occasional sensations of cold and warmth involving the face, neck and upper thorax. Polytomography of the sella turcica shows a double floor but no definite enlargement. Serum follicle-stimulating hormone (FSH) and luteinising hormone (LH) levels are markedly elevated, but serum prolactin is normal. The MOST LIKELY diagnosis is

A a gonadotrophin-producing pituitary tumour.

B neurofibromatosis.

C premature ovarian failure.

D non-hormone-producing pituitary tumour.

E craniopharyngioma.

OG-Q65

Which of the following statements concerning dysmenorrhoea is NOT correct?

A It is one of the most common gynaecological disorders.

B Primary dysmenorrhoea is not usually present during anovulatory cycles.

C Secondary dysmenorrhoea is by definition secondary to the onset of regular ovulation.

D Primary dysmenorrhoea is characterised by being relieved by inhibitors of prostaglandin synthetase.

E Placebo treatment provides symptomatic relief to 20–50% of patients.

OG-Q66

During an annual gynaecological examination, a 28-year-old woman, G2, P2, is found to have galactorrhoea. Breast examination is otherwise normal. Menses are regular at 28 day intervals. Serum prolactin level is 150 mU/L (50–750). The MOST APPROPRIATE management is

A reassurance that no treatment is necessary.

B bromocriptine (Parlodel®) therapy.

C oestrogen therapy.

D oral contraceptive therapy.

E mammography.

OG-Q67

Ovulation is MOST ACCURATELY CONFIRMED by which one of the following?

A Elevation of plasma progesterone in the luteal phase.

B Biphasic change in the temperature chart.

C Detection of a rise in plasma LH at midcycle.

D Alteration in cervical mucus.

E Plasma oestradiol peak at midcycle.

OG-Q68

A patient is MOST PROBABLY ovulating if she
- A has good breast development.
- B is having regular periods with some dysmenorrhoea.
- C is free of acne.
- D produces a moderate amount of white mucus.
- E has regular scanty midcycle bleeding.

OG-Q69

Which of the following is the MOST EXACT method of pin-pointing the TIME of ovulation?
- A Endometrial biopsy.
- B Serial assay of serum LH levels.
- C Basal body temperature.
- D Serial oestrogen estimations.
- E Examination of cervical mucus.

OG-Q70

A 27-year-old nulligravid woman is undergoing evaluation of infertility. Her last menstrual period commenced 14 days ago. Pelvic examination shows copious, clear, elastic cervical mucus. Which of the following statements concerning this patient is CORRECT?
- A She has normal ovulatory function.
- B She will ovulate within 36 h.
- C She is producing an effective amount of oestrogen.
- D A postcoital examination would presumably be normal.
- E She has a progesterone receptor deficiency.

OG-Q71

A 25-year-old woman presents with a 3 year history of primary infertility associated with oligomenorrhoea. General physical and pelvic examinations are normal; she has no expressible galactorrhoea. Her basal temperature charts confirm irregular cycles and they appear anovulatory. Her serum prolactin level is elevated. Which of the following could NOT be a cause of her hyperprolactinaemia?
- A Stress response.
- B Concomitant phenothiazine administration
- C The polycystic ovarian syndrome.
- D Chronic pelvic inflammatory disease.
- E A pituitary microadenoma.

OG-Q72

Which of the following statements about endometriosis is NOT CORRECT?
- A Malignant change is rare.
- B The diagnosis can be suggested by history and physical examination.
- C It is more common in women in their reproductive years than in postmenopausal women.
- D Infertility may be the presenting symptom.
- E The Fallopian tube is the most common site involved.

OG-Q73

Administration of clomiphene citrate may result in all the following EXCEPT

A   multifetal gestation.
B   vasomotor symptoms.
C   birth defects.
D   hyperstimulation.
E   inadequate luteal phase.

OG-Q74

Which of the following is MOST LIKELY to be the cause of dyspareunia in a 48-year-old woman?

A   Ovarian tumour.
B   Endometriosis.
C   Leiomyomata uteri.
D   Prolapse of the uterus.
E   Menopause.

OG-Q75

The AGE of menopause is

A   related to age of menarche.
B   related to age of last pregnancy.
C   increasing in well developed countries.
D   genetically determined.
E   delayed by oral contraceptive use.

OG-Q76

An absolute CONTRAINDICATION to oestrogen replacement after the menopause is

A   cholelithiasis.
B   severe liver disease.
C   decrease in serum low density lipoprotein (LDL) levels.
D   hypertension.
E   pancreatitis.

OG-Q77

During menopause, the severity of vasomotor symptoms (hot flushes) is directly correlated with each of the following EXCEPT

A   menopause before 40 years of age.
B   a low percentage of body fat.
C   low serum oestrone levels.
D   low serum levels of oestradiol bound to non-sex hormone-binding globulin (non-SHBG).
E   low serum levels of hypothalamic gonadotrophin-releasing hormone (GnRH) production.

OG-Q78

In order to maintain a normal calcium balance, a menopausal woman on oestrogen replacement requires what total of elemental calcium per day?

A   50 mg.
B   250 mg.
C   1 g.
D   5 g.
E   10 g.

OG-Q79

Menopausal dietary calcium supplementation, in the absence of oestrogen replacement therapy

    A has little impact on trabecular bone re-absorption.

    B is absorbed normally from the gastrointestinal tract.

    C is more protective against fractures in the presence of vitamin D.

    D is associated with a high risk of renal stone formation.

    E is best given at doses of 500 mg/day.

OG-Q80

All of the following statements regarding *Chlamydia trachomatis* infection are true EXCEPT

    A the organism is transmitted primarily by intercourse.

    B the majority of infected women are symptomatic.

    C the organism may cause salpingitis.

    D infected patients may demonstrate an acute urethral syndrome.

    E infertility may follow acute or chronic infections.

OG-Q81

A 21-year-old woman presents with florid vaginitis with a profuse, yellow, irritating, frothy and offensive discharge. The MOST APPROPRIATE next step would be to

    A give the patient an imidazole cream, such as clotrimazole.

    B culture for gonorrhoea and chlamydia.

    C culture for candida and trichomonas.

    D perform potassium hydroxide (KOH) smear and wet smear of vaginal discharge.

    E obtain venereal disease reference laboratory (VDRL) or fluorescent treponema antibodies (FTA-ABS) for syphilis.

OG-Q82

The micro-organism MOST FREQUENTLY responsible for septic shock in obstetrics and gynaecology is

    A *Proteus mirabilis.*

    B *Pseudomonas aeruginosa.*

    C *Staphylococcus aureus.*

    D *Bacteroides fragilis.*

    E *Escherichia coli.*

OG-Q83

Which one of the following statements concerning adenomyosis is CORRECT?

    A When multiple sections are examined, adenomyosis can be found in almost 100% of hysterectomy specimens.

    B Adenomyosis is more common in nulliparous than in multiparous women.

    C Adenomyosis is most often found in women in their fourth and fifth decades of life.

    D Adenomyosis usually coexists with endometriosis and is thought to be caused by invasion of the uterine serosa by endometriosis.

    E The glandular elements of adenomyosis are highly responsive to progestational suppression.

OG-Q84

A 40-year-old woman complains of increasingly heavy menstrual loss. Her uterus is irregularly enlarged to the size of an 8 weeks gestation with fibroids. Her cervical smear is normal and haemoglobin 14.0 g/dL. Your FIRST STEP in management should be

A   uterine curettage.

B   total hysterectomy.

C   progestogens premenstrually.

D   antiprostaglandin drugs.

E   myomectomy.

OG-Q85

A 45-year-old woman complains of a series of heavy irregular periods. Six months previously her menstrual pattern had been quite normal. On physical examination no abnormality was detected and a cervical smear was negative. Her haemoglobin value was 11.5 g/dL (11.5–16.5). What would be the MOST COMMON cause of this type of menorrhagia?

A   Endometrial carcinoma.

B   Anovulatory cycles.

C   Submucous fibroids.

D   Endometrial polyps.

E   Adenomyosis.

OG-Q86

A 25-year-old woman is found to have a 5 cm unilocular ovarian cyst. She is asymptomatic and is not pregnant. The BEST PLAN of management INVOLVES

A   a short course of oral contraceptives.

B   laparotomy with removal of the cyst.

C   laparoscopy to clarify the diagnosis and possibly aspirate the cyst.

D   tumour marker (CA-125) serial titres.

E   re-examination in 6 weeks.

OG-Q87

Which of the following is MOST APPROPRIATE when a clinically palpable ovarian enlargement is detected for the first time in a 58-year-old postmenopausal woman?

A   Treat with parenteral progestogens.

B   Take a Pap smear and review in 6 weeks.

C   X-ray to evaluate osteoporosis and collect urine for 24 h total oestrogen excretion.

D   Take a Pap smear and review in 6 months.

E   Admit to hospital for early surgical exploration.

OG-Q88

A 60-year-old woman complains of scanty vaginal bleeding and some lower abdominal discomfort. A large mass is palpable in the right side of the pelvis. Three years previously, pelvic examination had been normal. The MOST PROBABLE diagnosis is

A   endometrial carcinoma.

B   follicular cyst of the ovary.

C   a benign ovarian tumour.

D   degenerating uterine myoma.

E   carcinoma of the ovary.

OG-Q89

Which of the following is the MOST COMMON invasive malignancy found in the vagina?

A Clear cell adenocarcinoma secondary to diethylstilboestrol (DES) exposure *in utero.*

B Squamous cell carcinoma *in situ* of the vagina.

C Extension of disease from carcinoma of the cervix.

D Primary invasive squamous cell carcinoma of the vagina.

E Metastatic adenocarcinoma from the endometrium.

OG-Q90

Regular narcotic usage is commonly required for pain relief in gynaecological cancers. Its MOST TROUBLESOME side-effect is

A nausea.

B drowsiness.

C addiction.

D constipation.

E respiratory depression.

OG-Q91

A 33-year-old woman has a non-tender, vulval swelling which has been present unchanged for several months. It is spherical and is situated to the left of the fourchette with the posterior end of the labium minus stretched over it. The MOST LIKELY diagnosis is

A adenoma of Bartholin gland.

B Gartner duct cyst.

C Bartholin cyst.

D sebaceous cyst.

E carcinoma of the vulva.

OG-Q92

The MOST COMMON postoperative complication following major gynaecological surgery is

A vaginal vault haematoma.

B urinary tract infection.

C pneumonia.

D hydronephrosis.

E deep venous thrombosis of the calf.

OG-Q93

A 50-year-old Australian woman with a complaint of urinary incontinence

A is most likely to have a vesico–vaginal fistula.

B should have an anterior vaginal repair as the first step in management.

C is likely to have ureteric reflux.

D should have urodynamic studies carried out.

E will almost always have more than three children.

Psychiatry Questions

TYPE

A

Questions PS-Q1 to PS-Q51

- Type A questions consist of a stem and five responses
- **One** correct answer must be selected from five possible responses to the stem

PS-Q1

Benzodiazepines are known to affect MAINLY the intracerebral action of

A dopamine.
B noradrenaline.
C acetylcholine.
D gamma-aminobutyric acid.
E 5-hydroxytryptamine.

PS-Q2

Which of the following provides INDIRECT evidence in support of the dopamine hypothesis of schizophrenia?

A Small doses of amphetamines lead to clinical improvement in paranoid and grandiose delusions.
B Intravenous diazepam may cause catatonic schizophrenia.
C Chlorpromazine may cause parkinsonism.
D Imipramine may improve obsessional symptoms in patients with depression.
E Electroconvulsive therapy helps lower serum levels of phenothiazines.

PS-Q3

Childhood autism (autistic disorder) is CHARACTERISED by

A onset within the first 30 months of life after a period of apparently normal development.
B poor verbal communication but good non-verbal communication.
C an equal prevalence in both sexes.
D a high rate of deafness.
E all of the above features.

PS-Q4

The MOST COMMON cause overall delay in the development of normal speech is

A stammering.
B deafness.
C mental retardation (developmental disability).
D elective mutism.
E infantile autism.

PS-Q5

The TYPICAL clinical features of Down syndrome ('mongolism') INCLUDE

A sloping palpebral fissures.
B a cheerful, easy going temperament.
C hypotonia.
D varying degrees of intellectual impairment and developmental delay.
E all of the above features.

PS-Q6

Which of the following CHARACTERISTICS applies to Down syndrome ('mongolism')?

A In 95% of cases it is associated with trisomy 22.
B Temporal lobe epilepsy occurs in 40% of cases.
C Survival beyond age 40 is rare.
D Alzheimer-like changes in the brain develop in middle life.
E The most common chromosomal abnormality is translocation.

PS-Q7

Huntington chorea is an inherited disease with neurological and psychiatric symptoms and a variable age of onset. Its MODE of inheritance is

    A   unknown.

    B   autosomal recessive.

    C   autosomal dominant.

    D   sex-linked recessive.

    E   polygenic.

PS-Q8

Relatives of a 62-year-old woman, who migrated to Australia from a Greek island 36 years ago, have consulted you about her abnormal behaviour and beliefs. For many years she has been reclusive and isolated, at times she has appeared to be responding to voices, and lately she has been saying that her son, daughter and husband have been replaced by doubles and impostors. This abnormal belief is an EXAMPLE of

    A   querulant paranoia.

    B   Capgras syndrome.

    C   migration psychosis.

    D   Fregoli syndrome.

    E   de Clérambault syndrome.

PS-Q9

A delusion is an EXAMPLE of

    A   formal thought disorder.

    B   blunted affect.

    C   a false belief.

    D   auditory hallucinations.

    E   passivity experiences.

PS-Q10

A patient with schizophrenia TYPICALLY has

    A   a sociopathic personality.

    B   depersonalisation.

    C   auditory hallucinations.

    D   gender dysphoria.

    E   all of the above associations.

PS-Q11

A patient with schizophrenia TYPICALLY has

    A   passive–aggressive personality.

    B   illusions.

    C   delusions of reference.

    D   cataplexy.

    E   all of the above associations.

PS-Q12

According to World Health Organisation data, the MOST FREQUENT (97%) symptom of acute schizophrenia is

- A delusions of persecution.
- B auditory hallucinations.
- C lack of insight.
- D flattened affect.
- E ideas of reference.

PS-Q13

TYPICALLY an amphetamine-induced psychosis is PREPONDERANTLY

- A paranoid.
- B depressive.
- C grandiose.
- D confusional.
- E manic.

PS-Q14

The MOST CHARACTERISTIC feature of alcohol hallucinosis is

- A visual hallucinations.
- B tactile hallucinations.
- C delirium tremens.
- D auditory hallucinations.
- E confabulated memories.

PS-Q15

A young woman consults you about her 32-year-old husband. She has been concerned about a change in his behaviour following a serious head injury 6 months previously. He has become disinhibited, tactless and over-talkative; his mood is generally fatuous and his concentration and attention are reduced. He does not appear to have any insight into his psychological and cognitive deficits. The MOST LIKELY site of his brain lesion is the

- A frontal lobe.
- B non-dominant parietal lobe.
- C dominant parietal lobe.
- D temporal lobe.
- E corpus callosum.

PS-Q16

Depression can be ASSOCIATED with

- A anterior left hemisphere strokes.
- B aphasia.
- C Alzheimer disease.
- D Parkinson disease.
- E all of the above conditions.

PS-Q17

A 26-year-old man has been under your care after falling 10 m while rock climbing, sustaining bilateral compound tibial fractures and a fractured pelvis. Three days postoperatively, after open reduction and fixation of his tibial fractures, he becomes acutely breathless. A chest X-ray reveals a diffuse bilateral pulmonary infiltrate. He suddenly becomes confused and fearful, believing his food to be poisoned, and that the hospital staff are plotting against him and plan to murder him. The MOST LIKELY explanation for the change in his mental state is

- A aspiration pneumonia.
- B pulmonary embolism.
- C fat embolism syndrome.
- D subacute pancreatitis.
- E extradural haematoma.

PS-Q18

A 40-year-old school teacher has been receiving treatment for depressive symptoms following his wife's desertion. A week after being involved in a traffic accident in which a child was hospitalised with head injuries, he takes an overdose of fifty 25 mg imipramine tablets and a large amount of alcohol. He has previously refused referral to a psychiatrist or voluntary hospitalisation for assessment. Your INITIAL management, after successful medical treatment of his overdose, SHOULD BE to

- A increase his imipramine to 150 mg daily.
- B change him to a different tricyclic antidepressant.
- C contact his wife and try to persuade her to return home.
- D arrange involuntary psychiatric hospitalisation, if he still refuses voluntary admission.
- E refer him for alcohol counselling.

PS-Q19

A 38-year-old woman with many neurotic features who volunteers she is thinking of killing herself SHOULD BE

- A taken seriously and referred for treatment.
- B reassured that she will not do it.
- C given some support, but need not be taken too seriously.
- D considered a high suicide risk only if she is single.
- E given diazepam in adequate dosage.

PS-Q20

Despite overwhelming evidence to the contrary, a 19-year-old girl with anorexia nervosa insists she is overweight. This is an EXAMPLE of

- A an overvalued idea.
- B a delusion.
- C an obsession.
- D a rumination.
- E a phobia.

PS-Q21

Depersonalisation IS ASSOCIATED WITH

  A post-traumatic stress disorder.

  B schizophrenia.

  C agoraphobia.

  D ecstatic religious experience.

  E all of the above conditions.

PS-Q22

The MOST COMMON pattern for seasonal affective disorder is

  A onset in spring, recovery in summer.

  B onset in summer, recovery in winter.

  C onset in autumn, recovery in winter.

  D onset in winter, recovery in spring.

  E onset in spring, recovery in autumn.

PS-Q23

Diagnostic criteria for borderline personality disorder INCLUDE

  A identity disturbance, unstable relationships, inappropriate anger, impulsivity.

  B social withdrawal, depressed mood, magical thinking.

  C histrionic behaviour, high intelligence, reaction formation.

  D substance abuse, neurasthenia, repression.

  E recurrent self-harm, hypochondriasis, cognitive impairment.

PS-Q24

A 34-year-old married woman has sought your advice on chronic and fluctuating food intolerance, accompanied by nausea, vomiting spells, abdominal pain, bloating and diarrhoea. She tells you that she has been 'sickly' for most of the past 20 years of her life since puberty, and has had a lot of gynaecological investigations for severe dysmenorrhoea, excessive menstrual bleeding and dyspareunia. She has consulted a number of neurologists for trouble with walking, muscle weakness and fainting spells for which she was prescribed anticonvulsants, with little benefit. A cardiologist had prescribed a beta-blocker for episodes of palpitations accompanied by chest pain and breathlessness, and a rheumatologist had given her a trial of various anti-inflammatory drugs for small joint pain and lumbago with only temporary relief. Your physical examination revealed that she is apparently tense and anxious despite diazepam 15 mg daily and that she has abdominal scars from a previous appendicectomy and separate hysterectomy. The MOST LIKELY psychiatric diagnosis that this woman has is

  A somatisation disorder.

  B hypochondriasis.

  C conversion disorder.

  D Münchausen syndrome.

  E factitious illness.

PS-Q25

A 72-year-old man, who speaks no English, attends with his son who is able to explain that his father has just arrived in Australia as a refugee from Bosnia 1 month before. He tells you that his father is suffering from irritability, insomnia and nightmares connected with his experiences in the civil war. On further questioning, the father appears vague, concentrates poorly and cannot recall details of his recent experiences in Bosnia. The MOST LIKELY diagnosis is

A jet lag.
B culture shock.
C depression.
D post-traumatic stress disorder.
E dementia.

PS-Q26

A 65-year-old man, previously well adjusted, began to isolate himself and became suspicious of others after he had developed tinnitus and progressive loss of hearing. His only medication was methyldopa, 250 mg, t.i.d., which he had taken for 5 years for hypertension. The history SUGGESTS

A an early schizophrenic reaction.
B organic brain syndrome.
C cerebral arteriosclerosis.
D psychological reaction to deafness.
E a reaction to methyldopa.

PS-Q27

A 21-year-old ballet dancer is suspected of having anorexia nervosa. Which of the following would be CONSISTENT with this diagnosis?

A A history of binge eating.
B Hypokalaemia.
C Amenorrhoea.
D Obsessional personality traits.
E All of the above features.

PS-Q28

A 28-year-old sales assistant presents with difficulty sleeping. He recounts how he has great difficulty falling asleep, going over the events of the day in his head. When at last he gets to sleep, he wakes often during the night. He sometimes has nightmares and usually feels unrefreshed in the mornings. His sleep disturbance is CHARACTERISTIC of

A borderline personality disorder.
B major depression.
C schizophrenia.
D generalised anxiety disorder.
E nocturnal epilepsy.

PS-Q29

A 36-year-old accountant has sought advice for his increasing anxiety about a forthcoming speech he has to make at a social function. He has always had difficulty making oral presentations in front of his work colleagues, but lately he has felt that his boss has been scrutinising his work more closely and he has become extremely anxious about signing cheques or documents in public. He is a model employee, he knows his fears are groundless, but he has begun avoiding the staff canteen at lunchtime and has begun to drink alcohol during the day to steady his nerves. The MOST LIKELY underlying problem in this man is

A alcoholism.

B schizophrenia.

C social phobia.

D agoraphobia.

E panic disorder.

PS-Q30

Cognitive–behaviour therapy is a USEFUL treatment approach in

A chronic pain.

B social phobia.

C depression.

D bulimia nervosa.

E all of the above disorders.

PS-Q31

Exposure and response prevention are two behavioural approaches COMMONLY USED in the treatment of

A bulimia nervosa.

B social phobia.

C obsessive–compulsive disorder.

D agoraphobia.

E sexual dysfunction.

PS-Q32

A phobia

A is usually resisted by the sufferer.

B is an irrational delusion.

C frequently occurs in conjunction with schizophrenia.

D may respond to systematic desensitisation.

E is best managed initially with benzodiazepines.

PS-Q33

Vaginismus is spasm of the vaginal muscles which causes pain when intercourse is attempted. It is COMMONLY ASSOCIATED with

A schizophrenia.

B borderline personality disorder.

C major depression.

D obsessive–compulsive disorder.

E phobic anxiety.

PS-Q34

Postpartum psychosis TYPICALLY

    A begins with insomnia.

    B can be dominated by affective symptoms.

    C runs in families.

    D has a significant risk of recurring independently of further pregnancies.

    E demonstrates all of the above characteristics.

PS-Q35

Which one of the following SHOULD ALWAYS be suspended during the first trimester of pregnancy?

    A Benzodiazepines.

    B Fluphenazine decanoate.

    C Tricyclic antidepressants.

    D Methadone maintenance.

    E Lithium carbonate.

PS-Q36

A 22-year-old man walks into the Emergency Room with his head tilted sideways, his tongue sticking out and his eyes rolled up. With difficulty, he tells the doctor that he is stuck in this position and that it happened a few hours after getting a new medicine for his 'nerves'. At that point the doctor should ADMINISTER

    A chlorpromazine.

    B phenytoin.

    C haloperidol.

    D benztropine.

    E diazepam.

PS-Q37

Temporary reversal of anticholinergic-induced delirium OCCURS with an intravenous injection of

    A atropine.

    B succinyl choline.

    C benztropine.

    D physostigmine.

    E phentolamine.

PS-Q38

Lithium carbonate has been shown to be of THERAPEUTIC use in

    A the prophylactic treatment of bipolar affective disorder (manic–depressive illness).

    B the acute treatment of mania.

    C the treatment of resistant depression.

    D the treatment of aggression in the developmentally disabled (mentally handicapped).

    E all of the above conditions.

PS-Q39

Concerning the prophylactic management of bipolar affective disorder (manic–depressive illness)

A lithium carbonate is more effective in women than in men.

B lithium carbonate is more effective in patients under 45 years of age.

C lithium carbonate is less effective the longer it is used.

D lithium carbonate is neither habit forming nor addictive.

E all of the above statements are correct.

PS-Q40

Monitoring of plasma levels should be carried out routinely with

A tricyclic antidepressants.

B antipsychotic drugs.

C monoamine oxidase inhibitors.

D lithium.

E benzodiazepines.

PS-Q41

A 40-year-old man has been brought by ambulance to the Emergency Department some hours after an overdose of lithium carbonate. His two serum lithium levels taken 1 h apart are stable at 4 mmol/L (the normal therapeutic range is 0.5–1.2 mmol/L). Which of the following is ESSENTIAL to ensure recovery?

A L-Tryptophan.

B Parenteral diuretics.

C Hydration with sodium chloride.

D Haemodialysis.

E Oral charcoal.

PS-Q42

Fluoxetine is a recently available antidepressant drug which is neither tricyclic nor tetracyclic in structure. It shares with existing antidepressants the characteristic of altering biogenic amine function by SELECTIVE INHIBITION of

A monoamine oxidase.

B noradrenaline re-uptake.

C serotonin re-uptake.

D acetylcholine re-uptake.

E dopamine re-uptake.

PS-Q43

Clozapine is a psychotropic drug which has recently become available for use in Australia. It is used in the TREATMENT of

A refractory schizophrenia.

B bipolar affective disorder.

C obsessive–compulsive disorder.

D adjustment disorders.

E all of the above disorders.

PS-Q44

You are requested to visit a 17-year-old girl who is being nursed at home for suspected gastroenteritis. Her mother states that she seems very strange, yawns all the time and has been suspected of taking drugs. The patient has a 2 day history of nausea, running eyes and nose, colicky abdominal pains and twitches. Physical examination is normal. The drug that you SHOULD suspect is

A marijuana.

B D-lysergic acid diethylamide (LSD).

C heroin.

D cocaine.

E amphetamine.

PS-Q45

Which of the following occurs MOST COMMONLY during withdrawal from opiate narcotics?

A Rhinorrhoea.

B Drowsiness.

C Convulsions.

D Constipation.

E Headache.

PS-Q46

Electroconvulsive therapy (ECT) can be EFFECTIVE in

A acute schizophrenia.

B catatonic stupor.

C refractory mania.

D puerperal depression.

E all of the above disorders.

PS-Q47

Deinstitutionalisation of psychiatric patients REFERS to

A compulsory sterilisation.

B compulsory hospitalisation if they are suicidal.

C loss of the right to vote in elections.

D discharge to community based alternatives to hospital.

E transfer to prison hospitals.

PS-Q48

Transference, in the context of a psychotherapeutic relationship, REFERS to

A the payment of fees for private therapy.

B a form of resistance to change in therapy.

C the feelings a doctor or therapist has towards the patient based on childhood relationships.

D the feelings a patient may have about a doctor or therapist, based on the patient's childhood relationships.

E a form of insight gained by patients recovering from schizophrenia.

PS-Q49

Concerning reassurance as an important component of supportive counselling in the MANAGEMENT of chronic illness

A   reassurance is best given early on in the course of an illness to boost a patient's morale and hopes for a cure.

B   reassurance should only be offered when the patient's concerns have been fully understood and investigated.

C   it is always appropriate to reassure those patients who may otherwise get distressed or anxious if given bad news.

D   reassurance should only be used after relatives have been interviewed to determine the patient's state of mind.

E   all of the above statements concerning reassurance in counselling for chronic-illness are correct.

PS-Q50

A 45-year-old homosexual man with a 16 year history of bipolar affective disorder presents with an acute manic relapse. He willingly agrees to be hospitalised. As part of his organic workup, an HIV antibody screening test is done without his knowledge and is found to be positive. Which of the following is CORRECT?

A   Other inpatients should be informed of this man's HIV status and he should be nursed in a separate, sterile area of the ward.

B   He should be informed immediately of his infectivity, and pressed to reveal the names of his sexual partners, so that mandatory HIV testing can be performed on those who can be traced.

C   Lithium carbonate is known to lower immunity to infection, and he should be treated with AZT instead.

D   HIV antibody testing should not be performed routinely on patients, but only after obtaining their informed consent and after appropriate pretest counselling.

E   All of the above responses are correct.

PS-Q51

Concerning sexual relationships between doctors and patients

A   they are prohibited by medical codes of practice.

B   they are usually initiated by patients.

C   they are encouraged if both doctor and patient are single and attracted to one another.

D   they are permissible as part of a professional treatment programme for infertility.

E   all of the above responses are correct.

Commentaries for Multiple Choice Questions and Summary of Correct Responses

Medicine
Commentaries
and Summary of Correct Responses
TYPE
A

Commentaries ME-C1 to ME-C125

Correct Responses ME-Q1 to ME-Q125

ME-C1   CORRECT RESPONSE C

The lesions comprise multiple itching sores on the back of the hand and particularly between the fingers, which have evoked an artefactual component from scratching. Scabies should be suspected and a careful inspection should be made for the classical burrowing tracks of the responsible mite (*Sarcoptes scabiei*).

Treatment with gamma benzene hexachloride (Lindane®) is appropriate. The lotion is rubbed well into the lesions, left for 8–12 h, and then washed off thoroughly. Scabies remains an important cause of irritant skin lesions in neglected patients living under circumstances of deficient hygiene.

Erythromycin would not be the first choice for infective skin lesions, even those associated with acute bacterial infections. Neither topical nor oral steroids are appropriate therapy; and miconazole is an antifungal preparation suitable for tinea and candidiasis.

ME-C2   CORRECT RESPONSE D

The picture shows the lesions of a viral molluscum contagiosum infection with typical pearly nodules and umbilication. In chicken pox (varicella) the vesicles are widespread, tear-drop in appearance and polymorphic in evolution, with surrounding erythema. Herpes simplex virus infection produces small blisters (vesicles) which are closely grouped and often will show some ulceration. Viral warts (verrucae) are usually well demarcated with prickly roughened surfaces. Allergic reactions show oedema, erythema and sometimes vesicles with scratch marks from pruritus.

ME-C3   CORRECT RESPONSE A

The picture shows typical flexural eczema with some hypopigmentation due to pityriasis alba. ***The most appropriate treatment would be moisture and wet dressings.*** The lesions would be made worse by hot bathing, wool or nylon clothing, the application of tar cream or salicylic acid cream. These lesions are associated with penicillinase-producing *Staphylococcus aureus* infection, and appropriate antibiotics may also be indicated. Oral steroids are rarely used as the lesions often 'rebound' when the steroids are stopped.

ME-C4   CORRECT RESPONSE B

The picture shows the typical cysts and scarring of severe acne. ***Treatment of choice is isotretinoin (Roaccutane®) in a dose of 1 mg/kg/day for 16–20 weeks.*** Isotretinoin is a retinoid which inhibits sebaceous gland function and keratinisation; it is related to retinol (vitamin A). Because of significant adverse effects associated with its use, isotretinoin is reserved for patients with severe cystic acne unresponsive to conventional treatment. If this treatment is used in women of childbearing age they should have a pregnancy test before starting the treatment, be advised not to become pregnant during the treatment or for 4 weeks afterwards and be told that isotretinoin will produce deformity of the embryo especially between the 30th and 70th days.

Benzyl peroxide lotion would dry the skin out excessively, particularly as isotretinoin also dries the skin.

The use of tetracycline in combination with a vitamin A derivative elevates cerebrospinal fluid pressure and may produce benign intracranial hypertension. The two drugs should not be combined. Occlusive make-up will cause more blocking of the sebaceous follicles and could make the lesions worse. Cortisone cream will not help the condition, although it could act as a mild emollient.

ME-C5   CORRECT RESPONSE B

The photograph shows a domed nodular skin lesion with a necrotic plug of tissue in its central portion. The lesion looks typical of a kerato-acanthoma. These are keratinising lesions which grow more rapidly than the three common skin malignancies (basal cell carcinoma, squamous cell carcinoma and melanoma) from which they need to be differentiated. Kerato-acanthomas can reach a large size within a few weeks. They are characterised by a central plug of keratin which separates and sloughs to give a volcano-like crater. If the lesions are untreated, spontaneous healing and resolution may subsequently occur. Kerato-acanthomas are often difficult to distinguish clinically from malignant lesions, particularly from squamous cell cancers, and they can also be difficult to assess histologically on a small partial biopsy. *Thus, the preferred treatment of suspected lesions is total excisional biopsy* and the pathologist can usually give an accurate and confident diagnosis when presented with the whole specimen.

The requirement for total surgical excision is even more so after organ transplantation. Patients on immunosuppressive drugs have an increased tendency to develop carcinomas (skin cancers and pre-malignant hyperkeratoses are the most common). Furthermore, in immunosuppressed transplant patients, kerato-acanthomas do not always behave as benign self-resolving lesions, but can metastasise to nodes and via the blood stream in the same manner as aggressive squamous cell carcinomas. *Appropriate treatment is, therefore, surgical removal.*

ME-C6   CORRECT RESPONSE C

The telangiectatic lesions on the lower lip are typical of hereditary haemorrhagic telangiectasia (Osler–Weber syndrome). The disorder is inherited as an autosomal dominant. *Patients with this form of telangiectasia can present with iron deficiency anaemia due to bleeding telangiectases in the bowel* or with more urgent and acute gastrointestinal haemorrhage with haematemesis and melaena. Occasionally, intracerebral telangiectases can cause a cerebral haemorrhage. The syndrome is not associated with liver disease, small bowel tumours or polycythaemia. Chronic liver disease is associated with spider naevi. In the hereditary disorder of Peutz–Jeghers syndrome, brown melanin-pigmented lesions around the mouth and oral cavity are associated with benign small bowel polyps. Telangiectatic lesions are not produced by consumption of photosensitising drugs.

ME-C7   CORRECT RESPONSE D

The fundal appearances show a mixture of hard and soft exudates and focal haemorrhages. *The most likely cause is diabetes mellitus.* The fundal vessels that are visible do not show marked hypertensive silver wiring or nipping, and the presence of haemorrhages and acute exudates would reflect severe recent hypertension if this was the major cause. The optic disc, visible on the right, has clear margins with no evidence of papilloedema, such as might indicate an intracerebral metastatic lesion.

Alcohol amblyopia may have been suspected from the history of excessive alcohol intake, but the fundal appearances indicate diabetic retinopathy as the causative lesion of his blurred vision. *Toxocara canis*, a dog tapeworm that can infest humans and causes eye lesions, does not give this fundal picture.

ME-C8   CORRECT RESPONSE C

Deterioration in vision associated with misty vision is suggestive of cataract formation. Patients with early cataract formation may experience haloes around bright objects, as may also occur in angle closure glaucoma. This form of glaucoma is associated with visual impairment and pain. Chronic simple glaucoma is characterised by a gradual constriction of the visual fields without halo effects or misting.

A myopic is one who is short-sighted and the defect presents in early life. Patients with macular degeneration or diabetic retinopathy may have retinal defects that lead to deterioration or loss of vision, but without halo effects.

ME-C9   CORRECT RESPONSE D

All of the responses can complicate chronic otitis media, except for otosclerosis. Otosclerosis is a common cause of late onset deafness, and has no relationship with otitis media.

ME-C10   CORRECT RESPONSE B

Each of the five responses can present as a palpable solitary nodule in the thyroid. However, *most palpable and apparent solitary thyroid nodules are dominant nodules in a multinodular goitre, with the other nodules not being readily palpable.*

ME-C11   CORRECT RESPONSE B

Wernicke encephalopathy is characterised by an altered level of consciousness and brain stem signs, particularly ophthalmoplegia and nystagmus. Pathologically, these symptoms are due to petechial haemorrhages within the mid-brain and brainstem. Stiffness of the neck is not a phenomenon of Wernicke encephalopathy and would indicate meningeal irritation. Grand mal epilepsy (generalised motor seizures) is not associated with Wernicke encephalopathy, although it may occasionally occur in patients with this condition. Wernicke encephalopathy is due to thiamine deficiency usually associated with alcoholism, and alcohol-induced fits may occur during alcohol withdrawal. In the uncommon circumstance when fits are seen in Wernicke encephalopathy, they are due to an associated cause.

Extensor plantar responses would indicate an upper motor neuron lesion. In alcoholics with Wernicke encephalopathy other neurological disorders with upper motor neuron features may coexist; conditions such as central pontine myelinolysis or subdural haematoma. The finding of an extensor plantar response would, thus, indicate a coexisting disorder.

ME-C12   CORRECT RESPONSE E

Although numerous points have been proposed for distinguishing between a cerebral haemorrhage and a cerebral infarction, and it is possible to arrive at the probability of the correct diagnosis somewhat more reliably than by flipping a coin, these methods have no clinical validity when it is essential to know whether or not an individual patient has a cerebral haemorrhage. Thus before starting any therapy that may alter blood clotting or platelet aggregation in a patient with an acute stroke, the absence of haemorrhage should be ascertained by a cerebral CT scan.

The distinction between a cerebral haemorrhage and a thrombotic cerebral infarction is not absolute. Approximately 15% of infarctions become overtly haemorrhagic on CT scan within the first 48 h. This haemorrhagic transformation is most commonly due to petechial bleeding in the area of the infarction. Sometimes a clot of significant size develops within the area of infarction. In postmortem specimens petechial bleeding is seen in the majority of cerebral infarcts. This higher incidence is because smaller aggregations of red cells can be seen on direct vision or by microscopy than can be demonstrated on CT scan.

ME-C13 CORRECT RESPONSE C

Disorders of the cerebellum characteristically result in a reduced muscle tone, possibly due to decreased activity of gamma efferents. This results not only in decreased tone, but also in suppressed reflexes.

Increased tone produces either spasticity, due to a lesion of the pyramidal tract, or rigidity, due to extrapyramidal involvement. Lesions of the spinal cord corticospinal pathways involve the pyramidal tract and result in increased tone of the spastic type. Disorders of the basal ganglia produce rigidity, typically seen in Parkinson disease.

ME-C14 CORRECT RESPONSE C

The question deals with the treatment of a presumed symptomatic carotid stenosis of 25%. Recent studies have shown that operating on carotid stenosis of less than 30% does not produce any worthwhile clinical benefit, with the risks of the operation exceeding any reduction in stroke. Operating on a symptomatic stenosis of greater than 70% significantly reduces the incidence of stroke. *Current practice would be that a patient such as that described in the question would be treated with a platelet anti-aggregation agent such as aspirin.* The role of warfarin has not been demonstrated in this sort of patient although it is commonly used if aspirin fails. The INR quoted (3.5–4.0) is higher than that used in prevention of stroke. The range of 2.0–2.5 is preferred because of the lower risk of haemorrhage, particularly cerebral haemorrhage. Carotid endarterectomy, either immediate or delayed, is not indicated at this stage because of the mild degree of stenosis. Intracarotid streptokinase infusion has not been shown to decrease the risk of stroke in this sort of patient.

ME-C15 CORRECT RESPONSE A

The phenomenon described in this 50-year-old woman is a typical migrainous aura. Episodes of migrainous aura may occur without concomitant headache.

A transient carotid ischaemia would produce symptoms in one eye rather than a defect within the visual field on one side. The optic cortex and association cortex from which these symptoms arise are supplied by the posterior cerebral artery, which is a terminal branch of the vertebral artery. The progressive nature of the symptoms 'spreading' over the visual field would also be unlikely with transient cerebral ischaemia either in the carotid or vertebrobasilar territory, which is usually due to embolism from proximal atherosclerotic sites or the heart, and occasionally the result of thrombotic occlusions.

Retrobulbar neuritis does not last for a brief period of time and involves one eye rather than a visual field. The possibility of epilepsy producing the above phenomenon cannot be completely excluded as epilepsy arising in the occipital lobe may produce unformed visual hallucinations. However, compared with the incidence of migraine in the community, this is a very rare phenomenon.

ME-C16 CORRECT RESPONSE C

Unfortunately the diagnosis in this patient would be made too late to preserve his sight. *The most appropriate investigation to make the diagnosis would have been an erythrocyte sedimentation rate (ESR). Given this history, temporal arteritis is the most likely cause of both the headaches and the visual loss.* Characteristically there is a markedly raised ESR. The amount of recovery of visual loss in this situation is minimal. It is therefore critical to diagnose and treat temporal arteritis before visual loss occurs.

ME-C17 CORRECT RESPONSE E

The lesion causing a unilateral dilated right pupil that does not respond to light shone into that eye may be either in the sensory side (optic nerve) or the motor part (third nerve) of the reflex arc. The absence of a consensual reflex from that eye (contraction of the left pupil when the light is shone into the right eye) indicates that the lesion is on the sensory side of the reflex arc. The failure of the right pupil to respond consensually to light shone in the left (contralateral) eye confirms that there is also a motor lesion in the right eye. *There are, therefore, lesions of the right optic nerve and the right third nerve.* Involvement of both nerves is not uncommon in a periorbital fracture or tumour. Tests for eye movements in an unconscious patient (the Doll's Eye Manoeuvre) should not be done until the integrity of the cervical spine has been established. All other possibilities are inconsistent with the physical signs.

ME-C18 CORRECT RESPONSE D

The patient described has involvement of the left third nerve and the left pyramidal track and most likely both are involved at the level of the third nerve nucleus in the midbrain. *The most likely cause of the symptoms described would be a left midbrain infarct.* A midbrain infarct is most commonly a consequence of hypertensive cerebral vascular disease and may also arise from an embolus from a cardiac or proximal atherosclerotic lesion. The involvement of the third nerve excludes a lesion in the internal capsule, the medulla, the cervical cord and occipital lobe.

Rarely, a hemiparesis with a contralateral third nerve palsy can result from a hemisphere space-occupying lesion, which compresses the contralateral third nerve and the cerebral peduncle against the clinoid. These symptoms may be seen with a rapidly expanding intracranial tumour and with extradural or subdural haematoma.

ME-C19 CORRECT RESPONSE C

The picture is that of a man with recurrent episodes of vertigo and vomiting with progressive hearing loss. This is typical of Ménière disease. Acoustic neuroma rarely produces episodic vertigo and vomiting, although it does produce progressive hearing loss. Vertebrobasilar disease is not usually associated with vomiting and progressive hearing loss does not occur. In vertebrobasilar ischaemia involving the labyrinthine artery, acute severe hearing loss may occur in association with vertigo but vomiting is unusual. This is usually a single episode.

Vestibular neuronitis is characterised by recurrent episodes of vertigo becoming progressively less with each episode. Usually the symptoms last 6–12 weeks. It is not associated with progressive loss of hearing.

Benign positional vertigo rarely produces vomiting and does not produce hearing loss. It is characterised by recurrent episodes of positional vertigo usually occurring at approximately 12 month intervals. The majority of these patients are now thought to have debris impacted in the vestibular apparatus.

ME-C20 CORRECT RESPONSE E

A Horner syndrome may occur at any point along the central or peripheral path of fibres projecting to the cervical sympathetic outflow from the pons on the same side: through the lateral medulla down the lateral cervical spinal cord, at the C7-T1 level, in the stellate ganglion (inferior cervical ganglion) or in fibres running from the ganglion to the eye. The fibres from the inferior cervical ganglion follow the course of the common carotid, internal carotid and ophthalmic arteries. A lesion anywhere along this path may cause an ipsilateral Horner syndrome. The patient has an associated 10th nerve palsy (with loss of explosive cough and elevation of the palate on the right side), suggesting that there is a nuclear lesion involving the nucleus ambiguus (vagus nerve). *For these reasons, a right-sided brainstem infarction is the only site of the lesion that would explain the complete clinical picture.* A left capsular haemorrhage would not produce a Horner syndrome or a lower motor neuron vagal lesion. A meningioma at the foramen magnum could produce Horner syndrome, but the nucleus ambiguus is at a higher level. Thrombosis of the left posterior inferior cerebellar artery or a left cerebello–pontine angle tumour would produce symptoms on the left (ipsilateral) side.

ME-C21   CORRECT RESPONSE C

The clinical syndrome described is that of weakness of facial, palatal and neck muscles and dysphagia probably related to weakness of constrictors of the pharynx. There is also involvement of the periphery and weakness and slowness of hand grip. *The picture is typical of dystrophia myotonica.* This slowly progressive hereditary disorder may not become apparent until the age of 40. It is associated with a receding hairline and, in males, testicular atrophy. Later, cataracts and cardiomyopathy may develop.

Facioscapulohumeral muscular dystrophy usually presents at a younger age. It tends not to involve swallowing and to be more proximal in the limbs, such that there is weakness of the shoulder girdle, while the hands are clinically unaffected.

Myasthenia gravis may present with nasal speech and difficulty in swallowing. It would be very unusual to see a patient with a bulbar form of myasthenia gravis without ocular involvement indicated by a history of variable diplopia. Critical to the diagnosis of myasthenia gravis from the history is fatigability of muscles with a degree of weakness varying throughout the day, and tending to be worse towards the end of the day.

Bulbar palsy (i.e. lower motor neuron weakness of the cranial nerves originating in the medulla and pons) may present with nasal speech due to involvement of the vagus and weakness of the facial muscles due to involvement of the facial nerves. The neck muscles are not commonly affected except for the sternomastoid. Weakness of the hands would not be expected as part of a bulbar palsy. There is a rare form of Guillain–Barré peripheral neuropathy which involves predominantly cranial nerves. Usually there is ocular involvement (Miller Fisher syndrome).

ME-C22   CORRECT RESPONSE E

The symptoms described with bilateral sensory symptoms and involvement of sphincter control suggest acute compression of either the cauda equina or the lower end of the spinal cord. With the involvement of the bladder and bowel it is urgent to establish the cause of this compression. *For this reason, of the possibilities listed, urgent myelogram would be the most appropriate.* In large hospitals the preferred investigation now might be an urgent MRI of the thoracolumbar region.

Physiotherapy and spinal manipulation are most inappropriate for an acute compressive lesion and possibly hazardous. Strict bed rest with pelvic traction and epidural local anaesthesia may provide symptomatic treatment but the first important step in management is to establish the cause of the symptoms, followed by, if necessary, surgical decompression.

ME-C23   CORRECT RESPONSE C

The clinical syndrome described is that of a sensorimotor neuropathy that has been stable over a 2 year period. *Of the possibilities listed diabetic neuropathy is the one MOST LIKELY to produce this syndrome.* Sensory neuropathy is common in diabetics and involves both large and small fibres. Large fibre involvement results in reduced touch, joint position and vibration sense and in areflexia. Smaller fibre involvement causes loss of pain and temperature sensation and dysaesthesia.

Polymyositis is not associated with any sensory changes or symptoms and has muscle weakness only.

Charcot–Marie–Tooth disease does not present as a severe neuropathy in a 50-year-old man with only a 2 year history. Although mild forms of this disease may not become apparent until the age of 50, they do not produce an acute syndrome as described.

Acute postinfectious polyneuropathy (Guillain–Barré syndrome) presents as a predominantly motor neuropathy with the symptoms reaching their maximum in approximately 2 weeks and then progressively improving. It does not produce a prolonged sensory symptomatology.

Diabetic amyotrophy is characterised by a clinical presentation of pain, most commonly in the quadriceps muscle. When diabetic amyotrophy is due to a focal femoral neuritis, sensory symptoms may be experienced on the anterior surface of the thigh, but generalised bilateral symptoms in the legs and feet are not a feature.

ME-C24   CORRECT RESPONSE D

The vignette describes a typical presentation of a common condition: cervical spondylosis. The symptoms and signs fall into two groups. First, there are the symptoms in the leg of increasing stiffness and difficulty with walking and, on examination, there is bilateral spasticity, some weakness of hip flexion and brisk reflexes. This is consistent with a bilateral pyramidal lesion above the L2 (cord) level. In the upper limbs there is wasting of the biceps with depression of the tendon jerk, suggesting a C6 root lesion. These symptoms are very suggestive of cervical spondylosis at the C5–6 level with a disc protrusion and osteophytes compressing both the cord (producing cervical myelopathy) and the C6 nerve root. The C5–6 level is the most common level to find significant cervical disease. If not treated, the disorder may well continue with progressive development of cervical myelopathy resulting in increasing spasticity and weakness in the legs. Sensory involvement from this sort of lesion is uncommon. The mechanism of the pyramidal involvement is probably ischaemic from compression of the anterior spinal artery.

Bilateral weakness and spasticity in the legs may be seen in the legs in both multiple sclerosis and motor neuron disease. However, neither disorder would cause depression of reflexes. Depression of reflexes and wasting of muscles is not a symptom of multiple sclerosis, in which the weakness is upper motor neuron in type. Motor neuron disease is usually associated with brisk reflexes due to the concomitant upper motor neuron lesion and not with depression of reflexes. Brisk reflexes persist even when the muscles are wasted.

The picture in no way resembles Parkinson disease in that neither spasticity, weakness, nor reflex changes characterise this disorder.

Vertebrobasilar ischaemia may rarely produce bilateral spasticity, but will not produce wasting of muscles of the upper limb or depression of reflexes.

ME-C25   CORRECT RESPONSE D

The clinical picture describes the rapid onset of a motor weakness associated with depressed reflexes. This is typical of the onset of the Guillain–Barré syndrome. In the early phases there are relatively few sensory changes. As described in this patient the only sensory change manifest is that of depression of reflexes. Hysterical paralysis would not be associated with any organic signs such as depression of reflexes. Motor neuron disease does not produce a rapid onset of a symmetrical weakness and the reflexes would not be suppressed. Multiple sclerosis produces weakness by involving the pyramidal tracts and is associated with increased rather than decreased reflexes. Spinal cord compression may produce a focal weakness at the site of the compression due to involvement of the nerve roots at that level; but the weakness distal to the lesion will be pyramidal in nature and associated with increased rather than decreased reflexes.

ME-C26   CORRECT RESPONSE D

Mononeuritis multiplex is characterised by multiple, and focal, usually asymmetrical peripheral nerve lesions rather than a general involvement of all nerves. The only disorder in the list that produces this focal lesion of nerves is diabetes mellitus. It is thought that the primary mechanism in diabetes mellitus may be focal ischaemia in individual nerves. Infectious mononucleosis usually produces a Guillain–Barré-like syndrome. This is characterised by a polyradiculopathy with usually a symmetrical and predominantly motor deficit. Lead poisoning also produces a motor neuropathy, which is usually proximal. Myxoedema can produce a mixed sensorimotor neuropathy.

ME-C27   CORRECT RESPONSE A

Parkinson disease is most commonly 'idiopathic' in origin, by which we mean we do not know why the majority of patients develop this disorder. There are, however, several well recognised causes. Manganese intoxication, seen in the miners of that mineral, produces a parkinsonian-like syndrome. This is thought to be due to a direct effect on the substantia nigra. Phenothiazines, which block dopamine receptors, will produce tremor and increased tone of the parkinsonian-type. This may be partly reversible. Methyldopa is metabolised to alpha methyldopamine, which blocks central dopamine receptors, producing a parkinsonian syndrome. One of the post-carbon monoxide poisoning syndromes is characterised by an extrapyramidal disorder similar to Parkinson disease. The syndrome may also be seen in 'dementia pugilistica' in boxers and in a number of rare neurological conditions. Attempts to produce 'designer drugs' related to pethidine have resulted in the production of MPTP, which produces severe irreversible Parkinson disease.

Phenytoin intoxication does not produce parkinsonism. Phenytoin intoxication may cause cerebellar dysfunction and ataxia, but it does not produce parkinsonism.

ME-C28   CORRECT RESPONSE C

Post-herpetic neuralgia is fortunately a self-limiting symptom and the majority of patients will have no pain after 6 months. *Probably the most successful medication for controlling the pain is a tricyclic antidepressant such as amitriptyline.* Acyclovir, when given early during the vesicular phase of the illness, may limit the duration and severity of post-herpetic neuralgia, but it is of no value in treating the pain once it is established. Corticosteroids have also been recommended during the acute phase of Herpes zoster to reduce the incidence of post-herpetic neuralgia, but their effectiveness is doubtful. They are certainly of no benefit once post-herpetic neuralgia is established. Similarly, cimetidine has been tried but it has been found to be ineffective in the acute phase of Herpes zoster and neither cimetidine nor phenytoin are effective in post-herpetic neuralgia. The pain of post-herpetic neuralgia usually cannot be controlled by rhizotomy, indicating that it is central in origin.

ME-C29   CORRECT RESPONSE D

The clinical picture is that of a 60-year-old woman with well controlled rheumatoid arthritis who suddenly develops an acute arthritis. *The major concern in this situation, particularly in someone on corticosteroids, is that she has a septic arthritis.* This should be confirmed by a blood count and aspiration of the joint and should be treated immediately. After 35 years of rheumatoid arthritis and while on steroids, one would not expect an acute episode of monoarticular rheumatoid arthritis to occur. Gout may occasionally produce arthritis in the knee, although much more commonly it will involve the feet. However, gout in patients with rheumatoid arthritis is very rare. Osteoarthritis secondary to rheumatoid presents as pain and is confirmed by the X-ray findings. It will not present as an acutely swollen and tender joint. Similarly, while trauma may produce pain in the joint, one would not expect it to be warm and very tender unless a haemarthrosis is present.

ME-C30   CORRECT RESPONSE B

Rheumatoid factor will eventually become positive in approximately two-thirds of patients with rheumatoid arthritis. *It is strongly associated (more than 95%) with the presence of rheumatoid nodules.* It is not specific to rheumatoid arthritis and may be positive in patients with a variety of diseases, including systemic lupus erythematosus, Sjögren syndrome, chronic liver disease, sarcoidosis and a number of other conditions. It is found in approximately 5% of healthy persons in the general population and the percentage with a positive rheumatoid factor progressively increases with age. Thus, more than 10% of the population over the age of 65 years can be expected to show a positive rheumatoid factor. The presence of rheumatoid factor varies little with the activity of the rheumatoid disease, although patients with high titres of rheumatoid factor tend to have more severe and progressive disease than those with low titres.

ME-C31   CORRECT RESPONSE A

Ankylosing spondylitis reduces the mobility of the spine and the ribs and will reduce the lung vital capacity. It is most uncommon for the disorder not to involve the sacroiliac joints. Most of the spine, including its cervical region, is commonly involved.

Approximately 90% of patients with ankylosing spondylitis are male. X-ray changes in ankylosing spondylitis first appear in the sacroiliac joint with blurring of the cortical margins of the subchondral bone followed by erosion and sclerosis. In the lumbar spine there is a straightening of the lumbar lordosis and a reactive sclerosis in the anterior borders of the vertebral bodies. There is then a progressive ossification of the superficial layers of the annulus fibrosus. The intervertebral disc space is usually maintained, particularly when sclerosis develops in the annulus.

ME-C32   CORRECT RESPONSE D

Osteoarthritis can be seen secondary to rheumatoid arthritis after destruction of the joint by the rheumatoid process. In the hands, osteoarthritis most commonly affects interphalangeal joints and not the metacarpophalangeal joints. The other common symptom in the hand from osteoarthritis is pain on movement of the base of the thumb.

The disease process in osteoarthritis primarily involves the progressive thinning of cartilage. The X-ray appearance in the early stages may be normal, until the loss of articular cartilage makes the joint space narrowing evident. Later, there may be subchondral bone sclerosis, subchondral cysts and development of marginal osteophytes. With severe osteoarthritis there is bone remodelling, typically with expansion of the joints.

Morning stiffness is not a characteristic feature of osteoarthritis, but is typical of rheumatoid arthritis. Osteoarthritis is characterised by pain which comes on with use of the joint and is relieved by rest. Later in the disorder, pain, particularly in the hips, may occur at rest at night. Immobilisation is not the most appropriate treatment for osteoarthritis as this will produce only stiffening of the joints. Controlling pain with simple analgesics is usually the best and most effective treatment. There may be an inflammatory component at times in osteoarthritis, in which case non-steroidal anti-inflammatory agents may be added for a period of time, but they should not be used routinely for the treatment of this disorder.

ME-C33   CORRECT RESPONSE B

The characteristic radiological findings of osteoarthritis are narrowing of the joint space as cartilage is lost. There may be some osteophyte formation at the edges of the joints and some subchondral bone cysts. There is an increased density of bone ends as subchondral sclerosis develops. *Periarticular osteoporosis is inconsistent with osteoarthritis* and would suggest that an inflammatory arthritis, such as rheumatoid, is present.

ME-C34   CORRECT RESPONSE D

The clinical picture is that of a 73-year-old woman who develops a bilateral limb girdle pain. The onset of symmetrical limb girdle pain, particularly involving the shoulder, is most atypical of a degenerative arthritis. *The picture is, however, typical of polymyalgia rheumatica. The patient may also have temporal arteritis. The diagnosis would be confirmed by a markedly elevated erythrocyte sedimentation rate.* X-rays of the pelvis, serum levels of calcium, phosphorus and alkaline phosphatase are likely to be normal. The picture with bilateral limb girdle pain is atypical of the presentation of rheumatoid arthritis, particularly at this age. The latex rheumatoid factor is likely to be negative.

The possibility of associated temporal arteritis, with its attendant risk of blindness, make the rapid recognition and treatment of this condition crucial.

ME-C35   CORRECT RESPONSE D

Non-steroidal anti-inflammatory drugs (NSAID) can affect many organs because they are inhibitors of the cyclo-oxygenase (COX-1) enzyme. They can cause retention of sodium and subsequent oedema and can worsen pre-existing renal failure. They should not be used as the first line of treatment of osteoarthritis. The majority of patients with osteoarthritis respond well to simple analgesics such as paracetamol or paracetamol combined with dextropropoxyphene. While NSAID may certainly cause gastrointestinal symptoms, anti-ulcer therapy should not be used routinely as concomitant therapy. This only adds to the risks and costs of treatment. The use of anti-ulcer therapy could be considered with the onset of treatment (after appropriate investigation) if gastrointestinal symptoms are present at the time when treatment is initiated.

Gastrointestinal haemorrhage as a complication of NSAID administration is a systemic, not a local, effect. This is in part due to interference with prostaglandin metabolism. The use of suppositories does not diminish the risk of gastrointestinal haemorrhage.

Non-steroidal anti-inflammatory drugs are adequately absorbed when taken with food and food does not significantly alter their efficacy. Indeed, taking these medications with food may reduce the local gastrointestinal effects of NSAID.

ME-C36   CORRECT RESPONSE D

Of the disorders listed, squamous cell carcinoma of the lung is the most common cause of finger clubbing in the adult and clubbing may be the only clinical sign. Clubbing is rarely seen with tuberculosis. A patient with long-standing cor pulmonale occasionally has clubbing. It does not occur with sleep apnoea or recurrent pulmonary embolism. Other causes of clubbing include cyanotic heart disease and chronic pulmonary suppuration. The mechanism of clubbing is unclear; but it remains an important physical sign in association with a wide variety of circulatory and pulmonary disorders.

ME-C37   CORRECT RESPONSE B

The clinical picture described, that of accentuation of the first heart sound and loud secondary pulmonary sound with presystolic murmur is typical of mitral stenosis.

The classical features of mitral stenosis on auscultation of the cardiac apex region are: (i) a loud and usually palpable first heart sound; (ii) a presystolic murmur if the patient is in sinus rhythm; and (iii) an opening snap and a low-pitched, often palpable mid-diastolic murmur. The opening snap may be lost with a severely disorganised non-pliant valve. The mid-diastolic murmur may be difficult to hear at rest but usually becomes evident after exercise. It may disappear in the presence of severe pulmonary hypertension.

Pulmonary stenosis does not have a loud second sound. Aortic stenosis would not have a loud second sound or a presystolic murmur. Mitral incompetence causes a systolic murmur and is not characterised by a presystolic murmur. The changes in loudness of the heart sounds and the presence of a presystolic murmur are inconsistent with a functional heart murmur.

ME-C38   CORRECT RESPONSE B

A third heart sound may be detected in a variety of circumstances. It occurs 120–160 ms after the second heart sound, is low pitched and is best heard with the bell of the stethoscope. A third heart sound is a diastolic filling sound. *It is not dependent on atrial contraction and is not influenced by the presence of atrial fibrillation.* It is associated with rapid ventricular filling. It may be normal before the age of 30 years but should be assumed to be abnormal above 40 years of age, where it usually implies ventricular disease. It is commonly heard in acute left ventricular failure, as after acute myocardial infarction. It occurs in most cases of severe mitral regurgitation. Constrictive pericarditis is a rare cause where the third sound represents sudden cessation of ventricular filling.

ME-C39   CORRECT RESPONSE D

Addison disease may be associated with a mild bradycardia, but not a pulse rate of 32 /min, a rate which strongly suggests a significant degree of heart block. Iron deficiency that produces anaemia will tend to produce a mild tachycardia rather than a supraventricular tachyarrhythmia with block. Insulinomas can present with hypoglycaemia and syncope but are not associated with such a low pulse rate.

Structural disease of the cardiac conducting system (the 'sick sinus syndrome') could produce episodic heart block and dizziness but would be very uncommon in a woman of this age. *Sinus tachycardia with a 4:1 atrioventricular block would be the MOST likely cause.*

ME-C40   CORRECT RESPONSE E

The clinical picture is that of a 60-year-old man in cardiac failure due to complete heart block. *The correct treatment is to increase his heart rate immediately with a transvenous pacemaker. When the heart rate is increased the signs of cardiac failure will abate. He is at risk of sudden death so the insertion of a pacemaker should not be delayed.* The use of digoxin may increase the risk of asystole. Reducing the plasma volume with intravenous frusemide would reduce the filling pressure and further reduce the cardiac output. Abdominal paracentesis would reduce the filling pressure and blood volume and reduce the cardiac output.

ME-C41 CORRECT RESPONSE B

Systolic hypertension predisposes to stroke and one study (Systolic Hypertension in Elderly Persons (SHEP) Study) has now shown that a major (greater than 40%) reduction in stroke rate in the elderly can be achieved by reducing systolic blood pressure. Population studies have shown that systolic and not diastolic blood pressure is the best predictor of stroke risk.

The presence of a mildly elevated serum creatinine level and a past history of stroke are not contraindications to anti-hypertensive therapy. Indeed, effective treatment of hypertension may reduce the rate of deterioration in renal function. In patients with a history of stroke, treatment of hypertension reduces the incidence of recurrent stroke. Angiotensin-converting enzyme (ACE) inhibitors are quite effective in the elderly in reducing blood pressure. As yet there is no large trial that has shown that ACE inhibitors reduce the incidence of stroke. All antihypertensive primary prevention trials which have examined stroke incidence have used a thiazide diuretic with the addition, if necessary, of a beta-blocker.

ME-C42 CORRECT RESPONSE D

The haemodynamic changes that might be expected after a pulmonary embolus would include **raised right ventricular pressure** (blood unable to get into the pulmonary circulation) **and a raised systemic venous pressure** (backflow from an obstructed right-sided circulation). Low right atrial pressures and low right central venous pressures are suggestive of hypovolaemia. Low central and peripheral venous pressures with systemic arterial hypotension are also classic characteristics of hypovolaemic shock. High pulmonary venous pressure and pulmonary oedema suggests primary acute left heart failure. Mitral valvular disease with mitral valve incompetence causes high left atrial pressures.

ME-C43 CORRECT RESPONSE E

The abdominal segment of the aorta is the section of the arterial tree most frequently affected by atherosclerotic aneurysmal dilatation. The common site of rupture is in an **aortic aneurysm below the level of the renal arteries.** If the aneurysm extends to a higher level its surgical repair is more difficult and the likelihood of the complication of postoperative acute renal failure is increased.

ME-C44 CORRECT RESPONSE B

Causes of hypertension include fibromuscular hyperplasia affecting the renal arteries, *a disease of unknown aetiology most commonly detected in young women.*

Atherosclerotic plaques and strictures comprise the most common renal causes of hypertension overall; their frequency increases with age in both sexes.

ME-C45 CORRECT RESPONSE B

The relative reduction of movement of the chest on the right suggests the pathology is on that side. The percussion note is more resonant on the right and the breath sounds are softer. *These physical findings are consistent with a pneumothorax on the right.* With consolidation on the left, one would expect decreased movement on that side, bronchial breath sounds and crepitations. When there is a collapse on the left, one would expect decreased rather than louder breath sounds on the left. Consolidation on the right would be unlikely in the absence of decreased resonance. If there was a pleural effusion, the breath sounds would be decreased over the effusion and there may be bronchial breathing at the top of the pleural effusion.

ME-C46   CORRECT RESPONSE D

The question describes a number of typical physical findings in a patient with severe emphysema. There is inspiratory indrawing of the costal margins, diminished cardiac dullness and the breath sounds are faint. Commonly pulsus paradoxus (due to large oscillations of intrathoracic pressure) is present. *Diffuse expiratory rhonchi are not usually a feature of emphysema and would suggest a diagnosis of obstructive lung disease due to asthma or chronic bronchitis.*

ME-C47   CORRECT RESPONSE C

The most likely cause of persistent blood-stained effusion in a 50-year-old man is carcinoma of the lung. Neither coal miner's pneumoconiosis nor silicosis produces blood-stained effusions. Mesothelioma can produce a blood-stained effusion, but usually other signs of asbestosis are apparent and it is far less common than carcinoma of the lung. Pulmonary tuberculosis produces an exudative effusion with many lymphocytes but not a blood-stained effusion.

ME-C48   CORRECT RESPONSE D

The patient described has CO_2 retention and a low P_aO_2 and would benefit from controlled oxygen therapy. The pattern of blood gases described is that of respiratory failure ($P_aO_2 \leq 50$ mmHg, $P_aCO_2 \geq 50$ mmHg) and may represent acute, acute on chronic, or chronic ventilatory failure. The raised P_aCO_2 excludes hyperventilation. A P_aO_2 of 50 mmHg may not produce a sufficient degree of desaturation to produce obvious cyanosis. Patients with the blood gas values indicated do not necessarily require mechanical ventilation for hypoxia. A reduction in diffusing capacity affects primarily arterial oxygen tension, not CO_2 retention; indeed it is common to have a low P_aCO_2 due to hyperventilation.

ME-C49   CORRECT RESPONSE C

Chronic bronchitis is the most likely respiratory disorder of those listed to be associated with retention of CO_2. This occurs because of severe generalised airway narrowing.

In the majority of cases of acute asthma there is a reduction in P_aCO_2 due to hyperventilation. A raised P_aCO_2 is a sign that the episode of asthma is severe and life-threatening.

In lobar pneumonia, only one section of the lung is involved. There may be a reduction in arterial PO_2 because of blood shunted through the non-aerated lung but the remaining unaffected lung is quite adequate to remove CO_2.

In 'pure' (uncomplicated) emphysema the diffusing capacity of the lung is reduced. However, this primarily affects the transfer of O_2, rather than CO_2, which diffuses much more easily.

In chronic pulmonary tuberculosis the situation is similar to that of lobar pneumonia. There are usually sufficient areas of the lung unaffected by tuberculosis to exchange CO_2 adequately.

ME-C50   CORRECT RESPONSE C

Hypercapnia (elevated P_aCO_2) induces peripheral vasodilatation resulting in a hot, dry skin and retinal venous distension. The vasodilatation of the scalp vessels and intracranial extracerebral vessels are responsible for the headache of hypercapnia. Drowsiness is due to the direct cerebral effect of the elevated CO_2 or acidosis on the reticular formation. The muscle twitching is usually a peripheral phenomenon related to acidosis but myoclonic jerks of central origin may occur. *Cold, clammy skin is not a feature of hypercapnia.*

ME-C51   CORRECT RESPONSE D

In respiratory alkalosis there is an increased loss of CO_2 from hyperventilation. This reduces the $P_a\text{CO}_2$. The subsequent rise in pH is partly compensated for by an increased urinary excretion of bicarbonate and a *decrease in plasma bicarbonate. The correct response is reduction of $P_a\text{CO}_2$ and plasma bicarbonate.*

ME-C52   CORRECT RESPONSE A

The clinical circumstances described in the question would produce hypoventilation. *Hypoventilation produces a respiratory acidosis with a reduction in $P_a\text{O}_2$* (hypoxia) and an increase in $P_a\text{CO}_2$ (hypercarbia). One would expect an acidosis, not a normal pH, an increased $P_a\text{CO}_2$ and diminished oxygen tension. *A pH of 7.22, $P_a\text{O}_2$ of 70 mmHg and $P_a\text{CO}_2$ of 61 is consistent with hypoventilation.*

ME-C53   CORRECT RESPONSE B

The sputum in asthma is typically thick and tenacious so that the description of watery consistency is inconsistent with chronic asthma. Each of the other sputum descriptions is typical of the disorder indicated.

ME-C54   CORRECT RESPONSE B

It is usual to have a normal chest X-ray in a patient with pulmonary embolism. The other associations give results of investigations that are inconsistent with the diagnosis. With mild asthma it is common for the arterial $P_a\text{CO}_2$ to fall (due to hyperventilation) rather than increase. A raised $P_a\text{CO}_2$ is a sign of severe asthma and impending respiratory failure. The pleural effusion of cardiac failure is a transudate and the protein level is usually less than 2 g/dL. A protein level of 4 g/dL would suggest an exudate due to an infective or malignant process. Severe airflow limitation is associated with a marked reduction of the FEV_1. An FEV_1 of 80% of predicted is normal. Pulmonary embolism is usually diagnosed by a ventilation/perfusion lung scan. A normal ventilation–perfusion scan makes a pulmonary embolus unlikely.

ME-C55   CORRECT RESPONSE D

In a patient presenting with acute asthma who is clearly unwell, first assess the severity of the asthma and then look for any precipitating and other causes. The peak expiratory flow reading will give a good indication of the severity of the asthma. It would be inappropriate to send a febrile asthmatic patient to the Diagnostic Imaging department for an X-ray without first assessing the severity of the asthma. If the patient is well enough to cooperate, bedside peak expiratory flow should be done on presentation. The clinical picture with the soft vesicular breath sounds and expiratory wheeze could either be consistent with mild asthma and a chest infection or could indicate a life-threatening episode of asthma.

The arterial blood gases, particularly the $P_a\text{CO}_2$ level, will indicate whether this is a life-threatening episode of asthma. The next logical procedure would be a chest X-ray to detect infections, pneumothorax and other possible complications of asthma. *The most appropriate sequence is thus peak expiratory flow reading, arterial blood gases and chest X-ray.*

ME-C56   CORRECT RESPONSE B

In a patient with severe asthma, the most ominous sign is a raised arterial P_{CO_2} ($P_a_{CO_2}$ of 50 mmHg or above). This suggests the patient is at risk of cardiorespiratory arrest. It is common in moderate asthma for a reduction in arterial P_{CO_2} to occur because of hyperventilation. Hypoxia is common in severe asthma, but is less predictive of cardiorespiratory arrest. An FEV_1 of 0.8 L is not consistent with severe asthma. In patients with respiratory failure from asthma, usually wheezes become softer rather than louder. Variations in respiratory rate are of little help in judging the severity of asthma.

ME-C57   CORRECT RESPONSE D

The clinical picture is typical of the onset of acute lobar pneumonia. By far the most common cause is streptococcal (Streptococcus pneumoniae) *pneumonia.* Staphylococcal pneumonia and viral pneumonia tend to have multiple sites and do not have a lobar involvement. The chest X-ray in pulmonary embolism is commonly normal and is not associated with a productive cough and fever. Mycoplasma pneumonia can present as described above except that a productive cough is unusual and the chest X-ray usually shows more diffuse changes. It is, however, far less common than streptococcal pneumonia.

ME-C58   CORRECT RESPONSE B

In patients with Pneumocystis carinii *pneumonia the physical examination of the lungs is frequently normal.* Pulmonary examination may be normal even if the patient has cyanosis and tachypnoea. Pneumocystis pneumonia only occurs late in the course of HIV infection and is an AIDS-identifying illness. The chest X-ray is usually abnormal, showing bilateral diffuse infiltrates.

Diffusing capacity is commonly affected, resulting in arterial hypoxia. It is often difficult to diagnose *Pneumocystis carinii* pneumonia, as the organism cannot be grown from sputum culture.

ME-C59   CORRECT RESPONSE C

Mycoplasma pneumonia is sensitive to erythromycin and tetracycline, the former being the preferred treatment as tetracycline is contraindicated in children. *Mycoplasma is not sensitive to penicillin or amoxycillin.* Mycoplasma pneumonia occurs in young adults and cold agglutinins are commonly found in the blood. The white blood cell count is usually normal and the chest X-ray may show initially a lobar pattern of consolidation, which may then spread across lobar boundaries. The appearance of the chest X-ray usually suggests a much more severe pneumonia than the clinical state would indicate.

ME-C60   CORRECT RESPONSE E

The clinical vignette is very suggestive of pulmonary tuberculosis. *Acid-fast bacilli in sputum are highly suggestive, but not pathognomonic, for tuberculosis.* Non-pathogenic acid-fast bacilli may be found in the sputum of patients with inactive cavitating tuberculosis. BCG vaccination confers only a relative immunity to tuberculosis so that previous vaccination does not exclude this diagnosis. Other pulmonary disorders, such as Friedlander and staphylococcal pneumonia, may produce cavitation so the chest X-ray appearance, while suggestive, is not diagnostic. The Mantoux test is an intracutaneous test for hypersensitivity to tuberculin, indicating past or present infection with tubercle bacilli. A Mantoux test may become negative in the presence of active tuberculosis, particularly if the patient is very ill. An active tuberculous lesion may not excrete large quantities of acid-fast bacilli, so sputum smears can be negative.

ME-C61 CORRECT RESPONSE D

Anti-inflammatory drugs enhance the analgesic effect of opiates. When analgesics are necessary for severe pain, a regular oral dose of morphine is effective and has a lesser risk of addiction than the intermittent use of morphine. Currently, long-acting oral forms of morphine are preferred for long-term pain relief. Given in this way, severe respiratory depression is not usually a problem.

ME-C62 CORRECT RESPONSE E

The pulmonary second heart sound is increased in acute pulmonary embolism because of the increase in pulmonary arterial pressure. Typically, at the onset of significant pulmonary embolism there can be a period of syncope and dyspnoea. A pleural rub can develop within the first 48 h of the onset of a pulmonary embolus. *Consolidation is not present with uncomplicated pulmonary emboli so that bronchial breath sounds are not heard.*

ME-C63 CORRECT RESPONSE C

The clinical vignette is that of a patient with severe heart disease who presented with acute breathlessness. The presence of bilateral pulmonary emboli is confirmed by the ventilation–perfusion lung scan in association with normal lung fields on chest X-ray. *The correct treatment of pulmonary emboli in this situation is the immediate commencement of intravenous heparin with careful control of the dosage and commencement on warfarin.* The latter would normally be continued for 6 months. Identifying a source of emboli in the lower limbs is not particularly helpful in this sort of patient in that the emboli may have arisen from pelvic veins and identification of the site of an embolus will not alter and should not delay treatment. Bed rest and subcutaneous heparin is not adequate treatment for pulmonary emboli. Demonstration of the site of pulmonary emboli with pulmonary angiography would not alter the treatment and is unnecessary as the site is already known from the ventilation–perfusion scan. Intravenous thrombolytic therapy would not be the next most appropriate therapeutic step; however, if the patient developed progressive heart failure in spite of heparin, this measure could be considered.

ME-C64 CORRECT RESPONSE B

The Mantoux test is an indicator of delayed hypersensitivity and is read at 48 or 72 h. A negative result at 24 h is not helpful in diagnosis. *In a patient positive for HIV, a 5 mm induration at 72 h after the injection of 10 IU tuberculin is regarded as a positive result.* A positive Mantoux makes a diagnosis of tuberculosis more likely. However, it can be an indicator of past contact with tuberculosis and does not necessarily indicate active tuberculosis. The BCG vaccine should not be used for prophylaxis in patients positive for HIV. The probability of producing an immune response is reduced and its protective value is in doubt. There is also a concern because it is a live vaccine. Chemoprophylaxis is inappropriate. Chemotherapy should be started if active tuberculosis is present. The Mantoux test can become negative during the course of HIV, but may become positive if active tuberculosis is present. However, only approximately two-thirds of patients with HIV and active tuberculosis have a positive Mantoux. For this reason, careful microscopy of the sputum must be performed to exclude the possibility of tuberculosis.

ME-C65 CORRECT RESPONSE E

Dysphagia, commonly painful, is a typical symptom of monilial oesophagitis. It is due to local inflammation. Myasthenia gravis produces dysphagia when the striated muscle in the upper one-third of the oesophagus is involved in the disorder. Iron deficiency anaemia can be associated with an accompanying hypopharyngeal web in middle-aged women, causing sideropenic dysphagia (Plummer–Vinson syndrome). A small percentage of patients with Parkinson disease also complain of dysphagia, related to slow abnormal movements of the pharynx and the upper oesophagus.

Oesophageal varices are not associated with dysphagia. They are soft dilated venous channels easily displaced by food and liquid.

ME-C66 CORRECT RESPONSE E

Oesophageal motility disorders typically produce dysphagia for both liquid and solid food whereas dysphagia due to structural abnormalities such as a malignancy produces dysphagia predominantly for solid food. Diffuse oesophageal spasm can produce a crushing substernal pain which resembles cardiac pain. Sometimes this can be precipitated by drinking cold fluids. Both dysphagia and pain can respond to calcium channel-blocking agents. *The symptoms of diffuse oesophageal spasm are not usually progressive and can remain unaltered for some years or even regress.*

ME-C67 CORRECT RESPONSE B

The clinical picture is that of a young woman with reflux oesophagitis, absence of motility in the oesophagus and a past history of Raynaud phenomenon. A possible diagnosis is scleroderma. *The most appropriate treatment would be to continue medical treatment, changing from a histamine H_2 receptor antagonist (cimetidine) to a proton pump-blocking drug such as omeprazole.* Another histamine H_2 receptor antagonist (ranitidine) is unlikely to produce benefit if high doses of cimetidine have failed. Octreotide is a long-acting analogue of somatostatin, which inhibits release of numerous gastrointestinal hormones. It is ineffective in reflux oesophagitis. Dilatation of the lower oesophageal sphincter would be most inappropriate, as the cause of the dysphagia is the reflux oesophagitis, not an abnormality of the sphincter. The surgical procedure of fundo-plication would be inappropriate in a patient with scleroderma and could exacerbate the dysphagia.

ME-C68 CORRECT RESPONSE C

Oesophageal reflux (regurgitation of gastric content into the lower oesophagus) is common and its diagnosis is most usually dependent on taking a good clinical history. Endoscopy may reveal no abnormality, as reflux can be intermittent and only some patients have visually detectable oesophagitis. Endoscopy is, however, the most definitive method of diagnosing established oesophagitis due to reflux and is also most important in excluding other pathologies. A barium meal may or may not demonstrate reflux. Oesophageal manometry is usually normal, but infusion of acid in the distal oesophagus sometimes induces oesophageal muscle spasms. Nuclear scanning can elegantly quantitate reflux as a research investigation, but is not a requisite for diagnosis.

ME-C69 CORRECT RESPONSE E

Gluten-sensitive enteropathy, viral gastroenteritis in any ethnic group and Crohn disease may all show lactose intolerance with diarrhoea being produced following the ingestion of milk and other lactose-containing food. The intolerance is due to reduction in lactase in the intestinal mucosa. *Chronic pancreatitis, however, is not associated with intolerance to lactose, the primary problem being one of malabsorption of fat.*

ME-C70   **CORRECT RESPONSE E**

The anaemia of gluten-sensitive enteropathy is usually due to iron deficiency. The pretreatment biopsy shows a flat mucosa with absence of villi, but there is no inflammatory cell infiltrate with PAS-positive macrophages. Those changes occur in Whipple disease. Gluten is a specific protein in wheat and is not found in cornflour; so that cornflour need not be excluded from the diet. The response to a gluten-free diet is slow and some patients may take 24–36 months before clinical response is apparent. In some adults there may be little change in the intestinal histological features.

There is a substantial long-term risk of developing intestinal lymphoma in patients with gluten-sensitive enteropathy.

ME-C71   **CORRECT RESPONSE E**

The mode of presentation of Wilson disease is very variable and, in part, depends on the age of the patient. In younger patients the symptoms are usually neurological and they may present with dystonia and tic-like movements. In older patients cirrhosis is more common, with the patient presenting with jaundice or hepatic failure.

In the majority of adult patients there are diagnostic changes present in the eye with deposition of brown material around the periphery of the cornea: Kayser–Fleischer rings. These can usually be detected in a good light, but slit lamp examination is required to exclude them.

Reduced serum ceruloplasmin is a diagnostic test for Wilson disease, *but there is a poor correlation between the level and the clinical severity of the disease.*

ME-C72   **CORRECT RESPONSE D**

Hepatitis B is considered to be the most important aetiological agent for hepatocellular carcinoma worldwide. *Compared with non-carriers, hepatitis B carriers have a 90–100 fold increased risk of hepatocellular carcinoma.*

Alpha-interferon may be effective in clearing hepatitis B antigen (HBAg) from the serum, but it is not effective in clearing hepatitis B surface antigen (HBsAg) in chronic active hepatitis. Hepatitis B surface antigen is always positive by the time clinical jaundice occurs. The HBV-DNA polymerase activity is a more sensitive index of viral replication than the HB e antigen/e antibody status.

Only 1–5% of maternal–fetal transmission of hepatitis B occurs *in utero*; the greatest risk of transmission is at the time of delivery.

ME-C73   **CORRECT RESPONSE C**

Transmission of hepatitis B during birth is frequent if the mother is HBAg positive and less frequent if she is only HBsAg positive. The mother is most likely an asymptomatic carrier and no treatment is indicated on her behalf. Of infants with hepatitis B, less than 10% of cases have been acquired transplacentally. *The correct management is to prevent infection in the baby initially by hyperimmune globulin then to proceed with vaccination of the baby.*

ME-C74   **CORRECT RESPONSE B**

Patients with irritable bowel syndrome commonly complain of looser and more frequent stools and the passage of mucus with the stools. There is usually colicky abdominal pain and the feeling of abdominal distension. The pain is relieved by defaecation.

However, nocturnal diarrhoea associated with pain that wakes the patient up in the night suggests there is an organic cause and should be investigated further.

ME-C75   CORRECT RESPONSE A

Enterotoxigenic Escherichia coli *is the most common cause of 'traveller's diarrhoea'.* 'Traveller's diarrhoea' typically lasts only 48 h. *Giardia lamblia* may cause diarrhoea in travellers but this is a more prolonged illness with cramping abdominal pains. *Shigella* species, entamoeba and salmonella also produce more prolonged symptoms and are less common. The relative frequency of these infections varies and depends on the area in which they were acquired.

ME-C76   CORRECT RESPONSE D

The risk of developing bowel cancer is significantly increased in first degree relatives of patients with the disease. The risk rises from about one in 20 in the adult population over 50 years of age to approximately one in six if there is a first degree relative with bowel cancer. If one bowel cancer is present there is a three-fold increase in the risk of developing a subsequent bowel cancer. It is now thought that most colonic cancers arise in colonic adenomas so that patients with colonic adenomas have a significantly increased risk of bowel cancer. *The type of adenoma most likely to produce a cancer is a villous adenoma.* The risk of malignancy developing is also related to the size of the adenoma. There is an increased risk of developing carcinoma of the bowel both in patients with Crohn colitis and in those with ulcerative colitis.

ME-C77   CORRECT RESPONSE C

The correct response is to order a stool culture. A history of 2 weeks of bloody diarrhoea would be consistent with the first episode of ulcerative colitis *but an infective cause must be excluded by stool microscopy and culture.* Disorders such as *Campylobacter jejuni* infection, amoebiasis and even cytomegalovirus (CMV) enteritis in the immunosuppressed may have a macroscopic appearance indistinguishable from that of ulcerative colitis.

ME-C78   CORRECT RESPONSE E

The question lists four non-intestinal associations of ulcerative colitis. Pyoderma gangrenosum is a relatively painless ulcerating lesion usually occurring on the trunk. Approximately 5% of patients with ulcerative colitis develop ocular manifestations, such as uveitis and recurrent optic neuritis. These manifestations can be severe but usually respond to colectomy. Primary sclerosing cholangitis is characterised by portal tract inflammation with some bile duct proliferation; the lesion can be clinically insignificant, detectable only by elevated serum alkaline phosphatase and only rarely progresses to cirrhosis.

Vitamin B_{12} malabsorption can occur occasionally if the terminal ileum is involved by 'backwash' in ulcerative colitis. *Splenomegaly, however, is not associated with ulcerative colitis.*

ME-C79   CORRECT RESPONSE E

The clinical picture described is suggestive of a Shigella *infection. Numerous polymorphs are usually seen in the stool and the infection can be diagnosed by Gram stain and stool culture.* Cholera produces large quantities of watery ('rice water') stool and not a bloody diarrhoea. Antidiarrhoeal agents that slow gut motility are not recommended and are rarely indicated in infective diarrhoeas. They have little effect on the duration of the illness. When specific therapy is indicated this should be given instead (such as a quinolone antibiotic in the case of shigellosis). Cysts of *Entamoeba histolytica* can be seen in the stool without an active infection, particularly if the patient has been in an area in which amoebic dysentery is endemic. Bloody diarrhoea with cramping abdominal pains is more suggestive of colitis and is not typical of a *Campylobacter jejuni* infection, which is normally a self-limiting disorder. Antibiotics are thus not usually prescribed for infections with *C. jejuni*, especially in a patient of this age.

ME-C80   CORRECT RESPONSE B

Most cancers of the large bowel arise on the left side of the colon. They tend to present early with obstructive or other symptoms rather than pain. Usually at the time of presentation there are no liver metastases. *They arise most commonly from pre-existing adenomas rather than de novo in the mucosa, hence the importance of colonscopic screening in high-risk subjects.*

ME-C81   CORRECT RESPONSE B

Many cancers can produce ascites and the usual ones are primary neoplasms of the gut and female genital tract. Typically, ovarian cancer presents with abdominal swelling secondary to ascites. Colon and stomach cancer can produce ascites late in the disease, as can adenocarcinoma of the pancreas.

The ascites is secondary to tumour deposition in the mesentery, omentum and malignant invasion of the peritoneal tissues, with fluid secretion secondary to peritoneal irritation. The ascitic process is not related to obstruction of the gut lumen, or encroachment on hepatic venous return (in other conditions this could produce a transudative type of ascites). Hepatic metastases by themselves are not usually associated with ascites, unless they are very extensive.

ME-C82   CORRECT RESPONSE D

Of those patients who have pituitary dependent hypercortisolaemia due to a tumour, the majority have a microadenoma (less than 10 mm in diameter) and at least half the tumours are less than 5 mm in diameter. Because these tumours are not of a sufficient size to compress the optic chiasm, bitemporal field defects are an uncommon clinical finding in pituitary dependent hypercortisolaemia. Hypertension, proximal myopathy and diabetes mellitus are common findings with Cushing syndrome. Failure to suppress plasma cortisol following low-dose dexamethasone (0.5 mg, q.i.d.) is one of the diagnostic tests for Cushing syndrome.

ME-C83   CORRECT RESPONSE B

The one feature in the list not characteristic of acromegaly is a homonymous hemianopia. The visual field defect in acromegaly occurs because the expanding pituitary tumour compresses fibres of the optic nerves from both retinae which cross in the optic chiasm. These fibres originate from the medial (nasal) half of each retina, so that the resulting field defect is a bitemporal and not a homonymous hemianopia. Further, because the lowest crossing fibres are affected first and those arise from the lowest part of the retina onto which images originating above the line of visual fixation are projected, the defect is initially an upper bitemporal hemianopia.

The effect of growth hormone is to thicken the skin and increase the activity of the glands. Hypertension results from sodium retention and an increase in the plasma volume. There is an increase in the left ventricular mass, even if the patient is not hypertensive and cardiac failure, in the absence of any other form of cardiac disease, is common.

Insulin resistance occurs in approximately 80% of people with acromegaly. Approximately half of those with insulin resistance have abnormal glucose tolerance and approximately 20% have clinical diabetes mellitus.

ME-C84   CORRECT RESPONSE B

Although some of the symptoms in this clinical vignette are those of thyrotoxicosis, the rapid onset with thyroid pain and the palpable tender enlarged thyroid suggest thyroiditis.

The most reliable tests to distinguish between acute thyrotoxicosis and subacute thyroiditis are nuclear uptake tests. Reduced uptake of radioactive iodine is typical of subacute thyroiditis, compared with increased uptake in acute thyrotoxicosis. The serum thyroxine and T3 levels may not be high depending on the stage of the disorder. High antithyroid antibodies would suggest Hashimoto disease which is not consistent with the clinical picture. Subacute thyroiditis is thought to be a response to a viral infection rather than an autoimmune response. A low thyroid stimulating hormone with a flat response to thyrotropin releasing hormone can occur during the disease but this depends on the stage of the disorder and is thus not a reliable test for diagnosis.

ME-C85   CORRECT RESPONSE D

The clinical picture is that of a woman with amenorrhoea, galactorrhoea and a markedly elevated prolactin level. *This combination suggests a pituitary adenoma. Particularly in women, a microadenoma of the pituitary secreting prolactin is much more common than a macroadenoma.* The absence of symptoms such as headache or visual disturbance also suggests that the lesion was small. The drugs that commonly produce hyperprolactinaemia are those that are antagonistic to dopamine receptors, including phenothiazines and butyrophenones, those that deplete dopamine, such as methyldopa and reserpine, and oestrogens and opiates. All these drugs have a direct effect on the mechanism for the release of prolactin. Verapamil is not a drug implicated in prolactinaemia. In the perimenopausal state, prolactin levels are low, related to falling oestrogen levels. Craniopharyngioma destroys the pituitary and would if anything, reduce the production of prolactin rather than increase it.

ME-C86   CORRECT RESPONSE D

Osteoporosis is associated with a low bodyweight, smoking, high alcohol intake and premature menopause. Thiazide diuretics are useful in treating patients with high-turnover osteoporosis associated with hypercalciuria and secondary hyperparathyroidism. They do not cause osteoporosis. They lower the urinary calcium excretion and suppress parathyroid gland function.

ME-C87   CORRECT RESPONSE D

An ABO-incompatible blood transfusion typically results in fever, rigors and hypotension followed by back pain and, commonly, haemoglobinuria, the latter causing dark urine. While bilirubin is produced in excess from haemoglobin and the patient may be jaundiced, *the bilirubin is in unconjugated form and therefore does not appear in the urine.*

ME-C88   CORRECT RESPONSE D

The clinical presentation described is typical of acute leukaemia, particularly with pancytopenia and cervical lymph node enlargement. Idiopathic thrombocytopenia is not common in this age group, the white blood cell count and haemoglobin are usually normal and there is no cervical lymph node enlargement. A drug reaction may produce a thrombocytopenia, most commonly by immunological platelet destruction. Pancytopenia as described is uncommon as a drug reaction and would not normally be associated with enlarged cervical lymph nodes. Infectious mononucleosis can produce a mild neutropenia and thrombocytopenia but there is usually an absolute increase in the number of lymphocytes with abnormal forms. Thrombocytopenia is seen in both initial HIV infection and with AIDS, but pancytopenia is not common.

ME-C89   CORRECT RESPONSE E

The clinical vignette describes the sudden presentation of acute thrombocytopenia. This can follow a viral infection or blood transfusion. It can be seen in acute rheumatoid arthritis and can be induced by quinine in susceptible individuals. *However, there is no association between acute thrombocytopenia and the contraceptive pill.*

ME-C90   CORRECT RESPONSE C

The clinical vignette describes a macrocytosis and thrombocytopenia in a 60-year-old man with moderate to heavy alcohol intake. This is most likely mild liver disease from alcohol excess. Serum iron and ferritin can be disturbed in subjects who drink heavily and iron deficiency can result from gastrointestinal blood loss. However, the severe macrocytosis is the important clue here.

This is a common haematological pattern in an alcoholic. Macrocytosis may reflect a direct toxic effect of alcohol on the marrow, a deficiency in dietary folate or chronic liver disease. A low platelet count in subjects with very high alcohol intake usually represents a toxic effect on the marrow precursors in which case there is an acute recovery (sometimes to high levels) within days, on cessation of alcohol or during hospital admission. If the low platelet count persists it may be due to folate deficiency or hypersplenism.

Liver biopsy and bone marrow biopsy should not be undertaken without *first fully establishing the cause of the macrocytosis by blood tests: initially by serum folate and vitamin B_{12} levels.*

ME-C91   CORRECT RESPONSE E

Macrocytic anaemia occurs in hypothyroidism; the mechanism is not clear but may be related to either vitamin B_{12} or folate deficiency. However normocytic anaemia is more common than macrocytosis. Anti-epileptic medication, particularly phenytoin, interferes with the absorption of folic acid and will produce macrocytosis. Regional ileitis affects the terminal part of the ileum (which is the site of the absorption of vitamin B_{12}) and, thereby, may produce macrocytosis due to vitamin B_{12} deficiency. Chronic alcoholism is associated with macrocytic anaemia, most commonly due to the associated liver disease. There may be a relatively low folate in chronic alcoholism, which would also produce macrocytosis with a megaloblastic bone marrow. *Anaemia of chronic uraemia is usually normochromic and normocytic not macrocytic.* It is predominantly due to the inability of the kidneys to produce adequate amounts of erythropoietin.

ME-C92   CORRECT RESPONSE A

Macrocytic anaemia during pregnancy is most commonly due to a relative lack of folate. It should also not be forgotten that increasing the intake of folate during the first trimester to approximately three-fold the normal daily average intake significantly decreases the incidence of neural tube defects. The usual dose administered is 2.5 mg/day for the first 10 weeks of gestation.

Small bowel disease involving the terminal ileum (such as Crohn disease) can cause macrocytic anaemia in pregnancy, but would be a most uncommon cause. Increased vitamin B_{12} intake and chronic giardiasis do not cause macrocytic anaemia. Alcoholism, when associated with liver disease, is a common cause of macrocytic anaemia in older males, but in pregnancy would not be as common as folate deficiency.

ME-C93   CORRECT RESPONSE E

The clinical vignette describes a male patient with a mild microcytic anaemia. *The most appropriate initial course of action is to establish whether or not this is due to iron deficiency before proceeding with further investigations.* All the other responses listed may, under some circumstances, be appropriate, but not as the most appropriate initial step. If the anaemia is found to be due to iron deficiency it will be essential to exclude occult bleeding from the gastrointestinal tract.

ME-C94   CORRECT RESPONSE B

This patient's angina may have been precipitated by his iron-deficiency anaemia. This is likely to be the case when the ECG is normal.

An iron-deficiency anaemia in this man is probably due to chronic blood loss from the gastrointestinal tract. Two lesions that commonly present in such a fashion are chronic peptic ulcer and carcinoma of the right colon. The patient will require endoscopic or contrast examination of his upper digestive tract and colon.

Of all the options provided in the question, the most reasonable management decision would be to start with *examination of his large bowel by sigmoidoscopy and colonoscopy.* Most clinicians prefer to study the digestive tract endoscopically rather than radiologically, in order not to miss small mucosal lesions. In addition, the endoscopic approach will enable any suspicious lesions to be biopsied. Correction of the iron-deficiency anaemia, whatever the cause, would preferably be by oral iron.

ME-C95   CORRECT RESPONSE E

The clinical vignette is that of a woman taking a non-steroidal anti-inflammatory drug (NSAID) for 'rheumatic pains'. She then develops epigastric discomfort and is found to have an anaemia. The most likely cause is gastric ulceration and haemorrhage from the NSAID. *The most appropriate action would be to cease the piroxicam and control the pain with paracetamol alone while the cause of the anaemia and epigastric discomfort is being established.* Reducing the dose or changing to another form of NSAID will not result in healing of the gastric lesion. The effect of the NSAID is systemic (via the inhibition of prostaglandin synthesis) and not primarily local, so that suppositories can also produce gastric ulceration.

ME-C96   CORRECT RESPONSE E

The presence of abnormal liver function tests without jaundice would support the diagnosis of Epstein–Barr virus (EBV) infection. Splenic infarction is not a frequent complication of EBV infection. Eosinophilia would suggest a parasitic infection. Normally, the neutrophils are suppressed and the lymphocytes are elevated, with abnormal lymphocytes in EBV infection. A rash may occur with ampicillin in EBV infection but not with erythromycin. Cold agglutinins are typical of mycoplasma infections and not EBV.

ME-C97   CORRECT RESPONSE D

The primary effect of antidiuretic hormone is to increase the permeability of water in the distal tubules. As the distal tubule lies in an area of hyperosmolarity, there is a reabsorption of water, leading to more concentrated urine.

ME-C98   CORRECT RESPONSE C

Asymptomatic bacteriuria occurs in both males and females. It is common in pregnancy. In all instances it should be regarded as an indication of a urinary tract infection, investigated and treated. The majority of urinary tract infections arise from retrograde infection and not from haematogenous spread. *Patients with cystitis may not have a significant number of bacteria detected on urinary culture.* Adenovirus and herpes virus can cause cystitis with a sterile urine. There are a number of conditions which can cause sterile pyuria, including treated urinary tract infection, prostatitis, analgesic nephropathy, vesico–ureteric reflux, perinephric abscess, appendicitis and renal tuberculosis.

ME-C99   CORRECT RESPONSE C

The patient is acidotic with a pH of 7.28. *Her lowered P_aco_2 and bicarbonate indicate that the acidosis is metabolic (rather than respiratory) in origin.* With the raised chloride level, the anion gap has been decreased. In renal metabolic acidosis, the anion gap is increased.

Adults with profuse vomiting usually develop an alkalosis with elevated bicarbonate; and a lowered rather than normal potassium.

An infusion of bicarbonate would not contribute to the patient's treatment in that the bicarbonate is lowered secondary to the lowered pH. The primary treatment should be directed towards the cause of the acidosis.

ME-C100   CORRECT RESPONSE D

The most common cause for end-stage renal failure in Australia is chronic glomerulonephritis which accounts for approximately 32% of patients presenting for renal replacement therapy. There has been a rapid rise in the number of diabetics with end-stage renal disease and diabetics now account for 20% of patients with end-stage renal disease in Australia. Polycystic renal disease is another common cause of chronic renal failure, causing approximately 10% of end-stage renal disease in Australia. Analgesic nephropathy is on the decline in Australia, but still causes 5% of end-stage renal disease. Reflux nephropathy due to vesico–ureteric reflux is a common cause of chronic renal failure in childhood, but lags behind glomerulonephritis and diabetes as a cause of end-stage disease in adults.

ME-C101   CORRECT RESPONSE C

In patients with bilateral renal artery stenosis, the renin–angiotensin system may be responsible for the maintenance of renal perfusion. In this circumstance *the use of an angiotensin-converting enzyme (ACE) inhibiting medication to reduce blood pressure can significantly reduce glomerular filtration.*

Angiotensin-converting enzyme inhibitors inhibit the conversion of angiotensin I to angiotensin II and therefore lower angiotensin II levels. Because of the lower angiotensin II levels, plasma renin usually rises. The reduced angiotensin II level in the kidneys leads to a reduction in glomerular filtration rate (GFR) because the kidney distal to a renal artery stenosis is critically dependent on angiotensin II to maintain efferent arteriolar tone; if this falls then GFR falls.

Beta-blockers, calcium antagonists, nitrates and corticosteroids have no adverse effects on GFR.

ME-C102   CORRECT RESPONSE C

This scenario is a very typical story of a man presenting with renal colic with a stone being demonstrated in the lower part of the ureter. This is a common occurrence and the *most appropriate course of action is the relief of pain with paracetamol, paracetamol and codeine, or parenteral opiate, increasing urinary output by drinking more water and waiting expectantly for the stone to be passed. Usually the stone will be passed and this would be seen by repeating an X-ray within 2 days.* Advising the patient just to rest in bed does not facilitate the passing of the stone. Urological intervention with removal of the stone only becomes necessary in the relatively uncommon circumstance of the stone not being passed. The use of allopurinol presumes that the stone may be composed of uric acid (which is quite uncommon in this age group). A thiazide diuretic may be useful for long-term prophylaxis in patients with hypercalciuria, but not as acute therapy. The chemical composition of a stone and its aetiology should be established before recommending major changes in diet and specific therapies.

ME-C103   CORRECT RESPONSE D

The clinical picture presented would be consistent with renal colic and possibly with hydronephrosis. It is not possible to exclude renal stones on the basis of absence of passage of calculi. *The diagnosis of hydronephrosis should easily be established by renal ultrasound, which is the preferred first investigation.* If this shows no abnormality in the renal pelvis then a plain X-ray of the abdomen and intravenous urography may show a stone in the renal pelvis or in the line of the ureter. Cystoscopy and retrograde pyelography would not be the first line of investigation. These may be required at a later date but the diagnosis of both hydronephrosis and a urinary stone can be established by other simpler means.

Of patients with renal calculi, a significant number evince some renal excretory abnormality, such as hypercalciuria. However, it would be inappropriate to commence a low calcium diet without establishing hypercalciuria as the cause of renal stones; the majority of renal calculi occur without demonstrable abnormalities of calcium metabolism.

ME-C104   CORRECT RESPONSE C

The typical ECG changes of hypokalaemia are a flattening of the T wave and the appearance of U waves. *Tall peaked T waves are typical of hyperkalaemia.* Low serum potassium may result in cardiac arrhythmias, intestinal stasis and muscular weakness. These occur because an adequate concentration of potassium is necessary for the maintenance of cell membrane potential and release of neurotransmitters. Chronic potassium depletion causes impairment of renal tubular function resulting in polyuria.

ME-C105   CORRECT RESPONSE A

The clinical picture is the development over 3 days of a combination of meningitis with a well-defined rounded opacity in the lung. This combination in a young man is very suggestive of cryptococcosis with cryptococcal meningitis.

Sarcoidosis produces hilar lymphadenopathy and not rounded peripheral lesions in the lungs. The cerebral involvement of sarcoidosis usually produces a slow onset of a confusional state or basilar meningitis with multiple cranial nerve palsies, rather than acute meningitis. Primary pulmonary neoplasm could produce the lung lesion described but this would be unlikely in a young man. A cerebral metastasis from a primary pulmonary neoplasm would present as a space-occupying lesion rather than as an acute meningitic picture. Occasionally, a pulmonary neoplasm produces carcinomatous meningitis, but the symptomatology is usually that of a slowly progressive meningitis with the serial involvement of cranial nerves.

Disseminated tuberculosis and tuberculous secondary meningitis usually follow a much slower course with the gradual development of headache and drowsiness. Acute meningitic symptoms, such as marked headache and stiff neck, are either not present or minimal. Cerebral secondaries from melanoma present as multiple space-occupying lesions, but not as a carcinomatous meningitis.

ME-C106   CORRECT RESPONSE C

The clinical vignette presented is an example of the typical onset of acute post-streptococcal glomerulonephritis. As the disorder progresses it is common for hypertension and pulmonary oedema to develop, associated primarily with fluid overload. The diagnosis can be further supported by urine microscopy which, in acute post-streptococcal glomerulonephritis, usually shows hyalin and red cell casts. The normal treatment for a patient with acute post-streptococcal glomerulonephritis is diuretics and control of blood pressure. Bed rest is usual, but not required in mild cases without hypertension. The majority of patients will progressively improve without any further intervention. Close members of the family and associates would normally be screened for haemolytic streptococci and, if found, would be treated with antibiotics.

The antistreptolysin titre (ASOT) may not rise for 2–3 weeks after acute haemolytic streptococcal infection and, indeed, it may not rise at all; therefore, *the presence of a normal or low ASOT does not exclude the diagnosis of post-streptococcal glomerulonephritis.*

ME-C107   CORRECT RESPONSE A

Septic arthritis due to Staphylococcus aureus *is by the far the most common form of septic arthritis in a child under 5 years.* The other forms listed are uncommon.

ME-C108   CORRECT RESPONSE D

The most common initial manifestations of HIV infection are very similar to those of a mild influenza-like illness. Opportunistic infections do not occur until later in the disease process when there is profound immune deficiency. Meningitis, gastrointestinal and other symptoms are again less common as initial manifestations of infection.

Although some patients are unable to identify the time of HIV infection from symptomatic assessment, more do have evidence of an initial flu-like febrile illness.

ME-C109   CORRECT RESPONSE D

Meningitis in patients with AIDS is common and is usually due to Cryptococcus neoformans. In Australian-born patients the likelihood of tuberculous meningitis is low. The Human Immunodeficiency virus (HIV) can give a mild form of aseptic meningitis, both at the time of the initial seroconversion and at any time before the development of AIDS. However, the incidence of aseptic meningitis in a patient with established AIDS is low. Incidence of the common forms of bacterial meningitis, such as infections due to *Neisseria meningitidis* and *Streptococcus pneumoniae*, is not a problem in AIDS.

ME-C110   CORRECT RESPONSE B

Q fever is typically a respiratory tract infection with pneumonia, headache and malaise, acquired by abattoir workers from inhalation of the rickettsial organism Coxiella burnetii *from animal carcasses.*

ME-C111   CORRECT RESPONSE A

Tabes dorsalis, one of the varieties of tertiary syphilis, *is a condition where there is neurological evidence of posterior column demyelination.* This is the predominant lesion and results in a loss of vibration and position sense with subsequent damage to a variety of tissues and structures.

ME-C112 CORRECT RESPONSE A

Of the antibiotics listed, ampicillin is the one most commonly involved in the development of pseudomembranous colitis. Both oral and intravenous ampicillin can result in the overgrowth of *Clostridium difficile.* Metronidazole or vancomycin are used in the treatment of pseudomembranous colitis. It is unusual to have pseudomembranous colitis associated with trimethoprim–sulphamethoxazole or erythromycin; but any antibiotic can produce the syndrome. The propensity of an antibiotic to precipitate pseudo-membranous colitis is probably related to its spectrum of bacterial suppression.

ME-C113 CORRECT RESPONSE D

Bacteroides fragilis, *Giardia lamblia*, *Entamoeba histolytica* and *Trichomonas vaginalis* are sensitive to metronidazole. **Toxoplasma gondii *is not sensitive to metronidazole,*** but is sensitive to sulfadiazine, clindamycin and pyrimethamine.

ME-C114 CORRECT RESPONSE B

Ceftriaxone is effective against penicillinase-producing **Neisseria gonorrhoeae.** It is not effective against *Mycoplasma pneumoniae* or *Chlamydia trachomatis.* Both these organisms respond to tetracycline and erythromycin. *Giardia lamblia* and *Gardnerella vaginalis* do not respond to ceftriaxone, but do respond to metronidazole or related antibiotics.

ME-C115 CORRECT RESPONSE B

Drugs that have first order kinetics show a rate of reduction in the plasma concentration directly proportional to the plasma concentration. *This gives a constant elimination half life of the drug which does not vary with plasma concentration.* Logarithmic plot of the plasma concentration against time will be a straight line. First order kinetics do not imply only one metabolic pathway. Several metabolic pathways can be responsible for the elimination of the drug and providing each of them follows first order kinetics, the plasma level of the drug will follow first-order kinetics. Neither aspirin nor ethanol has first order kinetics and the half life is dependent on plasma concentration.

ME-C116 CORRECT RESPONSE D

Paracetamol does not produce easy bruising and has no effect on blood clotting or platelets. It is thus safe to give to patients who are on anticoagulants. Aspirin and indomethacin increase bruising because they reduce the aggregation of platelets through inhibition of the production of prostaglandins. Prednisone increases the fragility of capillaries, possibly by its effects on connective tissue. Easy bruising associated with warfarin is due to the reduced clotting of blood.

ME-C117 CORRECT RESPONSE E

Amoxycillin resistance in **Escherichia coli** *is usually due to a bacterial beta-lactamase breaking down the amoxycillin.* It can only be overcome by using specific inhibitors of beta-lactamase, such as clavulanic acid. Increasing the dose or adding in other antibiotics does not overcome the resistance. The resistance may develop rapidly and can be transferred between strains. Infections may occur at any site with beta-lactamase-producing organisms, so that amoxycillin will be ineffective in a urinary tract infection with resistant organisms.

ME-C118 — CORRECT RESPONSE D

Tetracycline is specifically effective in treating psittacosis; other alternatives would be erythromycin or chloramphenicol. Tetracycline is a bacteriostatic drug and while it may be effective for treating acute bronchitis, tonsillitis, *Klebsiella* urinary infections or gonorrhoea, it is not the preferred treatment of those infections.

ME-C119 — CORRECT RESPONSE D

Cimetidine affects the metabolism of a large number of drugs metabolised in the liver. Of those listed, propranolol, phenytoin, warfarin and theophylline are altered and the blood levels of these drugs may rise when cimetidine is given. *The metabolism of digoxin is, however, not affected.*

ME-C120 — CORRECT RESPONSE B

The statement that the incidence of birth defects in babies of mothers with epilepsy is approximately three-fold higher than in the normal community is correct. This applies whether they are on anticonvulsants or not, although some anticonvulsants appear to put the baby at higher risk. The most common abnormalities are minor musculoskeletal disorders, although sodium valproate has been recorded as increasing the incidence of neural tube defects.

Sodium valproate does not cause gingival hyperplasia; this is a typical side effect of phenytoin. It is usually more marked in younger patients. The preferred treatment of status epilepticus is not intravenous barbiturate, as this is likely to result in respiratory arrest. Commonly, small doses of diazepam are given intravenously, and if this fails to control the status epilepticus then intravenous clonazepam, phenytoin or, in the intensive care unit setting, midazolam are used.

There are several mechanisms for removal of phenytoin. One of these mechanisms saturates at serum levels within the therapeutic range so that the elimination of phenytoin is much slower at high plasma levels than at lower plasma levels. Proper management should include monitoring plasma concentration.

Phenytoin is ineffective for Petit-mal seizures. The preferred medication is usually sodium valproate.

ME-C121 — CORRECT RESPONSE E

Non-steroidal anti-inflammatory drugs (NSAID) reduce sodium excretion. Lithium is excreted by the same mechanism as sodium and the excretion of lithium is decreased by NSAID. *The features described, of ataxia, anorexia, nausea and tremulousness, are typical of lithium toxicity.* The correct therapeutic measure would be to cease NSAID and stop the lithium until the lithium level returns to the therapeutic range.

ME-C122 — CORRECT RESPONSE D

Stage 2 (node positive) breast cancer in premenopausal women is the only malignancy listed in the question in which survival has been clearly shown to be improved by adjuvant chemotherapy combined with surgery.

In oesophageal cancer chemoradiotherapy can cause remission of local disease; effects on long-term survival have not as yet been convincingly demonstrated.

After resection for gastric cancer, chemotherapy does not significantly improve survival; and chemotherapy has not been shown to be effective in management of melanoma.

Adjuvant chemotherapy after surgery is now widely used to diminish recurrence risks after resection of locally advanced colonic and rectal carcinoma (Dukes B and C). No effect on survival of Dukes A lesions has been demonstrated.

ME-C123   CORRECT RESPONSE E

Allergic rhinitis can be characterised by a large number of eosinophils present in a nasal smear. Pollen allergy can occur at any time of the year, although it is more frequent at the common flowering times of grass. Topical vasoconstrictors, while they work acutely, exhibit tachyphylaxis, such that with long-term therapy they become ineffective. Desensitisation and sublingual immunotherapy are not effective means of preventing allergic rhinitis.

ME-C124   CORRECT RESPONSE C

Smooth muscle antibodies are characteristic of chronic active hepatitis. They are not usually present in polymyositis or dermatomyositis and are not characteristic of hepatocellular carcinoma. They do not occur in Duchenne muscular dystrophy, which is due to a genetic defect and not due to an immune disorder.

ME-C125   CORRECT RESPONSE D

The clinical picture is that of a young man who has developed a tendency to suffer frequent episodes of normal bacterial infections. This is a typical picture of acquired hypogammaglobulinaemia. *Recurrent infections associated with acquired hypo-gammaglobulinaemia are largely prevented by recurrent intravenous infusions of immunoglobulin.*

Acquired immune deficiency syndrome is not characterised by an increased frequency of common bacterial infection. The plasma electrophoretogram may be normal in humoral immune deficiency. Congenital agammaglobulinaemia would have presented well before the age of 16 years. An isolated defect in cell-mediated immune function is not characterised by recurrent bacterial infections.

SUMMARY OF CORRECT RESPONSES

CATEGORY & QUESTION NO.	CORRECT RESPONSE	CATEGORY & QUESTION NO.	CORRECT RESPONSE	CATEGORY & QUESTION NO.	CORRECT RESPONSE
ME-Q 1	C	ME-Q 32	D	ME-Q 63	C
ME-Q 2	D	ME-Q 33	B	ME-Q 64	B
ME-Q 3	A	ME-Q 34	D	ME-Q 65	E
ME-Q 4	B	ME-Q 35	D	ME-Q 66	E
ME-Q 5	B	ME-Q 36	D	ME-Q 67	B
ME-Q 6	C	ME-Q 37	B	ME-Q 68	C
ME-Q 7	D	ME-Q 38	B	ME-Q 69	E
ME-Q 8	C	ME-Q 39	D	ME-Q 70	E
ME-Q 9	D	ME-Q 40	E	ME-Q 71	E
ME-Q 10	B	ME-Q 41	B	ME-Q 72	D
ME-Q 11	B	ME-Q 42	D	ME-Q 73	C
ME-Q 12	E	ME-Q 43	E	ME-Q 74	B
ME-Q 13	C	ME-Q 44	B	ME-Q 75	A
ME-Q 14	C	ME-Q 45	B	ME-Q 76	D
ME-Q 15	A	ME-Q 46	D	ME-Q 77	C
ME-Q 16	C	ME-Q 47	C	ME-Q 78	E
ME-Q 17	E	ME-Q 48	D	ME-Q 79	E
ME-Q 18	D	ME-Q 49	C	ME-Q 80	B
ME-Q 19	C	ME-Q 50	C	ME-Q 81	B
ME-Q 20	E	ME-Q 51	D	ME-Q 82	D
ME-Q 21	C	ME-Q 52	A	ME-Q 83	B
ME-Q 22	E	ME-Q 53	B	ME-Q 84	B
ME-Q 23	C	ME-Q 54	B	ME-Q 85	D
ME-Q 24	D	ME-Q 55	D	ME-Q 86	D
ME-Q 25	D	ME-Q 56	B	ME-Q 87	D
ME-Q 26	D	ME-Q 57	D	ME-Q 88	D
ME-Q 27	A	ME-Q 58	B	ME-Q 89	E
ME-Q 28	C	ME-Q 59	C	ME-Q 90	C
ME-Q 29	D	ME-Q 60	E	ME-Q 91	E
ME-Q 30	B	ME-Q 61	D	ME-Q 92	A
ME-Q 31	A	ME-Q 62	E	ME-Q 93	E

CATEGORY & QUESTION NO.	CORRECT RESPONSE
ME-Q 94	B
ME-Q 95	E
ME-Q 96	E
ME-Q 97	D
ME-Q 98	C
ME-Q 99	C
ME-Q 100	D
ME-Q 101	C
ME-Q 102	C
ME-Q 103	D
ME-Q 104	C

CATEGORY & QUESTION NO.	CORRECT RESPONSE
ME-Q 105	A
ME-Q 106	C
ME-Q 107	A
ME-Q 108	D
ME-Q 109	D
ME-Q 110	B
ME-Q 111	A
ME-Q 112	A
ME-Q 113	D
ME-Q 114	B
ME-Q 115	B

CATEGORY & QUESTION NO.	CORRECT RESPONSE
ME-Q 116	D
ME-Q 117	E
ME-Q 118	D
ME-Q 119	D
ME-Q 120	B
ME-Q 121	E
ME-Q 122	D
ME-Q 123	E
ME-Q 124	C
ME-Q 125	D

Medicine
Commentaries
and Summary of Correct Responses

TYPE

J

Commentaries ME-C126 to ME-C205

Correct Responses ME-Q126 to ME-Q205

ME-C126   CORRECT RESPONSE B,D

This vascular malformation involves the first, second and part of the third division of the trigeminal nerve. This is an example of the cutaneous component of the Sturge-Weber syndrome (cephalofacial angiomatosis). This malformation is associated with cortical calcification and cerebral angiomatous malformation. Epilepsy is common. Fifty per cent of these patients also have glaucoma. Growth of the lesion is commensurate with the growth of the subject and will not regress with time. *A CT scan of the head and skull is indicated and may reveal accompanying cortical calcification and cerebral vascular malformation.* Serum calcium, phosphate and alkaline phosphatase are normal. *Treatment with laser will reduce the extent of the vascular malformation and is the treatment of choice.* Low dose radiotherapy is contraindicated in a child.

ME-C127   CORRECT RESPONSE A,B,C

These well demarcated discoid lesions with an apparent inflammatory periphery are typical of a *Microsporum canis* fungal infection ('ring-worm'). Other possibilities are patches of discoid eczema, psoriasis or the herald patches of pityriasis rosea. However, fungal infection is most likely. *Appropriate treatment would be an imidazole antifungal cream (miconazole, clotrimazole) and systemic antifungals (griseofulvin).* Nystatin cream is mainly used for yeast infections, such as candidias, and is not indicated; topical steroids are not appropriate for fungal infections.

ME-C128   CORRECT RESPONSE B,C,D,E

The picture shows multiple well demarcated red plaques with some silver scales, typical of psoriasis. *Psoriasis is made worse by the use of lithium, beta-adrenergic blocking agents, antimalarial drugs* and non-steroidal anti-inflammatory medication. *Psoriasis can also be precipitated by the withdrawal of systemic steroids.* Antihistamines do not have any significant effect on psoriasis.

ME-C129   CORRECT RESPONSE A,C

The clinical vignette is that of the progressive onset of dementia. *The loss of memory and self-care skills in a 75-year-old could not be regarded as the normal ageing process.* Multi-infarct dementia is approximately one-third as common as Alzheimer dementia and, in the absence of any signs suggesting previous infarction or generalised cerebrovascular disease, would be an unlikely diagnosis.

Investigation of such a patient should include tests for reversible metabolic causes of dementia, such as hypothyroidism and B_{12} deficiency. *A CT scan is required to exclude intracranial lesions*, such as hydrocephalus and meningioma, which may present with the slow onset of dementia. However, there are no changes in the CT scan from which one can make the diagnosis reliably of Alzheimer disease. Although the possibility of concomitant depression should be considered in such a patient, the diagnosis should be made on the basis of symptoms and the clinical findings and not on a trial of medication.

ME-C130   CORRECT RESPONSE A,B

An altered level of consciousness or loss of memory can occur with vertebrobasilar insufficiency because of bilateral medial temporal lobe ischaemia. The blood supply of that area of the temporal lobe is from branches of the posterior cerebral artery.

Complex partial seizures by definition imply an altered level of consciousness of which the patient may have little memory. Another cause of amnesia for a period of 8 h is transient global amnesia. It occurs typically in men over 55, but can occur in women and may follow exercise. Whether or not this disorder is a form of vertebrobasilar insufficiency in which no other symptoms are apparent remains to be determined.

Internal carotid stenosis can produce a transient feeling of lightheadedness. However, it would be most unlikely to produce memory loss for 8 h. The areas concerned with memory are predominantly supplied by the posterior cerebral circulation.

In Wernicke encephalopathy, a confusional state is usually present, which lasts for longer than 8 h and the symptoms are more profound than a loss of memory. After recovery from the confusional state, the patient may have Korsakoff amnestic confabulatory syndrome. This is permanent in most patients, but there may be partial recovery over a period of many months with thiamine supplementation, good nutrition and abstinence from alcohol.

ME-C131   CORRECT RESPONSE A,B,C,D

A unilateral tremor, most commonly in the dominant side, is one typical mode of onset of Parkinson disease. Occasionally it may occur many years before the development of generalised Parkinson disease.

Dribbling and excessive salivation are also features of Parkinson disease. The dribbling is associated with a tendency to leave the mouth open and immobility of the mouth. There appears to be an excessive production of saliva in some patients; the mechanism for this is not clear.

The shuffling gait of Parkinson disease is very characteristic with the patient being generally flexed and taking small steps.

A tremor that occurs during relaxation of the arms and abates with activity is also typical of Parkinson disease. This serves to differentiate a parkinsonian tremor from benign essential tremor in which the tremor is always absent at rest and is made worse by muscle activity.

Distal weakness does not occur in Parkinson disease and its presence would suggest that there is another disease process.

ME-C132   CORRECT RESPONSE A,B,C,D,E

Myoclonic jerks, which are short sharp contractions of muscles, are associated with a number of disorders. *They occur during normal sleep. They can occur as a specific form of epilepsy or can occur in patients who have other forms of epilepsy. They occur in a number of forms of encephalitis, typically in the later stages of Creutzfeldt-Jacob disease and in other forms of subacute encephalitis. Multiple myoclonic jerks can also be a feature in patients with uraemia* and will respond to treatment for the uraemia.

ME-C133   CORRECT RESPONSE D,E

The middle cerebral artery supplies most of the convexity of the cerebral hemisphere. *A lesion on the left side would involve the areas concerned with speech and would thus produce dysphasia and would also involve most of the parietal lobe, resulting in a constructional apraxia.*

Diplopia arises from the nuclei of the cranial nerves, which are in the brainstem and are supplied by the basilar artery. Similarly, nystagmus is usually vestibular, brainstem or cerebellar in origin.

The areas involved with consciousness are deep in the thalamus and in the midbrain, are bilateral and are supplied by the vertebral artery and perforating branches of the vertebral artery. Even infarction of the entire territory of the middle cerebral artery does not alter the level of consciousness.

ME-C134   CORRECT RESPONSE A,E

Tremor that occurs only on activity and is not present at rest is usually either *benign essential tremor or exaggerated physiological tremor. Exaggerated physiological tremor occurs in hyperthyroidism.*

The tremor of Parkinson disease typically occurs at rest and is suppressed rather than augmented by activity. Several types of tremor are associated with multiple sclerosis: either a red nucleus tremor, which is a gross flapping tremor occurring while maintaining a posture, or an 'intention tremor' due to involvement of the cerebellum. 'Intention tremor' is not strictly a tremor in that it is a random rather than an oscillatory repetitive movement which occurs during attempts to produce precise movement.

ME-C135   CORRECT RESPONSE B

The response to painful stimuli in someone with a diazepam overdose indicates a moderate level of coma. *One would expect shallow and slow respirations due to the direct respiratory depression by diazepam.* A fixed dilated pupil would indicate a lateralised intracranial or high midbrain lesion and would not be consistent with diazepam overdose alone. Pinpoint pupils suggest a brainstem lesion, particularly a pontine haemorrhage and again would be inconsistent with coma solely due to diazepam overdose.

Bilateral extensor plantar responses may develop with profound coma in someone without a structural lesion of the nervous system. However, it is unlikely to be seen when the patient is responding to painful stimuli. If present at this level of coma, it would indicate a lesion of the central nervous system. The decerebrate posture may be seen in deep coma, but it is unlikely to be present in deep coma due to diazepam overdose, because the diazepam will suppress muscle tone.

ME-C136   CORRECT RESPONSE A,B,C

Optic neuritis classically produces a central scotoma in the affected eye. The lesion must be anterior to the optic chiasm.

An enlarged blind spot occurs with papilloedema. The blind spot is the representation in the visual field of the nerve head and when the nerve head swells the blind spot enlarges.

Constricted visual fields occur in glaucoma due to decreased peripheral perfusion because of the raised pressure and damage to nerve fibres in the optic cup.

Bitemporal hemianopia arises from involvement of the crossing fibres in the optic chiasm. An occipital infarct will produce a contralateral homonymous hemianopia.

Homonymous hemianopia can occur from a lesion anywhere from behind the optic chiasm, along the optic track, lateral geniculate body, the optic radiation or the optic cortex. Homonymous hemianopia cannot occur with lesions in front of the chiasm, such as an optic nerve glioma. An optic nerve glioma will produce a field defect or scotoma in one eye.

ME-C137   CORRECT RESPONSE D

Spastic paraparesis arises from bilateral involvement of the pyramidal tract. *This occurs in cervical spondylosis where the pressure backwards on the dura of a disc or osteophytes compromises the anterior spinal artery and produces an ischaemic lesion of the corticospinal and related tracts.* Both Guillain–Barré syndrome and lumbar canal stenosis produce lower motor neuron lesions and are not associated with spasticity. In Parkinson disease there is an increase in tone, but this is of the rigid type: it is constant throughout the range of movement and augments on inattention, whereas spasticity is characterised by a sudden 'catch' occurring during the first part of passive movement. Alzheimer disease primarily affects intellectual function and spastic paraparesis is not a function of that disorder.

ME-C138   CORRECT RESPONSE A,D,E

Three of the drugs listed are well known to induce peripheral neuritis. *Nitrofurantoin can cause a severe sensorimotor neuropathy, particularly if there is renal failure. Isoniazid can produce peripheral neuropathy, which is common in patients treated for tuberculosis.* The peripheral neuropathy may be improved with small doses of pyridoxine.

Vincristine produces a mild degree of neuropathy in most patients in whom it is used. In some patients it may produce a severe sensorimotor neuropathy requiring cessation of the drug.

ME-C139   CORRECT RESPONSE A,C,D

Mononeuritis multiplex is a disorder in which multiple individual peripheral nerves are involved in a disease process. *This can occur in polyarteritis nodosa where there are multiple infarcts in nerves. Scattered vascular lesions also occur in diabetes. In sarcoidosis, there can be invasion of individual nerves with granulomatous tissue, producing a mononeuritis multiplex picture.*

However, both thiamine deficiency and vitamin B_{12} deficiency produce a metabolic disorder affecting all nerves and, therefore, produce a generalised neuropathy. As the longer nerves are more likely to be metabolically compromised than shorter nerves, the symptoms are usually more marked peripherally.

ME-C140   CORRECT RESPONSE A,C,D

The small muscles of the hand (interossei, lumbricals, thenar and hypothenar muscles) are supplied by the *T1 nerve roots*, the fibres responsible for this motor supply passing through the lower trunk of the brachial plexus. Most of these fibres subsequently enter the ulnar nerve, others enter the median nerve.

Spondylitic compression of the T1 nerve root will produce wasting and weakness affecting all the small muscles of the hand (Klumpke paralysis).

An ulnar nerve lesion at the elbow will spare those small muscles of the thumb innervated by the median nerve and will also involve the ulnar-sided long deep flexors of the fingers.

Angulation of the lower trunk of the brachial plexus over a cervical rib will affect the lower trunk of the plexus, particularly the T1 fibres, to produce wasting of all small muscles.

Similarly, *apical carcinoma of the lung* may invade the lower part of the brachial plexus to cause a T1 lesion (Pancoast syndrome).

In the carpal tunnel syndrome, the median nerve is compressed at the wrist. The only small muscles supplied by the median nerve are the abductor and flexor pollicis brevis and opponens pollicis. Although weakness of abductor pollicis brevis is often detected, weakness of all the small muscles of the hand does not occur with a carpal tunnel syndrome, which affects only the median nerve at the wrist.

ME-C141   CORRECT RESPONSE C

Compression of the first sacral root will result in a loss of the ankle jerk. If there is associated weakness it will be of plantar flexion of the foot. Bladder function is mediated by the lower sacral nerves and would not be affected by an S1 root lesion. The knee jerk is mediated predominantly by the L4 nerve root and is not altered by an S1 lesion. Foot drop is due predominantly to weakness of the tibialis anterior muscle which is supplied from L5 through the common peroneal nerve. It is unaffected by an S1 root lesion. The quadriceps muscle is supplied by L2–3–4 (predominantly L4) and not by S1, so that the quadriceps is not weak with an S1 root lesion.

ME-C142   CORRECT RESPONSE B,C,D

Carbamazepine (Tegretol®) is an anticonvulsant commonly used as the initial treatment for epilepsy. It is thought to act by blocking sodium channels and decreasing the firing rate of rapidly firing neurons. *It is useful for complex partial seizures and generalised tonic clonic seizures. It is also an effective treatment for trigeminal neuralgia* with, in the first instance, more than half the patients responding. It does not however have an effect on cluster headache. The preferred treatment for Petit-mal seizures is sodium valproate or ethosuximide. Patients with Petit-mal seizures do not respond to carbamazepine.

ME-C143   CORRECT RESPONSE A

Prochlorperazine (Stemetil®) is effective in controlling the symptoms of vertigo. It is a purely symptomatic treatment and the response will last for approximately 8 h. There are serious side effects with long-term use. It may produce tardive dyskinesia which does not always regress on cessation of the medication. Unsteadiness of gait, except when it is due to vertigo, will not respond to prochlorperazine. Senile tremor and dizziness when standing do not respond to prochlorperazine. Prochlorperazine is not a treatment for Parkinson disease and may in fact cause parkinsonism.

ME-C144   CORRECT RESPONSE A,C

Osteoporosis occurs most commonly in postmenopausal women and is much less frequently seen in men. It is usually asymptomatic and *is usually associated with a normal serum calcium*. Osteoporosis is not a contraindication to antidepressive therapy, although certain drugs (such as phenytoin) can cause osteoporosis. The use of hormone replacement therapy decreases the risk of developing osteoporosis. Osteoporosis is not caused by oral contraceptives, in fact they increase bone mass.

ME-C145   CORRECT RESPONSE A,C

Gout can occur as a complication of haematological disease, especially when there is a rapid turnover of cells. *The two conditions listed in which gout is most likely to occur are polycythaemia vera and myelofibrosis.* Gout does not normally occur in chronic lymphocytic leukaemia unless there is an unusually rapid response to treatment and gout is not associated with portal hypertension or with systemic lupus erythematosus.

ME-C146   CORRECT RESPONSE A,C

A typical change of severe childhood nutritional rickets is increased prominence of the costochondral junctions. This usually persists into adult life. *There is also an increase in serum alkaline phosphatase.*

There is no haemorrhagic tendency with rickets nor is there hypertrophy of the gums. Both of these can be seen in vitamin C deficiency (scurvy). Rickets is associated with decreased serum calcium and nephrocalcinosis does not occur.

ME-C147 CORRECT RESPONSE B,C

In cardiac tamponade there is usually a tachycardia (not bradycardia), as the cardiac output is being maintained by increasing the heart rate with a fixed stroke volume. The clinical signs of cardiac tamponade are related to a fixed stroke output of the right ventricle (RV). *The jugular venous pressure (JVP) is usually raised, because of the reduced cardiac output from the restricted RV.* The JVP may rise with inspiration, due to increased venous return and a fixed RV output. The pulmonary arterial bed increases in volume with inspiration. As the output of the RV cannot increase, as occurs normally during inspiration due to increased venous return, the outflow from the lungs is decreased, so that the output from the left ventricle is decreased, *resulting in a fall in systemic blood pressure during inspiration.*

Because of the relatively low flow in the lung, if the chest X-ray is abnormal, it shows a reduction in vasculature rather than pulmonary oedema. A pericardial friction rub may be heard; a rub is less common when tamponade develops from an enlarging effusion, but its presence does not exclude an effusion.

ME-C148 CORRECT RESPONSE A,C

Mitral valve prolapse is more common in women. It may be (but is not always) accompanied by a systolic click and a late systolic murmur. Indeed, most mitral valve prolapses are diagnosed on echocardiography and not from physical signs. *A prolapsing mitral valve can be the site of infective endocarditis and can be the source of systemic embolism.* There is an increased prevalence of mitral valve prolapse in young patients with stroke. The volume of blood leaking into the left atrium is not haemodynamically significant and does not result in left ventricular hypertrophy.

ME-C149 CORRECT RESPONSE A,B,D

The pressure in the left ventricle is normally greater than that of the right so that *a shunt through the ventricular septum will be from left to right and the shunt can be diagnosed by cardiac ultrasound.* In the uncommon circumstance that pulmonary hypertension has developed and that the right ventricular pressure has risen to above that of the left, then such a shunt may reverse. Atrial fibrillation is not a feature of ventricular septal defect (VSD). It is associated with structural lesions which increase the pressure and sometimes the volume load on the left atrium. Because the flow through the lungs is the sum of the cardiac output and the shunt flow, there is dilatation of the pulmonary vasculature and increased lung markings on X-ray. Even when severe pulmonary hypertension develops, any reduction in pulmonary vasculature will be peripheral. In contrast to atrial septal defect, which is in a low pressure area, *bacterial endocarditis may complicate VSD.*

ME-C150 CORRECT RESPONSE A,B,E

The initial treatment of this patient should include reducing the pulse rate, controlling hypertension and treating the congestive heart failure. *Digitalis would be appropriate for controlling the heart rate. Angiotensin-converting enzyme (ACE) inhibitors could be used*, both to reduce the blood pressure and to help control the heart failure. They have the advantage over other antihypertensives in this situation in that *they will lower the blood pressure and reduce sodium and water retention.* Hypokalaemia is not a side effect of ACE inhibitors. A diuretic would normally also be used.

Given the presence of congestive biventricular failure, beta-blocking agents would not be the most appropriate initial therapy and digitalis is preferred to control atrial fibrillation. Recent studies have suggested that beta-blocker therapy, particularly the vasodilator beta-blockers (e.g. carvedilol), may have a place in the treatment of congestive heart failure.

ME-C151   CORRECT RESPONSE A,B,E

The clinical picture presented is that of myocardial infarction with hypotension and tachycardia. The appropriate treatment would be to *relieve pain with narcotics, to commence thrombolytic therapy*, preferably with tissue plasminogen activator (tPA), *raise the blood pressure and lower the pulse rate with carefully administered fluids.*

Vasodilators, which may reduce the load on the heart, will diminish the blood pressure and further increase the pulse rate and are not indicated. Diuretics are also not indicated because of the risk of further reduction in blood pressure.

ME-C152   CORRECT RESPONSE A,B,D

The patient has a number of predisposing factors to hypertension, particularly obesity and smoking. *He should be advised to stop smoking, moderate his intake of salt and alcohol*, reduce weight and undertake a programme of exercise. *Other risk factors of hypercholesterolaemia and diabetes should also be checked.* In some patients these measures may be sufficient to reduce the blood pressure to an acceptable level.

Although the urine should be tested for protein, detailed microscopic examination of the urine is unlikely to be helpful. A CT scan of his head would not be justified, unless there were signs suggestive of Cushing syndrome.

ME-C153   CORRECT RESPONSE A,C

The reduction in death from heart failure was one of the first major benefits demonstrated by large scale trials of the treatment of hypertension.

Although thiazide diuretics have been the major treatment used in large trials, they have the disadvantages of decreasing glucose tolerance and increasing cholesterol levels.

Adrenergic beta-blocking agents can exacerbate the symptoms of peripheral vascular disease and reduce claudication distance; and should be used with caution in symptomatic patients.

Population studies have shown that the risk of stroke correlates best with systolic, not diastolic, blood pressure and that lowering the elevated systolic blood pressure of patients with normal diastolic pressures still results in a major reduction in stroke incidence.

Some trials of hypertension treatment have shown a slight rise in mortality if the elevated diastolic blood pressure is lowered below 80–85 mmHg, a 'J' curve effect. However, the increased mortality appears to be in those patients who have a prior history of ischaemic heart disease. In otherwise well patients there is no good evidence that lowering the blood pressure below 130/80 mmHg carries any incresed risk. A systolic pressure of 130 mmHg or less gives the best protection from stroke. This issue is still controversial and is being addressed in clinical trials (e.g. the Hypertension Optimal Treatment Study).

ME-C154   CORRECT RESPONSE A,D,E

The patient has a well controlled blood pressure and medication should be continued to maintain blood pressure at this level. After a stroke the maintenance of a normal blood pressure significantly reduces the incidence of further stoke. *The pulse rate of 95 /min indicates that the atrial fibrillation is not well controlled and the patient should be digitalised.*

The probable cause of the stroke was embolism from the heart. The risk of recurrence in the first year is approximately 15%. *Warfarin reduces the risk of recurrent stroke in patients with atrial fibrillation by up to 85%,* aspirin by approximately 54%. *Warfarin is the preferred medication.* Combined therapy with aspirin is contraindicated because of the significantly increased risk of bleeding.

ME-C155   CORRECT RESPONSE B,C

Cessation of smoking certainly reduces vascular risk. Within 5 years of cessation, the risk of stroke is not statistically different from that of non-smokers. However, the cessation of smoking may not result in an immediate reduction in blood pressure as smoking may be inducing a mild vasodilatation. Indeed, a mild rise in blood pressure may occur on cessation, particularly if there is weight gain.

The family history of ischaemic heart disease, particularly in her mother, increases the risk of vascular disease.

The body mass index of 28 and hypertension per se *are likely to be associated with increased insulin resistance* and a glucose tolerance test may be abnormal. Thiazide diuretics are not appropriate as first-line therapy in this woman because they increase insulin resistance and may elevate the cholesterol level.

The most important therapeutic measures for her would be to reduce weight, lower plasma cholesterol, control blood pressure and to cease smoking. Only if these measures (coupled with drug treatment) fail, should further investigation be considered. A renal angiogram is not indicated at this stage as it is very unlikely to show a treatable abnormality.

ME-C156   CORRECT RESPONSE A,C,D,E

The question describes a man on *the verge of hypertensive heart failure, as indicated by the orthopnoea. Even though the ejection fraction is 60%, the end diastolic pressure in the ventricle is almost certainly increased. The likely diagnosis is significant diastolic heart failure.*

The left ventricular hypertrophy increases the risk of developing heart failure, myocardial ischaemia, myocardial infarction and stroke.

The most important treatment would be to decrease the blood pressure, thus decreasing the work of the heart. *As he is already on atenolol in an adequate dose, further increasing the dose is unlikely to be of benefit* and another antihypertensive of a different type should be added. Beta-blocking drugs are not contraindicated; indeed, if he has tachycardia and probable diastolic heart failure as noted, their continuation along with another anti-hypertensive agent may be of benefit.

In addition, a number of other measures should be introduced. *He should be advised to reduce his drinking and to lose weight, as both of these factors can contribute significantly to hypertension.*

ME-C157   CORRECT RESPONSE B,C,D

The onset of a systolic murmur and heart failure in acute myocardial infarction suggests acute mitral incompetence, *from either a ruptured papillary muscle, or a dysfunctioning papillary muscle or a ventricular septal rupture.*

Tricuspid regurgitation is not a complication of myocardial infarction, as infarction rarely involves the right ventricle. Left ventricular outflow tract obstruction is a chronic phenomenon that does not develop acutely immediately after myocardial infarction.

ME-C158 CORRECT RESPONSE C

A non-productive cough is a well recognised side effect of angiotensin-converting enzyme (ACE) inhibitors. It can occur at any time after the commencement of the therapy, but not commonly within the first weeks.

The development of a cough induced by an ACE inhibitor is not an absolute contraindication to further ongoing ACE inhibitor therapy and sometimes lowering the dose is effective in controlling the cough. However, changing to a different ACE inhibitor will not usually result in relief of the cough.

ME-C159 CORRECT RESPONSE A,B,C,E

A steady state plasma level is normally achieved after three or four doses of a drug given at the interval of its half-life. For this reason *digoxin given daily (with a half-life of 24 h) would take 3–5 days before a steady state level is achieved. A steady state plasma level of a drug can be achieved much more rapidly by using a loading dose.* In this case, the suggested loading dose of four-fold the maintenance dose would be very adequate to rapidly establish a steady state plasma level. *Verapamil increases the half-life of digoxin and reducing the dose of digoxin should be considered when using that drug.*

Atrial fibrillation in thyrotoxicosis can be very difficult to control and higher doses than usual may be required. *Digoxin binds to cholestyramine and this will reduce digoxin available for absorption.* When drugs that alter the half-life of digoxin are used it is advisable to measure digoxin levels until a stable steady state is reached.

ME-C160 CORRECT RESPONSE A,C

Severe central chest pain, radiating through to the back in a patient who has been hypertensive for years suggests an acute dissection of the aorta. The ECG changes would be consistent with this. The appropriate management would be *to control hypertension and arrange for an urgent CT scan of the chest.* Anticoagulants, anti-aggregants and thrombolytic therapy should be withheld until dissection has been excluded. Elevated enzymes do not exclude a dissection.

ME-C161 CORRECT RESPONSE A,B,D

Appropriate treatment for unstable angina is *the admission to a coronary care unit for monitoring and the administration of aspirin and heparin.* Thrombolytic therapy has no beneficial effect in unstable angina and an exercise test would at this stage be contraindicated.

ME-C162 CORRECT RESPONSE B,C,E

The clinical picture is that of a man with chronic airways obstruction who is hypoxic and acidotic but in whom the $P_a\text{co}_2$ is low. Given the low level of $P_a\text{co}_2$, he is not in acute respiratory failure.

This blood gas pattern could be related to superimposed acute left ventricular failure with pulmonary oedema decreasing his diffusing capacity for oxygen and associated hyperventilation lowering his $P_a\text{co}_2$. *The same situation could occur with acute bacteraemic shock.* Given that he has a low $P_a\text{co}_2$ and a low pH, *this is compatible with a primary metabolic acidosis and lactic acidosis could reasonably account for this.*

He is hypoxic with a low P_aCO_2 so that supplemental oxygen is unlikely to be dangerous in this man. Indeed his confusion and dyspnoea would be expected to improve with oxygen therapy. His deterioration is also unlikely to be due to administration of a sedative drug. The usual effect of a sedative drug is to decrease ventilation and produce a picture of respiratory failure with a raised P_aCO_2.

ME-C163   CORRECT RESPONSE B,D,E

Three possible causative agents for occupational asthma are listed. Toluene di-isocyanate, western red cedar dust and flour may all cause an asthma syndrome which has the typical pattern of occupational asthma (i.e. patients in whom the severity of asthma progressively increases during the working week).

Asthma induced by western red cedar dust may be absent for the first 2 or 3 days of the working week. The asthma improves or abates during the weekend, but recurs the following week. Neither silica (which produces the fibrosis of silicosis) nor asbestos (which produces a typical change of asbestosis and occasionally mesothelioma) produce asthma-like syndromes.

ME-C164   CORRECT RESPONSE D

The sensation of breathlessness or dyspnoea described by patients usually reflects the fact that they are aware of an increased effort required to breathe. Many patients with arterial hypoxaemia and cyanosis, raised P_aCO_2 and acidosis and altered diffusing capacity of the lung will have severe respiratory impairment, as judged by pulmonary mechanics and blood gases. However, they often do not experience any dyspnoea.

ME-C165   CORRECT RESPONSE B,E

The presence or absence of rhonchi is not a reliable indicator of airway obstruction. The sound is dependent upon the velocity of the airflow, which relates both to the volume of air moving through the bronchi and the diameter of the bronchi. In mild airway obstruction, the increase in flow rate due to the reduction in bronchial diameter may not be sufficient to produce rhonchi. In severe airway obstruction the flow may be so reduced that rhonchi are not produced.

Bronchial breathing is typically heard at the top of a pleural effusion. It is probably related to local collapse and the presence of a sound-conducting medium between the large airways and the surface of the chest.

Inspiratory stridor is atypical in asthma. In asthma, stridor is predominantly expiratory partly because of the tendency of the diameter of bronchi to be reduced during expiration. Inspiratory stridor is suggestive of an obstructive lesion higher in the bronchial tree.

Crepitations (crackles) are usually not heard throughout inspiration in the presence of airway obstruction. Crepitations are related to the opening and closing of alveoli, which are not primarily affected in airway obstruction. The disorder in which crepitations are characteristically heard throughout inspiration is idiopathic pulmonary fibrosis.

Bronchial breathing is heard over consolidated lungs. As indicated above, the auscultation of bronchial breathing is dependent on the presence of a sound-conducting pathway between a large bronchus and the surface of the chest wall.

ME-C166   CORRECT RESPONSE E

Bronchogenic carcinoma can present with hypokalaemia. This occurs typically with small cell carcinoma, due to the production of an ACTH-like hormone. The prognosis when hypokalaemia is present is usually poor.

It is not possible to exclude a carcinoma of the lung even with a normal chest X-ray. For example, clubbing and hypertrophic pulmonary osteoarthropathy can occur from carcinoma of the lung before it is visible on a chest X-ray. The diagnosis of carcinoma of the lung is often established by bronchoscopy. However, fine needle biopsy can also be used to sample tissue which is not within the range of the bronchoscope. If the carcinoma has metastasised to the lymph nodes, biopsy of a lymph node can also produce a definitive diagnosis.

In patients operated on for carcinoma of the lung in whom a curative lobectomy is attempted, only 30% survive 5 years and 15% survive 10 years. When patients who have a palliative resection are included the survival rate is even lower.

ME-C167   CORRECT RESPONSE D,E

Ninety per cent of all types of carcinomas of the lung, including small cell carcinoma, are associated with cigarette smoking. When a non-smoker develops carcinoma of the lung it is usually an adenocarcinoma. *At the time of diagnosis the majority of patients with small cell carcinoma have metastases beyond the hilar lymph nodes.* Because of metastases it is uncommon for a small cell carcinoma to be resectable and the 5 year survival rate after apparent curative resection is very low. The most common mode of treatment is combination chemotherapy, using several antimitotic drugs simultaneously. Various combinations are used; they may include cyclophosphamide, vincristine and cisplatinum. Single cytotoxic drug therapy is not regarded as appropriate. Radiotherapy can also be used, particularly for metastatic disease.

Both small cell and non-small cell carcinomas can produce hormones. The most common with a small cell carcinoma is an ACTH-like hormone and the non-small cell carcinoma can produce a parathormone-like prohormone. *Small cell carcinoma may also produce degeneration of the Purkinje cells of the cerebellum and several antibodies to cerebellar neuronal protein have been described.*

ME-C168   CORRECT RESPONSE C,D

Pulmonary sarcoidosis is most often characterised by hilar lymph node enlargement, which is usually bilateral. The next most common picture is of bilateral hilar lymph-adenopathy with diffuse parenchymal changes. Parenchymal changes without hilar lymphadenopathy are uncommon. One of the characteristics of the pulmonary lesions is that they do not cavitate.

Erythema nodosum is the typical skin manifestation of pulmonary sarcoidosis. It usually occurs on the anterior surface of the lower leg. Associated cutaneous anergy results in the tuberculin skin test and other related tests becoming negative.

In the majority of patients with pulmonary sarcoidosis, the disorder resolves spontaneously with or without the use of corticosteroids. Hypercalcaemia is a well recognised but uncommon complication of sarcoidosis. It does not indicate skeletal involvement and is probably related to increased absorption of calcium from the gut. Bone lesions are seen in approximately 5% of patients, usually in the form of rounded, well-defined punched-out lesions. These are most commonly in the hands and feet, but any bone may be involved.

ME-C169   CORRECT RESPONSE C,D,E

Idiopathic pulmonary fibrosis has a typical clinical picture in which the patient is usually cyanosed **with finger clubbing and** tachypnoeic with shallow respiration. **Examination of the chest usually shows widespread bilateral inspiratory crepitations** extending particularly into the midzones. Diagnosis can be made on the clinical signs and chest X-ray. **Alveolar washings usually show increased neutrophil and eosinophil counts.** Positive antinuclear and rheumatoid factors are not characteristic of idiopathic pulmonary fibrosis. However, a negative rheumatoid factor does not absolutely exclude rheumatoid as the aetiological cause of fibrotic lung disease.

Blood gases in idiopathic pulmonary fibrosis typically show hypoxia and hypocapnia, with a lowered P_aCO_2. This occurs because the altered diffusing capacity mainly affects the diffusion of oxygen. The patient hyperventilates to increase the plasma oxygen and at the same time lowers the P_aCO_2. When respiratory failure occurs, it is hypoxic and not hypercapnic.

ME-C170   CORRECT RESPONSE D

The treatment alternatives suggested in the answer of the treatment of chronic bronchitis are predominantly symptomatic. **The only measure shown which can prevent the progression of the disorder is the cessation of smoking cigarettes.** Even in severe bouts of chronic bronchitis survival can be improved by cessation of cigarette smoking.

ME-C171   CORRECT RESPONSE A,C,D

Barrett oesophagus is acquired (not congenital) intestinal metaplasia of the epithelium at the lower end of the oesophagus. **The normal stratified squamous epithelium is replaced by columnar epithelium. It is caused by gastro-oesophageal reflux and is a precancerous condition.** It is not reversible.

ME-C172   CORRECT RESPONSE A,B,C,D,E

Hepatitis A is a self-limiting form of hepatitis and **does not lead to chronic infection.** It is usually a mild form of hepatitis but **death can occasionally occur from a fulminant attack.** It is usually transmitted by the faeco–oral route and **not by the parenteral route. The excretion of the virus into the faeces diminishes at the time of onset of the the clinical disease. Close associates of the patient can be protected by an injection of gamma globulin, which will reduce the attack rate markedly if given within 2 weeks of exposure.**

ME-C173   CORRECT RESPONSE A

Delta hepatitis (hepatitis D) is caused by a defective virus and is dependent absolutely on the presence of hepatitis B for its infectivity.

Hepatitis C is a common cause of chronic continuing hepatitis. Cirrhosis may develop in up to 50% of patients with hepatitis C and there is a significant increase in hepatocellular carcinoma.

There is no difference between the effectiveness of plasma-derived vaccines and recombinant vaccines. Jaundice in hepatitis A is more common in children than in adults. Hepatitis A infection is not diagnosed in the acute phase by the presence of anti-HAV IgG antibodies. The presence of IgG antibodies occurs later in the disorder, 6 weeks to 9 months after the acute phase of the illness.

ME-C174   CORRECT RESPONSE A,B,E

There is no difference in the serum conversion rate for hepatitis B immunisation depending on the source of the vaccine. The vaccine is given by intramuscular injection.

Babies at risk should be vaccinated and also be given immune serum. The vaccine can be administered to chronic carriers without harm and recombinant vaccine can be used as a booster after primary vaccination with plasma-derived vaccine.

ME-C175   CORRECT RESPONSE C

Chronic pancreatitis normally presents with pain as the only symptom and with no physical signs. The serum amylase is normal or is mildly elevated. Some patients will have pancreatic calcification seen on the plain X-ray of the abdomen but this is not invariable. Chronic pancreatitis is most commonly associated with alcoholism. Acute pancreatitis has a greater association with cholelithiasis than does chronic pancreatitis. The finding of an abdominal mass is uncommon in chronic pancreatitis and if an abdominal mass is found it is usually a pancreatic pseudocyst following an episode of acute pancreatitis.

The diabetes associated with acute pancreatitis usually requires relatively low doses of insulin. In diabetes mellitus it is the peripheral insulin resistance which increases the requirement for insulin.

ME-C176   CORRECT RESPONSE A,B,D,E

All of the malignant tumours listed are chemosensitive except chondrosarcoma. *Decreased mortality as a result of chemotherapy has been demonstrated in small cell lung cancer, lymphoma, testicular cancer and breast cancer.* Chondrosarcoma is not sensitive to chemotherapy and excisional surgery is usually required for cure.

ME-C177   CORRECT RESPONSE B,D

Pseudomembranous enterocolitis is due to overgrowth of Clostridium difficile *with the production of a toxin, which can be found in the stool.* It is usually precipitated by the use of broad spectrum antibiotics and prolonged periods of treatment are not necessary to produce this disorder. *It responds well to oral vancomycin.*

ME-C178   CORRECT RESPONSE B,C,E

Gynaecomastia in the male is seen as a variant of normal ageing (senile gynaecomastia) and as a side effect of several drugs. *Spironolactone and histamine H_2 receptor antagonists are two such drugs that block the binding of androgens in target tissues.*

Gynaecomastia is also common in men with cirrhosis of the liver in which it is thought to be due to portal–systemic shunting of testosterone with peripheral conversion to oestrogen.

Gynaecomastia is not usually due to excessive prolactin and is not a common feature of raised prolactin levels: a much more common feature of raised prolactin in men would be loss of libido. The appropriate therapy for gynaecomastia is to reverse the cause where possible. Surgery may be required for cosmetic purposes. Testosterone is ineffective.

ME-C179   CORRECT RESPONSE A,B,C,E

A raised serum prolactin level occurs in patients with severe primary hypothyroidism due either to elevated TRH or decreased dopaminergic tone.

Pituitary tumours of mixed type may produce both prolactinaemia and acromegaly and *elevated prolactin can cause hypogonadism. If the acromegaly is treated by hypophyseal adenectomy, the prolactin level will drop and hypogonadism will be reversed; if the remaining pituitary is damaged in the process, the hypogonadism may remain.*

The neural pathway for release of prolactin is dopamine dependent and can be blocked with bromocriptine.

In the adult male, elevated prolactin is a very uncommon cause of gynaecomastia.

The most common cause of raised serum prolactin is a pituitary microadenoma (less than 10 mm). Such adenomas are too small to expand the pituitary fossa and are usually associated with a normal skull X-ray. Many microadenomas, however, can be detected by CT and MR scans.

ME-C180   CORRECT RESPONSE A,B,C,D,E

Autoimmune adrenalitis is now the most common cause of Addison disease. In the past, tuberculosis would have been the most common cause. The adrenals can be replaced by metastatic carcinoma or may be involved with amyloid, due to chronic infection, or rheumatoid arthritis. Meningococcal septicaemia can produce a bilateral haemorrhagic infarction of the adrenals with acute and often fatal hypoadrenalism.

ME-C181   CORRECT RESPONSE A,B,C,D,E

The characteristic sweating, nervousness and flushing associated with phaeochromocytoma is due to excessive circulating catecholamines. Urinary 24 h catecholamines are raised in at least 95% of cases and this test is the most suitable method of establishing the diagnosis. Because of elevated circulating catecholamines *fasting blood sugar may also be increased.*

The increased blood pressure associated with phaeochromocytoma may be intermittent or the blood pressure may be raised continuously, even if other symptoms are episodic.

ME-C182   CORRECT RESPONSE A,C

The clinical picture is of a woman who has developed a sore throat and a tender enlarged thyroid gland with signs of thyrotoxicosis. There are also signs of a recent viral infection and a history of infection in her children. *This is a typical picture of subacute thyroiditis and is not the picture of Graves disease.* The presence of hyperthyroidism is confirmed by the raised T3 and T4, with suppression of TSH. Antithyroid antibodies would not be expected to be high in subacute thyroiditis.

A thyroid scan in subacute thyrodiitis, in contrast to Graves disease, is likely to show a decreased uptake of radioiodine. The picture of somebody who is taking thyroxine surreptitiously would be quite different with a marked suppression of TSH and T3 levels. The disorder of subacute thyroiditis is usually self-limiting and treatment with radioiodine, particularly in a 25-year-old woman, would be quite inappropriate.

ME-C183   CORRECT RESPONSE A,C,E

High doses of oestrogen are associated with an increased incidence of arterial and venous thrombosis. This occurs particularly with 50 μg or higher daily doses of ethinyl oestradiol. The increase is particularly in the incidence of deep venous thrombosis. However, some evidence has suggested that high dose oestrogen oral contraceptives are also associated with a significant incidence of stroke; there is a lesser increase with the lower dose oestrogens and no significant change with progesterone contraceptives. Hormone-replacement therapy with oestrogen patches appears to be associated with a slight decrease in the incidence of stroke and other thrombotic complications.

Migraine can become more frequent after high doses of oral contraceptives. Once the headaches have been precipitated it may take up to 6 months after cessation of treatment for the headaches to regress.

A small rise in blood pressure has also been noted with high dose oestrogen contraceptives. High doses of oestrogen, however, do not produce frigidity or depression, and usually suppress rather than induce dysmenorrhea.

ME-C184   CORRECT RESPONSE B,D,E

With ageing there are alterations in the male sexual response. *There is a need for more direct stimulation of the penis to achieve an erection. The time between successive erections (refractory period) is increased and the volume of semen is decreased.* However, there is neither an alteration in the ability to enjoy sexual activity nor a tendency to ejaculate prematurely.

ME-C185   CORRECT RESPONSE A,B,E

The erythrocyte sedimentation rate (ESR) reflects rouleaux formation in red cells. This is effected predominantly by proteins adhering to red cells. *An increased ESR can, therefore, be expected in IgG myeloma and acute inflammation, such as in subacute bacterial endocarditis and gout.*

In both congestive cardiac failure and polycythaemia rubra vera, the ESR is typically lowered rather than raised.

ME-C186   CORRECT RESPONSE B,C,D,E

The majority of urinary stones pass within 48 h of presenting with symptoms and do not require extracorporeal lithotripsy.

Renal stones composed of calcium oxalate and phosphate may be associated with an increased urinary calcium, as can occur with prolonged immobilisation or in hyperparathyroidism.

In the majority of instances, however, kidney stones occur in the absence of demonstrable abnormality in calcium metabolism.

Excessive consumption of ascorbic acid, usually more than 1 g/day, can result in renal stones.

A number of renal stones, particularly stones growing slowly in renal calyces, are asymptomatic.

ME-C187   CORRECT RESPONSE B,D,E

Neurofibromatosis type II (von Recklinghausen disease), which is characterised by bilateral acoustic neuromas and a tendency to astrocytomas and gliomas, has an autosomal dominant inheritance.

Congenital spherocytosis, which is due to a defect in the red cell membrane protein is also autosomal dominant in 80% of cases. The adult form of polycystic disease of the kidney is inherited as autosomal dominant, whereas the infantile and childhood forms are autosomal recessive traits.

Glucose-6-phosphate dehydrogenase deficiency is normally an X-linked recessive and alpha$_1$-antitrypsin deficiency is an autosomally recessive inheritance.

ME-C188   CORRECT RESPONSE A,B,D,E

Mildly raised serum calcium can occur with excessive consumption of calcium-containing medication. Some antacid preparations contain a significant amount of calcium and continued ingestion of these with other calcium foods, such as milk, may raise the serum calcium above normal levels.

Mild hypercalcaemia can also occur as calcium is released from bones with disuse, *as during prolonged recumbency and immobilisation.*

Oral contraceptive preparations have no significant effect on serum calcium. They have a protective effect against the development of osteoporosis.

Carcinoma of the breast, together with a number of other tumours, can produce hypercalcaemia. This can occur through two mechanisms: more commonly due to a parathormone-like compound secreted by the tumour; alternatively, it may be due to multiple bone metastases with release of calcium from bone erosion. It is always important to exclude carcinoma as a cause of hypercalcaemia in elderly patients.

Hyperparathyroidism typically produces raised serum calcium. Differentiation of hyperparathyroidism from other possible causes of hypercalcaemia requires concomitant estimation of parathormone of glandular origin. Most cases of primary hyperparathyroidism are curable by surgery.

ME-C189   CORRECT RESPONSE A,B,C,E

Tetracyclines are primarily bacteriostatic and are thought to act by the inhibition of protein synthesis. They are not the drug of choice in any type of staphylococcal infection, particularly in osteomyelitis, when a bactericidal antibiotic should be used. They should also not be used in pregnant women or in children as they may cause permanent discolouration of the teeth in the child.

Doxycycline, up to 100 mg/day, is effective prophylaxis for chloroquine-resistant Plasmodium falciparum *malaria. The combination of tetracycline for 3–6 weeks and streptomycin for 2 weeks is effective treatment for brucellosis. Q fever* (Coxiella burnetii) *responds to both tetracyclines and chloramphenicol, but the former is preferred for safety reasons.*

Non-gonococcal urethritis is thought to be most commonly caused by Chlamydia trachomatis *and this can be effectively treated with tetracycline.*

ME-C190   CORRECT RESPONSE B,D,E

Patients with neutropenia are at risk of developing common bacterial infections. *Of the organisms listed* Staphylococcus, Pseudomonas *and* Klebsiella *are the most likely.*

Pneumocystis is associated with immune deficiency, most commonly AIDS; and the incidence of *Mycoplasma pneumoniae* is not increased in either immune deficiency or neutropenia.

ME-C191   CORRECT RESPONSE D

Hydatid disease represents one phase in the life of the tape worm *Echinococcus granulosa.* The definitive (primary) host for the worm is the dog, where the tiny 5 mm worm resides in the duodenum. The worm releases eggs and if these are eaten by human or sheep (intermediate hosts), the embryo escapes from the egg, penetrates the intestinal mucosa and forms a unilocular cyst, usually in the liver. The larvae can produce daughter cysts within the original cyst. The ingestion of scolices within these cysts by dogs eating sheep offal completes the life cycle. The scolices grow into tapeworms in the dog's alimentary tract; and the cycle of carnivore to herbivore to carnivore is completed.

It is only by ingesting the eggs released by the tapeworm in the dog faeces that hydatid disease can develop in the intermediate host, so that *faeco–oral transmission from a dog excreting parasite ova is the means of transmission to humans.* Contact with hydatid material from eating lamb liver or other food sources will not result in hydatid disease. Such material contains scoliceal larvae which will develop into tape worms only in the primary host; not eggs which will develop into cysts in an intermediate host. The tape worm infesting pigs is *Taenia solium*; in this instance humans contract the disease by eating infested pork and develop an intestinal tapeworm as a primary host.

ME-C192   CORRECT RESPONSE A,C,D,E

Levodopa in high doses produces confusion. Before the stage of confusion develops, patients will usually complain of nightmares then visual hallucinations.

Amantadine has very similar side effects to levodopa. It does not, however, produce choreiform movements in high doses. Amantadine probably facilitates the release of dopamine. The most common side effect seen would be visual hallucinations.

Propranolol is a beta-blocker which crosses the blood–brain barrier and nightmares are common side effects of centrally acting beta-blockers.

Haloperidol, along with all butyrophenone and phenothiazine types of drugs, can produce tardive dyskinesia. There are a number of possible explanations for this; possibly the induction of additional dopamine receptors is the most plausible.

Chlorpromazine and related drugs block dopamine receptors and, as a result, they can produce parkinsonism. Tremor, bradykinesia, akathisia and increased tone are seen with chlorpromazine. The disorder is usually self-limiting, abating within 6 months of the cessation of the medication. The treatment of patients with chlorpromazine-induced parkinsonism with levodopa is usually ineffective.

ME-C193   CORRECT RESPONSE A,B,C

Digitalis (digoxin) is effective in controlling ventricular rate in atrial fibrillation by slowing conduction through the AV node. The effect of digitalis is potentiated both by hypokalaemia and hypercalcaemia. Paroxysmal atrial tachycardia with block may develop under these circumstances. The most common situation in which this arises is with hypokalaemia occurring in the treatment of heart failure with thiazide diuretics and digitalis.

Atrial fibrillation is not a common toxic side effect of digoxin, but a common significant side effect is the development of ventricular ectopic beats. For this reason, the appearance of pulsus trigeminus, due to ventricular ectopic beats, is not a sign of good digitalisation but one of digitalis intoxication.

ME-C194   CORRECT RESPONSE C,E

Angiotensin-converting enzyme (ACE) inhibitors, while they should be used with care in patients with renal artery stenosis, are not contraindicated in the presence of renal disease or diabetes. Diuretics can be added to further reduce blood pressure and reduce oedema and are not contraindicated with ACE inhibitors, the two drug classes being complementary. Treatment of cardiac failure with diuretics, control of atrial rate with digoxin and control of blood pressure with diuretics should be the initial treatments for cardiac failure. Subsequently, ACE inhibitors can be used if there is not an adequate response to these measures. There may be other indications to use ACE inhibitors. *They have been shown to reduce the incidence of subsequent ischaemic events after myocardial infarction in patients with impaired left ventricular function.*

Persistent non-productive cough, which may start months after the commencement of ACE inhibitors, is a troublesome adverse reaction. Reducing the dose or changing the type of ACE inhibitor may only occasionally stop the coughing, although all ACE inhibitors have been shown to produce cough. An additional complication is angioedema, with a dramatic sudden swelling of the tongue or areas of skin. All current ACE inhibitors have this adverse reaction, which is thought to be due to the reduction in the production of kinins.

ME-C195   CORRECT RESPONSE B,D,E

High doses of steroids can, in the short term, be associated with changes in mood. The change in mood is quite variable and there may be either euphoria or marked depression.

Because of the mineralicorticoid side effects of all steroids, *mild hypokalaemia can occur.* The glucocorticoid effects *can cause mild hyperglycaemia* and diabetes can be precipitated by high doses of corticosteroids.

Iatrogenic Cushing syndrome requires prolonged medication with steroids to develop the typical picture of steroid facies, obesity, striae and hypertension. Similarly, osteoporosis follows prolonged use of steroids.

ME-C196   CORRECT RESPONSE A,C,E

High doses of steroids can produce *insomnia* and an increase in appetite. *The mineralocorticoid effect of prednisolone results in the retention of sodium and water. There is a small but definite risk of avascular necrosis of bone.*

Prednisolone and related steroid medications have a catabolic effect; there is a loss of muscle bulk and sometimes overt weakness as the typical picture of steroid myopathy develops.

ME-C197   CORRECT RESPONSE A,C,E

Intravenous amphotericin B frequently produces severe and dangerous side effects and should only be used for potentially fatal fungal infections when the benefit outweighs the risks. Most frequent side effects are fever, headache, nausea and vomiting and diarrhoea. There is usually pain and phlebitis at the site of the infusion and *a normochromic, normocytic anaemia can develop. Renal impairment is common, with rising creatinine and urea, hypokalaemia and renal tubular acidosis.* The changes may not be reversible, particularly if large doses are used.

Although there are many adverse reactions to amphotericin B, optic neuritis and hypercalcaemia are not among them.

ME-C198   CORRECT RESPONSE A,D

Of the drugs listed *both digoxin and gentamicin are excreted in part unchanged by the kidney and the dose should be modified in the presence of renal failure.* The other drugs are metabolised prior to renal excretion and while care should be taken with using them in patients with liver failure, they are usually not a problem in patients with renal failure.

ME-C199   CORRECT RESPONSE A,B,C

Major tranquillisers can produce a number of abnormal movements. These fall generally into three groups. *Episodes of dystonia, such as oculogyric crises, can occur after only one dose as an idiosyncratic reaction.*

After prolonged use of major tranquillisers *parkinsonian features may appear due to dopamine receptor blockade. The most common sign is a resting tremor in the hands.*

Inability to sit or stand still (akathisia) can occur after the first dose of a major tranquilliser and may last for 1–2 days. It does not necessarily occur again if the patient is challenged with a similar drug.

Flapping tremor (asterixis), which is actually a momentary relaxation in muscle tone rather than a positive muscle contraction, typically occurs in liver failure, but is not a feature of major tranquillisers.

Action myoclonus is most commonly seen as a post-hypoxic syndrome and is not a phenomenon of major tranquillisers.

ME-C200   CORRECT RESPONSE A,B,C,E

Palliative radiotherapy can reduce tumour size with relief of superior vena caval obstruction and bony pain and can reduce tumour fungation. With chronic debilitating haemorrhage, the reduction of vascularity in response to radiotherapy may stop the haemorrhage.

In paraplegia whether or not a response is obtained by radiotherapy depends on the responsiveness of the tumour and the duration of the paraplegia. If the paraplegia is evolving progressively, is not yet complete and the tumour is radiosensitive, then there is a reasonable chance that the paraplegia may respond to radiation. However, if the paraplegia has progressed to the stage where there is no movement and particularly if an established paraplegia has been present for some days, it is unlikely radiotherapy will produce any improvement.

ME-C201   CORRECT RESPONSE A,B,C,E

Long-term immunosuppression (e.g. with azathioprine, cyclosporine, cyclophosphamide, steroids or other agents) is associated with a variety of complications. *Cancer (and, particularly in Australia, skin cancer) is the most serious; but an increased infective risk is also present, for both bacteria and viruses,* due to diminished humoral and cellular immunity. *Aseptic bone necrosis* (particularly of weight-bearing joints) and *cataracts* are especially liable with high steroid dosage. Renal tract calculi are not influenced by immunosuppression.

ME-C202   CORRECT RESPONSE A,C,D

Most patients with HIV/AIDS have some involvement of the central nervous system, either directly related to the HIV virus or from secondary infection. Some abnormality is found in the cerebrospinal fluid in 90% of those with HIV/AIDS. There are three forms of peripheral nerve involvement. *There is an acute demyelinating neuropathy, similar to the Guillain–Barré neuropathy.* This occurs early in the course of HIV. A mononeuritis multiplex picture, due to a necrotising arteritis, may be seen, usually when there is significant immunosuppression. *Approximately two-thirds of patients with AIDS have electrophysiological evidence of a neuropathy with axonal types of changes and approximately half of these have symptoms of a sensorimotor neuropathy.* Myopathy with proximal weakness, related to zidovudine, HIV or the generalised wasting syndrome may also be seen.

Dementia is an AIDS-identifying illness and eventually develops in approximately two-thirds of affected individuals. Typical of dementias, there is no change in the level of consciousness or alertness. Alteration in these suggests a toxic confusional state due to other causes. Parkinsonism and trigeminal neuralgia are not features of HIV or AIDS.

ME-C203 CORRECT RESPONSE B,C

Immune thrombocytopenic purpura (ITP) has, by definition, a reduced platelet count. In children it commonly follows a viral infection. In the adult (usually a woman between the ages of 20 and 40), a clear antecedent history of a viral infection is less common. Thrombocytopenic purpura may occur with HIV infection, both in the early stages and as a complication of AIDS. Antibodies are formed to platelets and it is the destruction of platelets at a rate faster than they can be replaced by the megakaryocytes which reduces the platelet count and not a reduction in the number of megakaryocytes.

Immune thrombocytopenia can occur as a reaction to a number of drugs, including quinine, penicillin and heparin. Although the primary treatment is usually the administration of steroids, the destruction of platelets can also be suppressed by intravenous gamma globulin. This treatment is expensive and its effect is relatively short lived. In the adult, splenectomy would be considered in chronic ITP which is poorly controlled by other means; however, it is not the first line of treatment.

ME-C204 CORRECT RESPONSE D

Whether or not the creatinine is elevated with renal involvement in systemic lupus erythematosus (SLE) depends on the type of renal involvement. Most patients with SLE have immunoglobulins deposited in the kidney. Patients with mild focal or mesangial nephritis may have normal creatinine. However, those with diffuse proliferative nephritis can develop renal failure. The presence of haematuria and proteinuria are more sensitive indicators of renal disease than serum creatinine.

Antinuclear antibodies (ANA) are at best only a screening test for SLE. Testing for ANA may be positive in normal people and the incidence of this rises with age. Testing is also positive in other immune diseases, chronic inflammatory disorders and with some viral infections.

Sclerodactyly is a feature of systemic sclerosis and digital infarcts are common in that disorder. They are only seen occasionally in SLE.

Most patients with SLE have joint involvement with intermittent arthritis. The predominant symptom is pain, with relatively few physical signs. *The joint symptoms and signs are symmetrical and usually involve the proximal interphalangeal (IP) and the metacarpophalangeal (MP) joints. Joint deformities and bone changes on X-ray are uncommon.*

Recurrent pleurisy is common in SLE, although the possibility of pulmonary infection must always be excluded.

ME-C205 CORRECT RESPONSE B,E

A high fever is atypical of an allergic reaction and would suggest another underlying diagnosis. *The presence of dysphonia indicates that there is oedema involving the larynx and pharynx and that there is an imminent risk of upper respiratory tract obstruction — thus urgent hospitalisation is mandatory.* The most common cause of severe acute urticaria is food allergy, with shell fish, crustaceans and nuts being the most common. Urticaria from an inhaled antigen is uncommon. Hereditary angioedema involves the deeper layers of the skin and subcutaneous tissue and produces localised non-pitting oedema. Urticaria involves the superficial layers of the skin and produces wheals. It is a typical response to food allergy. The form of allergy described can be life-threatening and *the pursuit of the specific allergen is mandatory*, with subsequent avoidance being an essential part of management.

SUMMARY OF CORRECT RESPONSES

CATEGORY & QUESTION NO.	CORRECT RESPONSE	CATEGORY & QUESTION NO.	CORRECT RESPONSE	CATEGORY & QUESTION NO.	CORRECT RESPONSE
ME-Q 126	B,D	ME-Q 157	B,C,D	ME-Q 188	A,B,D,E
ME-Q 127	A,B,C	ME-Q 158	C	ME-Q 189	A,B,C,E
ME-Q 128	B,C,D,E	ME-Q 159	A,B,C,E	ME-Q 190	B,D,E
ME-Q 129	A,C	ME-Q 160	A,C	ME-Q 191	D
ME-Q 130	A,B	ME-Q 161	A,B,D	ME-Q 192	A,C,D,E
ME-Q 131	A,B,C,D	ME-Q 162	B,C,E	ME-Q 193	A,B,C
ME-Q 132	A,B,C,D,E	ME-Q 163	B,D,E	ME-Q 194	C,E
ME-Q 133	D,E	ME-Q 164	D	ME-Q 195	B,D,E
ME-Q 134	A,E	ME-Q 165	B,E	ME-Q 196	A,C,E
ME-Q 135	B	ME-Q 166	E	ME-Q 197	A,C,E
ME-Q 136	A,B,C	ME-Q 167	D,E	ME-Q 198	A,D
ME-Q 137	D	ME-Q 168	C,D	ME-Q 199	A,B,C
ME-Q 138	A,D,E	ME-Q 169	C,D,E	ME-Q 200	A,B,C,E
ME-Q 139	A,C,D	ME-Q 170	D	ME-Q 201	A,B,C,E
ME-Q 140	A,C,D	ME-Q 171	A,C,D	ME-Q 202	A,C,D
ME-Q 141	C	ME-Q 172	A,B,C,D,E	ME-Q 203	B,C
ME-Q 142	B,C,D	ME-Q 173	A	ME-Q 204	D
ME-Q 143	A	ME-Q 174	A,B,E	ME-Q 205	B,E
ME-Q 144	A,C	ME-Q 175	C		
ME-Q 145	A,C	ME-Q 176	A,B,D,E		
ME-Q 146	A,C	ME-Q 177	B,D		
ME-Q 147	B,C	ME-Q 178	B,C,E		
ME-Q 148	A,C	ME-Q 179	A,B,C,E		
ME-Q 149	A,B,D	ME-Q 180	A,B,C,D,E		
ME-Q 150	A,B,E	ME-Q 181	A,B,C,D,E		
ME-Q 151	A,B,E	ME-Q 182	A,C		
ME-Q 152	A,B,D	ME-Q 183	A,C,E		
ME-Q 153	A,C	ME-Q 184	B,D,E		
ME-Q 154	A,D,E	ME-Q 185	A,B,E		
ME-Q 155	B,C	ME-Q 186	B,C,D,E		
ME-Q 156	A,C,D,E	ME-Q 187	B,D,E		

Surgery
Commentaries
and Summary of Correct Responses

TYPE

A

Commentaries SU-C1 to SU-C107

Correct Responses SU-Q1 to SU-Q107

SU-C1 — CORRECT RESPONSE A

The single most important factor in the determination of the overall prognosis of a patient with a malignant melanoma is the depth of invasion, as measured by the thickness of the lesion. Those less than 0.76 mm thick are less likely to metastasise, while those of greater thickness will do so with a frequency exceeding 30%. This measurement is part of the Breslow classification, which categorises the metastatic potential of a malignant melanoma according to its thickness. The other classification is that devised by Clark, in which the level of dermal or deeper invasion determines the likelihood of malignant spread.

SU-C2 — CORRECT RESPONSE C

This malignant melanoma has a depth of 0.5 mm on microscopy (Breslow). The critical thickness of a malignant melanoma is approximately 0.76 mm. Lesions thinner than this are less likely to metastasise, while patients with lesions of greater thickness stand a more than 30% chance of developing secondary disease. The resection margin is also important. In this patient the resection margin of 1 mm is very close and a *wider excision of the primary tumour would be advised*, with subsequent regular follow-up. A 1 cm margin of excision is probably adequate for most of these thin tumours. The draining lymph nodes should be kept under review; excision is not recommended as prophylaxis but is reserved for suspicious enlargements.

Melanoma is not a radiosensitive tumour and adjuvant radiotherapy is not applicable.

SU-C3 — CORRECT RESPONSE A

A full thickness burn, such as would be expected from a molten metal splash injury, involves destruction of all epithelial elements of skin and appendages. Healing, if left to proceed by natural processes, would be by sloughing of the dead skin and gradual re-epithelialisation of the resulting ulcer. The best treatment of the local wound is therefore *early excision and primary wound closure*, especially when the wound is small and well defined, as described. Larger wounds, which leave a significant defect after excision need closure by skin grafting or local flap rearrangement, but these techniques are unnecessary in the case described. For primary closure, the circular defect after excision is converted into a fusiform defect in the direction of skin cleavage lines (longitudinally in the mid-thigh); the margins are mobilised and the wound closed without tension.

SU-C4 — CORRECT RESPONSE A

An unstable burn scar with recurrent ulceration is liable to neoplastic change, developing into a squamous cell carcinoma. Such a malignant ulcer is called a Marjolin ulcer. The other tumour types either do not complicate chronic ulcerating scars or do so very rarely.

SU-C5 — CORRECT RESPONSE E

The photograph (Figure 11) shows a black lesion on the lower eyelid. A malignant melanoma must be excluded. If you are a plastic surgeon, remove the lesion; if not, *refer the patient to a plastic surgeon*. Anything less than total excision is clearly inappropriate.

SU-C6 — CORRECT RESPONSE E

The bluish glistening domed cystic lesion in the mucous membrane of the lip is typical of a benign mucoid cyst from obstruction of a mucoid salivary gland. The lesions can be enucleated or unroofed if persistent and symptomatic.

Squamous cell carcinomas affect the mucocutaneous junction of the lower lip in smokers and in individuals exposed to sunlight, as do basal cell carcinomas. These are usually older patients.

'Sebaceous' (epidermoid) cysts are lesions of hair-bearing skin. They contain desquamated keratin, not sebum. Syphilitic lip lesions comprise chancres (primary), snail-track ulcers (secondary) and gummata (tertiary).

SU-C7   CORRECT RESPONSE B

The photograph (Figure 13) shows a mucous (synovial) cyst of the finger.

Mucous (synovial) cysts of the finger are subcutaneous cystic lesions analogous to ganglia and are found over the dorsum of the distal phalanx just beyond the joint and overlying the germinal nail bed. They may cause (as here) local distortion of nail growth and can be situated in the midline or laterally (as here). Like ganglia they grow slowly, may regress spontaneously and tend to recur if inadequately excised.

Osteoarthritis of the distal interphalangeal joint causes Heberden nodes, firm bilateral swellings over the dorsum of the interphalangeal joints themselves, named after an 18th century English physician.

Gouty tophi also overlie the joint line and often exhibit yellow urate deposits shining through the skin.

Chronic paronychia is usually fungal (monilial) or staphylococcal and causes a crescentic swelling of the whole nail fold.

Chronic suppurative arthritis is seen more commonly in the toes in diabetics and is clinically related to the joint line.

SU-C8   CORRECT RESPONSE E

Lipomas are soft benign solid tumours of fat cells and may be found in any part of the body containing fat. They usually occur in the subcutaneous fat layer, but may be subfascial or intramuscular or in many other sites.

They are not premalignant. Retroperitoneal malignant fatty tumours (liposarcomas) occur; but these are malignant from the onset.

As very little subcutaneous fat is present in the scrotum, lipomas almost never occur there (apart from lipomatous deposits within the spermatic cord). Scrotal sebaceous cysts, however, are very common.

Lipomas are usually freely mobile and are not attached to the overlying skin (a useful differentiation from sebaceous cysts, which always show an attachment to overlying skin). However, in areas like the back of the neck or trunk, where the skin is less mobile and more intimately attached to the underlying fat, this subcutaneous mobility may be impaired and the lipoma may be tethered to the overlying skin.

The outstanding physical characteristic of the lipoma is its lobulated contour, which again is a useful differentiating feature from the spherical smooth contour of the sebaceous cyst.

SU-C9   CORRECT RESPONSE D

The photograph (Figure 14) shows a well circumscribed lesion which appears to arise from within the epidermis and contains a punctum in the centre. These are the features of an epidermoid ('sebaceous') cyst and the back is a common site for such lesions. An epidermoid cyst may be mistaken for a malignant lesion, particularly if noisomely infected. Such a lesion is known as Cock peculiar tumour.

The lesion illustrated is, however, classic in appearance of a non-complicated keratinous epidermoid cyst. Excision is advisable because inflammatory complications due to secondary infection can occur, leading to suppuration and abscess formation. The patient should be advised that **the lesion is benign but should be excised because it may become an abscess.**

'Sebaceous' cysts are of dermal origin and are thus attached to the skin. They are related to the pilo-sebaceous follicle and can occur in hair-bearing skin at any site. The most common sites are the scalp, scrotum and back. The yellow cheesy material within the cyst is desquamated keratin, not sebum.

SU-C10   CORRECT RESPONSE B

Each of the lesions listed is potentially or actually premalignant, **except for the intradermal naevus. The intradermal naevus is a benign, mature melanocytic naevus with no malignant potential.** Benign melanocytic naevi are of three major types and are classified according to the position of the melanocytes (naevus cells) in relation to the epidermal layers. Intradermal naevi account for the majority of benign hairy congenital moles. Junctional naevi have the naevus cells at the junction of the basal epidermal layers and dermis. With intradermal naevi, the naevus cells are entirely within the dermal layer. Compound naevi combine junctional and intradermal pathology. Malignant change from a pre-existing naevus to a malignant melanoma is believed to occur from the junctional component. The other lesions can all be precursors or early manifestations of squamous cell carcinoma.

Leucoplakia is a whitish lesion found in the oral cavity associated with squamous cell carcinoma. Bowen disease is a condition of squamous cell carcinoma *in situ* involving the skin and foreshadows invasive squamous carcinoma. Chronic radiation dermatitis leads to squamous cell skin cancers. Solar keratosis is a discrete horny plaque of the skin occurring on exposed areas such as the face and back of hands and is a common precursor of squamous cell carcinoma.

SU-C 11   CORRECT RESPONSE B

The photograph (Figure 15) illustrates multiple seborrhoeic keratoses (seborrhoeic warts). These are very common papular skin lesions which are seen particularly on the trunk and face with increasing frequency from middle age onwards. *The site of the lesions depicted, the variegated pigmentation from brown to black, the verrucous greasy surface and their occurrence in crops of lesions at varying stages of development, are all classical.* 'A blob of sealing wax stuck on the skin' is an often-used and apt description. They are entirely benign, but if infected or traumatised they may require removal because they can mimic a more suspicious lesion, such as a pigmented basal cell carcinoma or melanoma. Hutchinson melanotic freckle is a name given to a variant of superficial spreading melanoma, usually a solitary macular lesion with a variegated but smooth surface and usually seen on the face of elderly women, where the freckle may grow very slowly for years before assuming a nodular malignant form.

Solar keratoses are firm, hyperkeratinous plaques seen on sun-exposed surfaces, such as the dorsum of hands, ears and face.

Mycosis fungoides ('fungus-like') is a misleading term. It describes a rare involvement of the skin with lymphoma, giving an irregular eczematous dermatitis progressing to form plaques.

SU-C12   CORRECT RESPONSE E

The most likely diagnosis is a parotid pleomorphic adenoma. Swellings of the parotid, as they enlarge, displace the ear lobe outwards as in this photograph (Figure 16), a sign best observed from behind. Most parotid lumps are benign slow-growing tumours. The most common parotid tumour is the benign (but locally recurrent if inadequately excised) pleomorphic adenoma ('mixed' parotid tumour). These tumours classically exhibit slowly expansile painless growth and do not cause facial nerve paralysis even when large.

Tumours of the submandibular gland are more commonly malignant than are those of the parotid. They present as submandibular swellings, lower and more anteriorly than parotid swellings and do not displace the ear lobe.

A less common benign parotid tumour is the adenolymphoma (Warthin tumour) which also grows slowly and progressively. Carcinomas of the parotid are of various types (anaplastic undifferentiated, adenoid cystic tumour, malignant 'mixed' tumour (pleomorphic adenocarcinoma), mucoepidermoid cancer and others). They usually have a relatively short history. They infiltrate the facial nerve causing facial palsy and spread by local invasion and also by lymphatics. Parotid calculus presents as an acute and painful swelling precipitated by anticipation of food.

SU-C13   CORRECT RESPONSE C

Parotid swellings are usually benign pleomorphic adenomas (mixed parotid tumours). Whether in the superficial or deep lobe, these benign tumours displace but do not invade the facial nerve. An adenolymphoma (Warthin tumour) is a similarly benign tumour and the inflammation of chronic parotitis also does not cause facial paralysis.

A facial nerve palsy in a patient with a parotid swelling implies a malignant infiltrating tumour. An adenoid cystic carcinoma is one such tumour.

SU-C14   CORRECT RESPONSE B

When a patient presents with a history of a neck lump, the first step in physical examination is to establish that the 'lump' is not a normal anatomical structure, mistaken for an abnormal lump by the patient.

Structures that can mimic abnormal lumps include bones, cartilages, muscles and vessels. They include the thyroid and cricoid cartilages in the midline, the greater horn of hyoid bone in the anterior triangle, masseteric muscle hypertrophy over the jaw, a prominent carotid artery bifurcation in the anterior triangle, the sternomastoid tendon and a prominent sternoclavicular joint low in the neck, the lateral mass of the atlas high in the posterior triangle and the anterior tubercle of the transverse process of the sixth cervical vertebra low in the posterior triangle. The thyroid gland forms a fullness in the lower throat, but is not normally palpable other than in very thin individuals.

The most common significant neck swelling is an enlarged lymph node, particularly of the deep cervical group at the level of the jugulo–digastric (tonsillar) node. A malignant node is likely to be firm or hard. *Of the structures mentioned, the greater horn of the hyoid bone, which is in the anterior triangle, close to the deep cervical nodes, would be most likely to mimic a malignant node.*

SU-C15   CORRECT RESPONSE E

A branchial cyst exhibits all of the characteristics outlined. A branchial cyst usually presents as a cystic lump in the neck *protruding into the anterior triangle from under the anterior border of sternomastoid in its upper third.* Although thought to be of developmental origin, they are uncommonly found at birth and *present in early or mid-adulthood,* often when associated infection causes enlargement. *They are usually lined by squamous epithelium* and their wall often contains lymphoid tissue. Branchial cysts are most likely to be confused with upper cervical lymph node swellings. Aspiration is usually diagnostic, confirming the cystic nature of the lump and the presence of cholesterol crystals, with re-entrant angles, on microscopy. Treatment is by surgical excision.

SU-C16   CORRECT RESPONSE A

The two common carcinomas of the thyroid are papillary and follicular cell tumour. They tend to occur in young adults and present as a painless lump in the thyroid gland. Medullary tumours are rare, produce calcitonin and may present with symptoms of hypocalcaemia rather than a swelling in the neck.

Papillary tumours are usually solitary and spread preferentially to the lymph nodes, in contradistinction to follicular tumours, which can be multifocal and spread through the bloodstream to bone. *Papillary tumours are slow growing and are influenced by thyroid stimulating hormone.* These tumours exist in isolation and are not associated with other endocrine abnormalities. The preferred treatment of a papillary carcinoma of the thyroid is surgical excision.

SU-C17   CORRECT RESPONSE E

You should also ask the patient if he had just had a meal or had suffered similar episodes in the past. The history of sudden onset of pain, with the photograph (Figure 17) showing a swelling in the region of the left submandibular salivary gland is virtually pathognomonic of submandibular duct obstruction by stone. Submandibular calculi are much more common than calculi in the parotid, the submandibular secretions being more viscous.

The diagnosis can be clinched by examining inside the mouth and feeling the stone in the submandibular duct on *bimanual palpation of the floor of the mouth.* This will also confirm that the swelling is an enlargement of the submandibular salivary gland, which has a superficial cervical portion and a deep lobe extension best felt bimanually.

The presence of a submandibular duct stone can be confirmed by an intra-oral X-ray. This view shows the calculus best. With X-rays of the mandible or neck the stone is often obscured by the bony mandible.

Although cervical lymph node enlargements are very common causes of neck swellings and are often secondary to pharyngeal and tonsillar pathology, such swellings will most commonly affect the tonsillar (jugulo–digastric) node, which is lower and more posterior than the swelling shown.

SU-C18   CORRECT RESPONSE C

A ranula is a cystic transilluminable swelling bulging the oral mucosa in the floor of the mouth. The name derives from the fanciful resemblance of the swelling to a frog's belly. Ranulas can present in childhood or adulthood. *They are believed to result from obstruction of a minor salivary duct* and are usually simply treated by unroofing or fenestration into the oral cavity. They are not associated with inflammation of the major salivary glands, they occur in the floor of the mouth and not the lip. Only very occasionally do they extend into the upper neck ('plunging ranula') and they do not cause a neck sinus such as occurs in congenital branchial fistula.

SU-C19   CORRECT RESPONSE C

The correct response is *venous obstruction from retrosternal extension of the thyroid neck mass. The picture gives a striking illustration of facial congestion with venous flushing on arm elevation* (Pemberton sign). Venous obstruction at the thoracic inlet by a retrosternal upper mediastinal mass is accentuated on elevation of the arms (as in reaching upwards for objects on a shelf or hanging up washing). Impaction of the mass in the thoracic inlet causes further obstruction of innominate vein and vena cava and light headedness and syncope may be associated with venous distension. The usual cause, as in this instance, is retrosternal extension of a thyroid neck mass. The diagnosis of retrosternal extension is often first suspected when the lower border of the thyroid mass is not easily visualised on swallowing.

Traumatic asphyxia is an uncommon sign of interstitial extravasation of blood into congested tissues of the head and neck when acute venous obstruction is caused by a prolonged compressing injury of the chest; for example, after burial by earthfalls.

Carotid vascular steal syndromes occur when an arterial atherosclerotic stricture (e.g. in the carotid or vertebral system) is associated with reversal of blood flow. Increased flow occurs on demand to an arterial branch in parallel (such as the arm with muscular exertion) so that blood is shunted downwards from the carotid or vertebral to the brachial artery. The conductor Toscanini was said to have suffered a minor stroke from this cause while vigorously conducting.

Medullary thyroid carcinoma is the least common of the differentiated thyroid carcinomas (follicular, papillary, medullary). It originates from the parafollicular 'C' cells which secrete calcitonin. Serotonin is a vasoactive peptide associated with the carcinoid syndrome.

Paralysis of the sympathetic trunk causes Horner syndrome (ptosis, miosis, anhidrosis, enophthalmos, stuffy nostrils).

SU-C20   CORRECT RESPONSE C

Unconscious patients are best placed on their sides to minimise the risk of airway obstruction or inhalation of vomitus. The supine position is not the best position for transportation of an unconscious patient; the patient should preferably be transported on the side. Before moving the patient should be checked for cervical spine injuries and a cervical collar should be applied before the patient is 'log-rolled' onto the side by a suitable technique. All the other responses are correct and relevant to an unconscious patient lying supine.

SU-C21   CORRECT RESPONSE C

Any patient with a significant head injury must be assessed according to the Glasgow coma scale. The three components of the scale are best motor response (to verbal command or a painful stimulus), best verbal response and eye opening. In most systems the scale is scored out of 15, as indicated in the table below. A coma scale score of 3 indicates a patient in deep coma, with neither eye opening, nor motor nor verbal response to painful stimuli.

Glasgow coma scale; score range 3–15.

Eyes open:	
Spontaneously	4
To verbal command	3
To pain	2
No response	1
Best motor response:	
Obeys commands	6
Localises pain	5
Flexion withdrawal	4
Abnormal flexion	3
Extension	2
No response	1
Best verbal response:	
Oriented	5
Confused	4
Inappropriate words	3
Incomprehensible sounds	2
No response	1

In the assessment of a patient with a head injury, the most important clinical observation is a change in the rating. In the examination of such patients, all the observations stated in the question must be made and the *most important will be any change in the level of consciousness, as assessed by the Glasgow coma scale.*

SU-C22   CORRECT RESPONSE C

A chronic subdural haematoma is defined as one in which any associated neurological deficits occur more than 2 weeks after the head injury that produced the haematoma. The injury is often minor, without a skull fracture, and may have gone unnoticed by the patient. These lesions typically occur in the elderly where there may be shrinkage of the brain, allowing space for the haematoma to fill while producing few symptoms. The condition is frequently seen in alcoholics, where clotting defects and head injuries are common. The bleeding occurs when vessels spanning the cerebral cortex and the dural sinuses are torn. *Headache is common and the slow progression of symptoms can lead to a diagnosis of dementia.* The natural history of chronic subdural haematoma is often to increase progressively in size due to osmotic absorption of fluid as the haematoma breaks down.

The diagnosis can be confirmed on a CT scan and treatment is to aspirate the liquefied haematoma through burr holes. Corticosteroids and diuretics are of no benefit.

SU-C23   CORRECT RESPONSE E

Division of the ulnar nerve above the wrist is a common sequel of lacerations and knife wounds. Sensory and autonomic loss affects little and ring fingers. Motor loss affects all the muscles of the hypothenar eminence (abductor, flexor and opponens of the little finger), all the interossei (four dorsal and four palmar), the lumbrical muscles to the little and ring fingers and the adductor of the thumb.

Paralysis of interossei is demonstrated by an inability to spread the fingers apart while the hand is held flat on the table.

Opposition of the thumb to the index finger involves predominantly median nerve-innervated thenar muscles and is not a discriminatory test for ulnar nerve function. Opposition of the thumb to the little finger exposes the deficiencies of oppositional movement of the little finger; this deficiency is most marked in the later sequelae of a chronic ulnar nerve palsy with an ulnar claw hand involving little and ring fingers.

Flexion of the distal interphalangeal joints of the ring and little fingers (fourth and fifth digits) is a function of the flexor digitorum profundus tendons to these fingers. These are supplied by the ulnar nerve, but the nerve supply enters the muscle higher in the forearm. A lesion of the ulnar nerve just above the wrist would not affect the function of these muscles. A laceration may directly injure the tendons themselves, but these disabilities are not due to the injury to the nerve. Division of tendons of the long deep finger flexors would be likely to also involve division of the tendons of flexor digitorum superficialis (flexors of the proximal interphalangeal joints) and the wrist flexors (flexors carpi ulnaris, radialis and palmaris longus).

Flexion of the wrist is not relevant to ulnar nerve injury at this site because the nerve supply to flexor carpi ulnaris (from ulnar nerve) also arises high in the forearm.

Extension of the wrist is not affected by ulnar nerve injury. All the wrist extensors are supplied by the radial nerve or its posterior interosseous branch.

SU-C 24   CORRECT RESPONSE B

The deformity is an ulnar claw hand, typical of an established ulnar nerve palsy.
Hyperextension at the metacarpo–phalangeal joints of the little and ring fingers is accompanied by flexion at interphalangeal joints: the deformity is due to lumbrical paralysis to these fingers. The lumbricals reverse the deformity by their action: they flex metacarpo–phalangeal joints and extend interphalangeal joints as in the pincer grip, for holding a pen or chopsticks. The claw deformity is accentuated when the patient attempts to extend the fingers actively, as in the photograph (Figure 20). Wasting of hypothenar muscles and interossei is also apparent, typical of a late lesion.

Congenital finger contracture (clinodactyly, camptodactyly (literally bent finger)) affects the little finger only and is a fixed flexion deformity at the metacarpo–phalangeal joint often associated with a shortened, curved finger.

Dupuytren contracture is also a fixed deformity. It causes flexion contracture at metacarpo–phalangeal and proximal interphalangeal joints associated with subcutaneous fibrous bands, often causing skin puckering. Ring and little fingers are most often affected; the thumb is least often affected. The disease is due to nodules and later fibrosis affecting the palmar fascial aponeurosis.

Rheumatoid arthritis can cause a host of deformities, initially mobile and later becoming fixed.

Those commonly affecting the fingers are ulnar deviation and flexion deformities with subluxation at metacarpo–phalangeal joints, 'boutonniere' with flexion at proximal interphalangeal joint due to erosion of the central extensor tendon slip, 'swan-neck' (the reverse deformity to boutonniere) due to erosion and weakening of the volar plate of the joint capsule of proximal interphalangeal joint and mallet finger or dropped finger due to extensor tendon rupture at distal interphalangeal and metacarpo–phalangeal joints respectively.

Volkmann contracture gives a finger deformity due to ischaemic contracture of the long flexor tendons. The fingers are clawed as in ulnar nerve palsy, but usually to a greater degree and involving all the fingers and thumb. Metacarpo–phalangeal hyperextension occurs due to the pull of the stretched long extensor tendons on these joints. The deformity is affected by wrist movement. Wrist extension increases flexion of the fingers and vice versa.

SU-C25   CORRECT RESPONSE D

This question is an uncomplicated exercise in anatomy. The root supply to the peroneal muscles controlling eversion of the foot and which also contains the reflex arc for the ankle jerk reflex, is **sacral 1** by way of the tibial nerve, which sends motor branches to the soleus and gastrocnemius muscles, and by the superficial peroneal nerve to the peronei. The sensory dermatome of the sacral 1 root gives innervation to the postero–lateral aspect of the leg and foot down to and including the little toe and sole of foot.

SU-C26   CORRECT RESPONSE D

Volkmann ischaemic contracture is an ischaemic muscle necrosis due to acute vascular occlusion affecting the muscles of the volar forearm compartment: the flexors of the fingers and thumb and wrist. *Each of the responses is a potential cause of such vascular occlusion, but the most common association is with supracondylar humeral fractures in children, displacements of which can injure the brachial artery.*

Fractures of the medial or lateral epicondyles are not usually associated with vascular injury. An elbow dislocation can cause vascular occlusion; but less commonly than a supracondylar fracture.

Fractures of both bones of the forearm and fractures round the wrist need to involve both radial and ulnar arterial branches to cause vascular occlusion. Ischaemic necrosis from these injuries is less common than with a supracondylar fracture.

SU-C27   CORRECT RESPONSE E

Successful resuscitation of patients with multiple skeletal and soft tissue injuries is initially focused on correction of hypovolaemia and maintenance of the airway and of ventilation. With effective and early circulatory support, renal failure is uncommon and when it ensues, is often a component of multi-organ failure associated with uncontrolled sepsis. Renal failure can be treated effectively with combinations of haemodialysis, peritoneal dialysis and haemofiltration, so that death from renal failure *per se* is rare. Death from hypovolaemic shock may occur if initial resuscitation is delayed or in the face of uncontrollable blood loss, but after initially successful resuscitation hypovolaemic shock would be a rare cause of death.

Septic shock is an important late development due to inadequately controlled septic complications of the injuries. Septic shock will require vigorous treatment with a range of intravenous fluids, appropriate antibiotics, inotropic support and monitoring of right and left heart function and pressures. Identification of a persisting source of sepsis requiring surgical excision or drainage is also of major importance. Septic shock itself may, if irreversible, occasionally cause death; more commonly systemic sepsis can be fatal despite control of shock because of persistent end organ failure affecting multiple systems, of which the lung is often the most significant. Massive pulmonary embolism is an important cause of death after severe trauma, especially when the embolus is massive and unheralded. Monitoring of venous flows with Duplex–Doppler studies, early thrombolytic therapy for established embolism and percutaneous insertion of inferior vena caval filters have all aided in treatment. *However, the most common mode of death in patients with overwhelmingly severe multisystem trauma, in whom fat embolism syndrome is a potential sequel and who often develop multiple organ failure and adult respiratory distress syndrome is ventilatory failure.* The lung tends to bear the brunt of the effects of multiple end organ failure, with progressive loss of compliance and hypoxia despite increasing oxygen concentrations of inspired air. Vigorous treatment with prolonged mechanical ventilatory support combined with control of sepsis is necessary. Complete recovery can occur after prolonged acute post-traumatic lung failure, but uncontrollable lung failure with associated sepsis remains the most common direct cause of death in such patients.

SU-C28   CORRECT RESPONSE C

The patient has sustained a rupture of the supraspinatus tendon (complete rotator tendinous cuff tear). Age-related degeneration of the rotator cuff of shoulder tendons, particularly the supraspinatus component, is usual as a precursor to rupture. The clinical vignette is classical, with a full range of passive abduction but failure to initiate and complete active gleno–humeral abduction (even with active contraction of deltoid muscle), unless the initial part of the movement through the first 90° is assisted.

The condition is distinct from the painful arc syndrome, which can be caused by an incomplete tear of the tendinous cuff.

Rupture of the long head of the biceps tendon gives a characteristic bunched deformity of the biceps muscle on elbow flexion; the short head is not usually affected.

The subscapularis tendon is stripped from the glenoid and scapula in recurrent dislocation of the shoulder.

Slipping of the upper humeral epiphysis would not be a consideration in a man aged 55. It is also rare in children, as distinct from the important syndrome of slipped upper femoral epiphysis in children and in adolescents.

SU-C29   CORRECT RESPONSE D

The most likely explanation for the swelling in this man's arm is a rupture of the long head of the biceps muscle, as indicated by the photograph (Figure 21), which shows a deformed biceps muscle. Rupture of the tendon of the long head of biceps within the bicipital groove usually follows long-standing avascularity and degeneration and occurs spontaneously in older patients after unaccustomed exercise. The history and appearance are classical, with bunching and deformity of the biceps muscle accentuated by contraction during elbow flexion. Functional disability is usually minor and active treatment is not usually indicated. The short head of biceps brachii remains normal and functional.

There is no history of trauma, so a haematoma or false aneurysm would not be expected. Variceal dilatation of the upper limb veins is unusual and the photograph shows that the swelling lies deep to the superficial veins.

SU-C30   CORRECT RESPONSE B

Fractures of the neck of the humerus in elderly patients frequently occur through the surgical neck and usually result in impaction with minimal displacement. If this is the case, manipulation is not required and *all that is needed is to rest the arm in a sling, starting shoulder exercises as soon as it is comfortable for the patient to do so.*

In the less common situation, if there is a significant degree of displacement and angulation exceeding 45°, then open reduction and fixation may be required. Bed rest and traction would rarely be used. Hanging casts and shoulder spicas are not appropriate in the management of these injuries.

SU-C31   CORRECT RESPONSE D

Fractures of the carpal bones tend to occur in fit active young adults and the usual bone involved is the scaphoid. The fracture is often undisplaced. A scaphoid fracture can be difficult to diagnose and should be suspected in any wrist injury where damage to another structure is not evident. Because of the difficulty in identifying fractures in this region, oblique views of the carpal bones should be requested, with the wrist in midpronation and anteroposterior views with the wrist in maximum ulnar deviation. These fractures may still not be visible on the initial X-rays and if the degree of pain and tenderness (in the anatomical snuffbox) suggests a fracture which is not initially revealed by X-ray, the patient should be treated as if a fracture is present: the wrist immobilised in plaster and the X-ray repeated out of plaster after 2 or 3 weeks. A 'sprained wrist' is often, in fact, a scaphoid fracture.

Scaphoid fractures occur through the tubercle, the waist or the proximal third of the bone. The latter fractures cause most concern **because the blood supply of the proximal (not distal) fragment can be interrupted with the risk of avascular necrosis.** Reduction of the proximal fragment and adequate immobilisation are of paramount importance. Internal fixation or bone grafting may sometimes be required to ensure stability and continuity of the fractured segments or for the late complication of avascular necrosis.

SU-C32   CORRECT RESPONSE B

Of those listed, the most common late complication to consider in an elderly patient with a Colles fracture would be stiffness of the wrist and fingers. All of the other complications are uncommon, with the exception of joint stiffness. Therefore, in the elderly patient, and particularly if there is minimal deformity, treatment is aimed at early mobilisation and return of function. Union is not usually delayed, although varying degrees of malunion can occur.

SU-C33   CORRECT RESPONSE D

Pain in the knee may be due to a problem within that joint or referred pain from the hip. *The clinical vignette here is most typical of a slipped upper femoral epiphysis (adolescent coxa vara),* which should be suspected in any patient aged between 10 and 20 years with pain in the hip or knee associated with a limp. The limb tends to lie in external rotation with limitation of abduction, internal rotation and flexion.

Osteochondritis dissecans causes local avascular necrosis of a portion of the articular surface of bone with its overlying cartilage, ultimately causing separation of the fragment to form a loose body within the joint. The cause is unknown; adolescents and young adults are most often affected. The knee joint is most commonly involved with necrosis of a segment of the medial condyle of the femur. Examination usually reveals a joint effusion.

Perthes disease (osteochondritis juvenalis of the femoral head epiphysis) affects children from 5–10 years, with softening and potential deformity of the femoral head. Symptoms of pain in the affected hip are accompanied by painful limitation of all hip movements.

Congenital dislocation of the hip should be diagnosed on neonatal screening. Diagnosis after the age of 10 years would be suspected by persistent problems with walking, shortening of the leg at the hip and impaired abduction in flexion.

Osgood–Schlatter disease (osteochondritis juvenalis of the knee, apophysitis of the tibial tubercle) causes pain below and in front of the knee in adolescents, with prominence and tenderness of the tibial tubercle.

SU-C34 CORRECT RESPONSE C

Fractures and dislocations due to falling on an outstretched hand tend to have different likelihood and frequencies according to age. In a 7-year-old child, common injuries due to such a fall include a variety of forearm injuries: fracture of both bones of the forearm, displacement of the distal radial epiphysis due to breaks involving the epiphyseal plate and metaphysis or greenstick fractures of individual forearm bones.

At a higher level, stress transmitted to the elbow and arm can lead to supracondylar humeral fractures, another common injury of young children. All of the above are likely fractures in a 7-year-old child.

Colles fracture, on the other hand, is a fracture of the lower radius with classical displacements, which is more common in middle or late adulthood, particularly affecting osteoporotic bones in women. *Thus, Colles fracture is the least likely fracture of those listed to occur in a 7-year-old child.*

SU-C35 CORRECT RESPONSE C

Chronic leg ulcers are a common problem in our community. Most patients are middle aged or elderly and the ulcers are secondary to chronic ambulatory superficial venous hypertension. Venous hypertension is either the result of primary incompetence of the superficial veins and their communicating branches with the deep system ('perforators'), or secondary to obstruction of the deep venous system. The ulcers associated with venous hypertension are typically situated around the ankle and are surrounded by the other characteristic changes of long-standing deep venous insufficiency, namely skin pigmentation, dependent oedema, a scaling dermatitis and subcutaneous fat atrophy and induration.

The next most frequent form of ulceration is that associated with diabetes mellitus. Poor peripheral circulation and sensory impairment combine to give ulceration, typically over pressure points, such as the skin of the sole of the foot over the first metatarsal head.

Other important causes of chronic leg ulceration include arterial insufficiency and infections.

In the case described in the question *the young man sustained a fractured femur, which may have been complicated by deep venous thrombosis of that leg. Deep venous thrombosis in such instances is often occult.* Deep venous thrombosis may later be followed by the development of superficial varicose veins, as well as by *late ulceration, secondary to perforator vein incompetence.*

SU-C 36 CORRECT RESPONSE A

The photograph (Figure 22) of the right flank and lateral abdominal wall shows dilated tortuous subcutaneous veins running between groin and axilla, indicating collateral venous channel dilatation due to inferior vena caval obstruction. The venous dilatation visible in the erect position indicates that venous flow is upwards in these collaterals of the systemic venous system.

Portal venous obstruction with portal hypertension also causes dilated subcutaneous abdominal wall veins, but these radiate centrifugally from the umbilicus due to portal–systemic collaterals developing between the intra-abdominal portal circulation and the subcutaneous abdominal wall veins. The veins run cephalwards and caudally (caput Medusae) to drain into superior vena caval and inferior vena caval fields, respectively.

Obstruction by thrombosis of the external iliac vein could also produce venous collaterals bypassing the groin, but not of such extent nor running so high, and usually involving mainly collaterals via the pelvis and perineum between external and internal venous systems.

A fistula between aorta and inferior vena cava is usually due to aortic aneurysm and can lead to distal aortic ischaemia, but not to collateral channels such as are visualised.

Axillo–femoral arterial bypass grafts are used for aortic obstructive lesions, but a recent graft would not be so tortuous in appearance.

SU-C37 CORRECT RESPONSE A

Occlusions of the superficial femoral artery commonly occur near the adductor hiatus and may be asymptomatic. When symptoms do occur, they are usually those of pain or aching in the calf, experienced on walking. Calf claudication at 50 or 100 m would be a common finding. Claudication distance may improve with the development of collaterals; but the disease may also progress, particularly if the patient continues to smoke.

If the patient has rest pain or has developed gangrene, then the degree of superficial femoral arterial obstruction and distal ischaemia has reached a critical level and surgical intervention will be required to save the limb. *If the patient has claudication affecting the thigh, the obstruction must be at the level of the common femoral artery or higher, with associated involvement of the deep femoral artery.*

SU-C38 CORRECT RESPONSE D

Acute arterial occlusion causes sudden pain, pallor and coldness of the limb with associated paralysis of ischaemic muscles.

Acute arterial occlusion suddenly stops blood entering the limb and, *therefore, would not be expected to cause oedema, a sign of fluid excess.*

Oedema is a manifestation of acute venous (not arterial) obstruction.

SU-C39 CORRECT RESPONSE C

The clinical features suggest an acute arterial embolus from an intracardiac mural thrombus. This is a surgical emergency requiring, in the first instance, *intravenous heparin administration* to minimise the development of intravascular propagating thrombus adjacent to the embolus. This should be *followed by urgent operative embolectomy.* Arteriography wastes time; anticoagulant treatment or embolectomy alone are less appropriate, as is conservative expectant treatment.

SU-C40 CORRECT RESPONSE C

Venous thrombo-embolism often presents clinically in the second week after surgery. Risk factors include immobility and venous stasis, obesity, trauma to the delicate calf venous sinusoids, increasing age, increased blood coagulability after surgery and operations known to be at high risk (cancer surgery, hip surgery). Clinical features of deep vein thrombosis are notoriously unreliable, but the combination of leg swelling and calf tenderness, fever and tachycardia is very suggestive of the diagnosis. *Anticoagulant treatment with heparin is the most important aspect of treatment,* which should be instituted immediately while preparations may be made for confirming the diagnosis by venography or by venous Duplex–Doppler flow studies. The other treatments are either ancillary (elevation of the foot of the bed, elastic stocking support) or reserved for repeated life-threatening emboli (insertion of caval filter or ligation of the draining leg vein).

SU-C41   CORRECT RESPONSE D

Acute superficial thrombophlebitis complicating varicose veins is best treated by analgesia, *by supportive compressive bandaging to relieve local pain and enhance deep venous flow and by continuing ambulation to diminish the risk of extension of thrombosis to the deep venous system.* Bed rest is inappropriate and increases the risk of progression to deep venous thrombosis.

The use of systemic anticoagulant therapy is usually reserved for suspected or established progression of disease to the deep venous system, such as would be the case with thrombophlebitis of the long saphenous vein in the upper thigh.

The differentiation of superficial thrombophlebitis requiring ambulation, deep venous thrombosis requiring anticoagulant treatment and cellulitis requiring antibiotics and rest can be sometimes difficult; however, in the case described, superficial thrombophlebitis without extension to the deep venous system is the likely diagnosis.

SU-C42   CORRECT RESPONSE B

Vasovagal syncope (fainting) can follow prolonged standing, acute blood loss or other upsetting and unpleasant stimuli.

Vasovagal syncope involves a massive sympathetic response, associated with pooling of blood in the peripheries which leads to a reduction in cerebral perfusion. The patient will have cold, clammy, pale skin; but blood is pooled in deeper vasodilated muscle vessels. The peripheral pulses are weak and a reflex vagal bradycardia is accompanied by a reduced cardiac output and fall in blood pressure. In contradistinction to most forms of shock, *the heart rate in vasovagal syncope* decreases *rather than increases*. This is a very helpful sign in distinguishing vasovagal syncope from other and more serious, causes.

A vasovagal attack may be fatal if the person remains in the upright position, such as may occur in the crush of a crowd, the cramped surroundings of a privy or as in execution by crucifixion. The situation is rapidly remedied by lying the patient down and elevating the legs, which allows the essential redistribution of blood flow to the cerebral circulation.

SU-C43   CORRECT RESPONSE D

The haemodynamic response to increasing blood loss is not incrementally linear. Compensatory secondary neuro-endocrine responses of venoconstriction and redistribution of blood flow ensure that acute loss of 5% (approximately 250 mL) or 10% (approximately 500 mL) of blood volume in an adult can be tolerated without significant changes in blood pressure or pulse rate. Blood donors give up to 500 mL without ill effects. With increasing losses over approximately 20%, compensatory mechanisms cannot maintain blood pressure despite a maximal increase in peripheral resistance. The patient described has severe hypotension (70/30 mmHg) and gross tachycardia and has established severe haemorrhagic shock. *Clinical shock due to haemorrhage implies a loss of at least 30% of blood volume (1.5–2 L); the best response is thus approximately 40% of blood volume (a loss of 2–2.5 L), rather than 20%.* Acute loss of 80% of blood volume (4–5 L) would be expected to cause even more catastrophic haemodynamic effects and to affect consciousness and orientation.

SU-C44   CORRECT RESPONSE D

All of the responses are relevant indicators of the effectiveness of resuscitation. *Restoration of cerebral circulation is the most vital aim and to indicate this the restoration of normal size and reactivity of the pupils is the best of the indicators listed.* Electrocardiography denotes electrical activity of the heart but not its functional efficacy. The presence of the femoral pulse shows that the relevant limb is being perfused. Return of normal colour to skin and mucous membranes is influenced by ambient temperature; returning responses to external stimuli are also helpful but do not necessarily indicate cortical reperfusion.

SU-C45   CORRECT RESPONSE C

The clinical syndrome of acute back pain in a man of this age associated with hypertension, symptoms and signs of distal arterial ischaemia and an aortic murmur is very suggestive of a dissecting aortic aneurysm.

Myocardial infarction is not usually associated with asymmetrical pulses nor is back pain a feature. Emboli affecting the abdominal aorta and its branches most significantly and seriously involve the mesenteric vessels. Mesenteric vascular infarction can present as an acute abdomen and may be accompanied by lower gastrointestinal bleeding. A pulmonary embolus often mimics myocardial infarction; and large emboli are associated with refractory shock due to massive vascular obstruction. Spontaneous pneumothorax presents with chest pain and dyspnoea and is most common in young adult males or in patients with chronic obstructive airway disease. Classical physical signs are diminished air entry and tympanitic percussion on the affected side.

SU-C46   CORRECT RESPONSE E

The diagnosis most suspected in this man is acute aortic dissection (dissecting aortic aneurysm).

Aortic wall dissections can be classified into those involving the ascending (10%) or descending (90%) aorta. Each may be acute or chronic.

Transaminase determination and haematocrit are not specifically helpful in diagnosis of aortic dissection, although both can be abnormal in mesenteric infarction.

Chest X-ray is useful and rarely normal in patients with aortic dissection and can be enhanced by CT scanning. It may show aortic dilatation, mediastinal widening, cardio-megaly or pleural effusion: electrocardiography is also a useful test: Electrocardiographic abnormalities (left axis deviation, arrhythmias) are common in aortic dissection. An ECG is even more important by excluding changes diagnostic of myocardial infarction, with which aortic dissection is most often confused. Chest X-ray and ECG will, therefore, be helpful in supporting the diagnosis of dissection and in excluding other pathology, respectively. Neither chest X-ray nor ECG, however, is specific for the diagnosis of dissection. *Aortography is the MOST specific diagnostic test.* Aortography will localise the origin of the dissection, either distal to the left subclavian artery (the usual site) or in the ascending aorta. Patients presenting with suggestive chest pain and an abnormal X-ray should thus proceed to aortography or contrast-enhanced CT scan.

SU-C47   CORRECT RESPONSE D

By the time a patient with bronchogenic carcinoma develops obstruction of the superior vena cava or hoarseness of the voice the disease has become so locally advanced, with invasion of adjacent structures, that it is inoperable. *Pulmonary osteoarthropathy is a paraneoplastic stigma which, in itself, does not reflect on the operability of a lung cancer.* Performing a lobectomy or pneumonectomy on a patient with very poor exercise tolerance would be hazardous and such a clinical picture is also suggestive of advanced disease. A blood-stained effusion indicates pleural involvement and makes any attempted resection merely palliative.

SU-C48   CORRECT RESPONSE B

Postoperative collapse with chest pain and dyspnoea at 1 week is strongly suggestive of a large pulmonary embolus but other causes must be considered.

All of the responses may contribute helpful diagnostic information, *but the ventilation–perfusion lung scan is the most specific*. This would be expected to show ventilatory/perfusion imbalance, with one or more areas of unperfused but ventilated lung tissue.

SU-C49   CORRECT RESPONSE A

The timing of the fever, within the first 24 h of surgery, makes pulmonary atelectasis associated with sputum retention the most likely cause. A urinary tract infection most commonly occurs in postoperative patients more than a day after contamination is introduced by urethral catheterisation. Wound infection does not usually become clinically manifest until several days after operation.

Manifestations of deep venous thrombosis (DVT) can occur early if the patient has been confined to bed prior to surgery; however, more classically, symptoms and signs of DVT are delayed until the second week after an operation such as elective gastrectomy. Superficial thrombophlebitis affecting intravenous cannulae begins as a chemical aseptic inflammation and is more likely if the intravenous drip is left for more than 48 h in the one site. It is uncommon within 24 h of cannula insertion.

SU-C 50   CORRECT RESPONSE A

The ultrasound of the abdomen shows a longitudinal cut of the gall-bladder with three gallstones, each demonstrating echogenicity and acoustic shadowing. Gallstones often present clinically with recurring episodes of severe pain (biliary 'colic') which may be situated in the right or left hypochondrium or epigastrium, or retrosternally, the latter site requiring to be distinguished from pain of oesophageal or cardiac origin. *Symptomatic gallstones are best treated by cholecystectomy.*

Endoscopic retrograde cholangiopancreatography (ERCP) and endoscopic papillotomy are not normally used to investigate and treat gallstones unless biliary duct stones are suspected. Non-surgical management of symptomatic gallstones is not appropriate, unless associated disease makes the small risk of operation greater than the risk of complications.

Bile salt dissolution using bile acids or lithotripsy are associated with high recurrence rates or life-long therapy and would not be applicable in the case described.

SU-C51   CORRECT RESPONSE C

Perhaps 10% of patients with peptic ulcer disease suffer a complication of the disease. Over the past two decades the incidence of gastric outlet obstruction and perforation has dropped dramatically, but the incidence of bleeding has remained constant. This is despite the increased awareness of the problem and the frequent prescription of potent antisecretory drugs.

Most patients admitted to hospital with a bleeding duodenal ulcer will settle on their own accord and the bleeding will cease spontaneously. Of all the patients admitted with bleeding duodenal ulcers, less than 10% will continue to bleed or rebleed and so come to surgical intervention.

Indications for early surgical intervention include major initial blood loss with shock, continuation of bleeding and rebleeding. The most sensitive indicator of recurrent haemorrhage in a patient who has been adequately resuscitated is postural hypotension (a fall of more than 10 mmHg when the patient is sat up). A fall in haemoglobin is less sensitive and may only reflect haemodilution after resuscitation. Any patient who has required more than 10 units of blood should be seriously considered for surgery and the older the patient the more alert the clinician must be (the elderly tolerate major haemodynamic changes less well than young patients). *Age over 60 years is thus a common and important consideration in early surgical intervention; and is the most important consideration among those listed.* The size or site of a bleeding duodenal ulcer does not sway the management decisions nor does the sex of the patient, the blood group of the patient or the secretory status.

SU-C52 CORRECT RESPONSE E

This man has had an episode of acute pancreatitis and now has a complication of the disease. The two complications to be considered are a pancreatic abscess and a pseudocyst. If he had an abscess the patient would probably be much sicker and the epigastric mass would be tender.

A persistent elevation of serum amylase is a common finding with a pseudocyst, but the presence of the pseudocyst is best confirmed by abdominal imaging.

Imaging can be done by ultrasound or by the more sensitive and less operator-dependent investigation of a CT abdominal scan.

Plain X-ray is not usually rewarding and oral cholecystography is not relevant to the diagnosis of a peripancreatic mass.

An ERCP may sometimes show communication of a major pancreatic duct with the pseudocyst, but is invasive and may introduce infection.

SU-C53 CORRECT RESPONSE A

Chronic fissure-in-ano is characterised by pain, bleeding and constipation. The pain and bleeding occur at the time of defaecation and the spasm triggered by the passage of a constipated stool causes a lingering burning perianal pain which can last several hours. The patient may have times when the fissure heals and so goes through cycles of pain and remission.

Diagnosis is best made by careful inspection of the anal verge. On inspection of the anal verge a sentinel pile is found adjacent to the chronic ulcer, which is usually in the midline posteriorly. A fibrotic tender ulcer is seen and can be felt on digital examination of the anal canal. If the ulcer is in an acute phase, the degree of tenderness and anal spasm will prohibit digital examination.

SU-C54 CORRECT RESPONSE D

Most perianal abscesses form as a result of local sepsis. They should be treated by simple incision, deroofing and drainage. *The large majority will heal without complication and the patient will not have any further troubles.* In a minority of patients a perianal fistula due to a persistent internal communication, recurrent abscess formation, or identification of an underlying chronic lesion, such as Crohn disease, will require further investigation and treatment.

SU-C55 CORRECT RESPONSE A

This man has ischaemic bowel from mesenteric ischaemia. Formation of mural thrombus is a well recognised event after myocardial infarction and occasionally segments of clot may be dislodged into the systemic arterial circulation. The mural thrombus usually develops on the wall of the left ventricle. When dislodged, the clot may find its way to the brain or the legs or the embolus may occlude the superior mesenteric artery. Patients with ischaemic bowel develop generalised abdominal pain and sometimes pass fresh blood per rectum. Physical findings are often relatively slight with initially minor tenderness and guarding.

Abdominal X-ray can sometimes show pathognomonic features of ischaemia, such as gas within the bowel wall but more commonly, as in this patient, just shows distended small gut. Slight elevations of temperature and of serum amylase are often found and can cause confusion with other possible diagnoses.

Although the other conditions listed can mimic mesenteric vascular ischaemia, the development of persisting abdominal pain and tenderness in an elderly patient with a source of embolus requires this complication, which has a very high mortality, to be thought of as first diagnosis.

SU-C56   CORRECT RESPONSE B

Lesions in the ano–rectum such as haemorrhoids, fissure, polyps or cancer can present with bleeding on defaecation. With haemorrhoidal bleeding small amounts of bright blood may be noted on the toilet paper, in the toilet bowl or on the surface of the faeces; and may present as a drip or squirt of blood.

Apart from a full history to pick up associated symptoms (alteration in bowel habit, pain, tenesmus, pruritus) assessment must always include inspection of the anal verge, digital rectal examination and proctosigmoidoscopy. These examinations establish the presence or absence of fissure or haemorrhoids and examine the last 25 cm of the alimentary canal (where a large proportion of polyps and cancers are found). *In a patient aged 32 years with no additional symptoms, an established diagnosis of haemorrhoids and no additional pathology observed on rigid sigmoidoscopy, treatment of his haemorrhoids as the cause is appropriate.* Further investigations will be required if symptoms are not relieved by this treatment.

In older patients and in patients with additional bowel symptoms suggesting a higher lesion, colonoscopy would also be required. Air contrast barium enema is less sensitive than colonoscopy in picking up small mucosal lesions. Contrast enema is particularly helpful in diagnosing extramural spread of pathology, such as fistulae.

SU-C57   CORRECT RESPONSE D

Although all the responses are symptoms of acute pancreatitis, the one most likely to be the INITIAL symptom is acute pain.

The importance of the pattern of the *'march of symptoms'* is often rightly stressed in the diagnosis of common causes of abdominal pain.

Pain is often a first symptom in acute inflammatory abdominal conditions (pancreatitis, appendicitis, cholecystitis, diverticulitis). Sweating is sometimes a prodromal or early symptom of haemorrhage, as is faintness or syncope. When vomiting precedes abdominal pain, the cause is unlikely to be appendicitis and suggests gastroenteritis or other causes. Constipation preceding abdominal pain occurs often in large bowel obstruction.

SU-C58   CORRECT RESPONSE D

Surgery is indicated for benign gastric ulcers for failed medical treatment and for complications (bleeding, stenosis, perforation). Gastric ulceration must be assumed to be malignant unless repeated endoscopic reviews demonstrate that the ulcer heals and (most importantly) that it does not subsequently recur. Relief of symptoms is no indication that the ulcer has healed.

Surgery preferably removes the ulcer to obtain histological diagnosis and tries to minimise risk of recurrence. *Partial gastrectomy, which includes removal of ulcer and of antrum with reduction of parietal cell mass, satisfies these criteria and is the usual operation performed*. Gastrointestinal continuity is restored by Billroth I (gastroduodenostomy) or Billroth II (gastrojejunostomy) anastomoses.

Vagotomy, either truncal or highly selective, is the usual operative treatment for benign duodenal (not gastric) ulcer. Truncal vagotomy requires an associated gastric drainage procedure, either pyloroplasty or gastrojejunostomy.

SU-C59   CORRECT RESPONSE B

The pain of intestinal obstruction of small or large bowel is felt in the mid or lower abdomen centrally. Pain is felt and described as intermittently cramping or gripping. Each spasm of pain has a sine wave crescendo/diminuendo sequence with relief between regularly recurring spasms. This is classical intestinal colic.

Change in character of colic to a constantly persisting generalised pain suggests the presence of strangulated (ischaemic) bowel. The other responses are clinical manifestations of bowel obstruction, but are not discriminatory of strangulation.

SU-C60   CORRECT RESPONSE B

The history of prolonged biliary pain, associated with signs of right upper abdominal peritonitis and systemic manifestations of fever and tachycardia, suggests a diagnosis of acute cholecystitis, which would usually be secondary to gallstones. *Abdominal ultrasound is indicated and is the most helpful diagnostically of the investigations listed.* Ultrasound will diagnose gallstones with high sensitivity and specificity and can give information regarding concomitant oedema of the gall-bladder wall, distension of the organ and the presence of pericholecystic collections. It can also indicate whether the extrahepatic and intrahepatic bile ducts are dilated, which in the presence of gall-bladder stones would suggest an associated bile duct stone. Ultrasound is also helpful in excluding associated pathology in liver, kidney and pancreas.

Cholecystography by the oral route is more time consuming than ultrasound and is unsuitable for the immediate diagnosis of acute abdominal pain, especially when associated with nausea and vomiting. It has been largely replaced by ultrasound as the preferred imaging investigation for the diagnosis of gallstones.

Liver function tests (LFT) are often also done in assessment of patients with acute cholecystitis; and abnormal LFT with elevated bilirubin, GGT and alkaline phosphatase in the presence of acute cholecystitis will suggest a bile duct stone. Liver function tests are not themselves diagnostic of cholecystitis. Abdominal plain X-ray will reveal radiologically opaque gallstones in a minority (approximately 15–20%) of patients with gallstones and is therefore much less diagnostically helpful than ultrasound. Other biliary pathologies occasionally seen on plain X-ray include a soft tissue gall-bladder mass, air in the gall-bladder wall (emphysematous cholecystitis) or in the biliary tree (indicating an enteric biliary fistula or previous sphincterotomy of the duodenal ampulla).

Serum amylase would be expected to be elevated only if associated pancreatitis existed with acute cholecystitis, suggesting an additional bile duct stone impacted at the ampulla. The patient's history suggests cholecystitis rather than pancreatitis, so that amylase would not be expected to be as helpful as an initial diagnostic test as would tests seeking the former diagnosis.

SU-C61   CORRECT RESPONSE B

Ulcerative colitis affects only the colon. Crohn disease can affect the entire gastrointestinal tract. Both of these inflammatory bowel diseases of unknown cause can be associated with diarrhoea. Both are chronic relapsing diseases, both are influenced by the general anti-inflammatory effects of steroid therapy and both have extra-intestinal manifestations.

Granulomas are a distinguishing feature of Crohn enteritis (granulomatous enteritis is a synonym for Crohn disease). Crohn enteritis is a transmural disease causing acute or chronic ulceration with cobblestoning, deep fissuring and strictures. Ulcerative colitis is predominantly a mucosal disease with cryptitis and non-specific inflammatory changes progressing to ulceration and sometimes to acutely dilating megacolon with perforation. Strictures and fistulae are rare in ulcerative colitis, whereas they are common in Crohn enteritis.

SU-C62   CORRECT RESPONSE A

Haematemesis and melaena can be due to any of the causes listed; *but the most common cause and the MOST likely diagnosis in the patient described is a bleeding duodenal ulcer.* This is also supported by the previous dyspepsia and abdominal tenderness.

Oesophageal varices associated with portal hypertension and liver disease are less common but can cause severe haematemesis and melaena. Diffuse gastritis is another less common cause, which can be associated with sepsis, analgesics and NSAID. Carcinoma of the stomach rarely causes gross haematemesis nor does ampullary carcinoma. Early endoscopic confirmation of the cause of the bleeding is an important principle in management.

SU-C63   CORRECT RESPONSE A

This swelling has the classic features of an inguinal hernia. Inguinal hernias typically appear at the external ring, through which both direct and indirect inguinal hernias protrude to cause clinical swellings. Reducible hernias classically have an expansile impulse when the patient coughs or strains. If of sufficient size, indirect inguinal hernias may descend down the spermatic cord and into the scrotum. Direct inguinal hernias rarely, if ever, extend into the scrotum. An inguinal hernia in a 14-year-old boy is much more likely to be indirect than direct, but delineation of indirect from direct inguinal hernias is usually only possible with certainty at operation. Inguinal hernias, particularly if indirect, often contain bowel and left untreated there is a risk of strangulation–obstruction of the bowel within the hernial sac. *All patients with symptomatic hernias should be advised to have them treated by surgical repair, particularly a 14-year-old boy.* The other investigations mentioned are irrelevant to the management of inguinal hernia in a young patient.

SU-C64   CORRECT RESPONSE E

The correct answer is *to inspect the anal verge with a view to establishing the diagnosis.* The most likely cause of this woman's symptoms is an **anal fissure.** Acute pain during defaecation associated with bright red bleeding is characteristic of an anal fissure. During the initial consultation it is important to inspect the perineal region carefully and to identify the lower margin of the anal fissure, which is most commonly situated posteriorly in the midline. Sphincter spasm is usually marked, making adequate rectal examination by the finger or by instruments difficult or impossible without general anaesthesia. Attempting to dilate the anus at first consultation would induce considerable pain. The patient should be treated by an early examination under anaesthesia at which stage the anus can be dilated and proctosigmoidoscopy can be performed to check that no higher lesions are present.

SU-C65   CORRECT RESPONSE D

Surgery on this patient is planned for two reasons. First, she is getting symptoms of mucous diarrhoea from the lesion. Second, villous adenomas are premalignant and, therefore, need to be completely excised, even if biopsies have not shown any evidence of malignancy. The prime concern in this woman about to undergo surgery should be to maximise her fitness for surgery. She has chronic congestive cardiac failure and, apart from a tumour which will cause excessive losses of potassium in the stool, is taking medications (diuretics) which could also contribute to electrolyte disturbances and hypokalaemia. Her serum electrolytes must be measured and **the *potassium levels checked and any hypokalaemia should be corrected prior to surgery.*** Digitalis dose monitoring is done by clinical assessment and electrocardiography rather than by serum digoxin levels; a preoperative haemoglobin level is advisable but less likely to be influential in preparation for surgery than the serum potassium; the serum chloride is not likely to contribute in this scenario, and the serum calcium, apart from the chance of finding asymptomatic hypercalcaemia and hyperparathyroidism, also would not be expected to aid surgical planning.

SU-C66   CORRECT RESPONSE A

There are many causes of calcification of abdominal structures. Any of the disease processes mentioned in the question can produce calcification. Although gallstones are common, they do not usually contain sufficient calcium to allow them to be radio-opaque. Chronic pancreatitis is not common and while fibroids are common, they do not often calcify. Similarly, aneurysms may calcify, but not as often as a *lymph node previously infected with tuberculosis.* Worldwide, tuberculosis is a common and important disease. Many individuals become exposed to the bacterium and although they may not develop the full-blown disease, subclinical infection is frequent and is often detected only as calcification on chest or abdominal radiographs.

The following photographs show examples of calcified stones in the gall bladder (Figure 41), a calcified uterine myoma (Figure 42) and tuberculous lymph nodes (Figure 43).

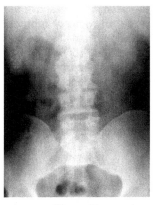 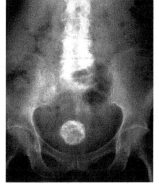 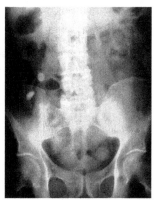

Figure 41   *Figure 42*   *Figure 43*

SU-C67   CORRECT RESPONSE B

Acute onset of left iliac fossa pain in a patient of this age would suggest a diagnosis of *acute diverticulitis.* Diverticulosis of the large bowel is common in the Australian community and frequently complicated by *local infection and paracolic abscess* formation. The patient is febrile, supporting a diagnosis of sepsis and has radiological evidence of small bowel dilatation, which can occur due to adherence of small bowel to the area of the paracolic abscess.

A urinary calculus is not usually associated with evidence of small bowel dilatation and urinary symptoms are often also present. Appendicitis would produce pain in the right iliac fossa and the two other conditions are relatively uncommon.

SU-C68   CORRECT RESPONSE A

Any of the complications listed in the question may occur after splenectomy. Subphrenic abscess formation is uncommon, as is prolonged paralytic ileus. A pancreatic fistula would also be a rare event. A deep venous thrombosis may occur after any operation and is made more likely after splenectomy by thrombocytosis. **Chest problems (left lower lobe atelectasis) are more common than any of the preceding complications.**

SU-C69   CORRECT RESPONSE C

Transient paralytic ileus may occur after any abdominal operation. Paralytic ileus may also be associated with conditions producing peritoneal inflammation or irritation, such as acute pancreatitis or retroperitoneal haemorrhage. The more massive the degree of retroperitoneal haemorrhage and the more prolonged the peritoneal inflammation, the greater the chance of prolonged ileus. Of the operations listed, the one with the greatest potential for prolonged paralytic ileus after surgery is **surgery for resection of a ruptured abdominal aortic aneurysm.** Paralytic ileus following the other operations listed is either expected to be absent (inguinal hernia repair) or transient and unlikely to persist beyond the first day or two after operation. Prolonged paralytic ileus after operations such as gastrectomy or repair of an oesophageal hiatus hernia or removal of an inflamed appendix would cause one to suspect a complication of surgery, such as an intraperitoneal abscess.

SU-C70   CORRECT RESPONSE C

Scrotal swellings can be acute or chronic and painful or non-painful.

The most important single diagnostic test is to determine whether the swelling is confined to the scrotum or is part of an inguinoscrotal swelling (can the examiner get above the swelling?). **An inguino-scrotal swelling is MOST likely to be an indirect inguinal hernia extending into the scrotum.** The major exception to the above statement is when an apparent inguinoscrotal swelling is actually a combined inguinal lump contiguous with and difficult to separate from an additional scrotal lump (e.g. an inguinal hernia together with a hydrocele). The distinction is made easy if the inguinal hernia is reducible, leaving the scrotal lump for separate assessment.

Common causes of purely scrotal lumps are hydroceles (swellings affecting the tunica vaginalis), epididymal cysts, testicular neoplasms and inflammations of epididymis and testis.

Hydroceles and epididymal cysts are usually transilluminable. Hydroceles partly surround the testis. Therefore, large tense hydroceles often obscure and conceal the underlying testis. Evaluation of the testis may be impossible until the hydrocele fluid is drained.

Hydroceles can be primary (without associated scrotal pathology) or secondary to lesions of testis or epididymis. Thus, a hydrocele in a young patient may be indicative of an underlying testicular neoplasm.

The appendix of the testis (hydatid of Morgagni) is a vestigial small swelling above the superior pole of the testis.

Tuberculous epididymo-orchitis is a chronic and relatively uncommon inflammation, usually presenting as a chronic and firm epididymal swelling.

SU-C 71   CORRECT RESPONSE E

The prolonged history over a 2 month period, together with the physical findings, suggest a lymph node swelling in the right groin. *In searching for a primary site it is important to remember to examine the perineum and especially the anal canal.*

The lymph drainage of the testicle is to para-aortic nodes. A saphena varix is unlikely to cause a firm lump. A strangulated hernia must be distinguished from a lymph node swelling but, in addition to the absence of a cough impulse, the swelling would be tense and tender.

SU-C72   CORRECT RESPONSE E

The correct response is **Staphylococcus aureus.** An appendiceal abscess is usually associated with bowel organisms, of which Gram-negative bacilli (*Escherichia coli*) and anaerobic organisms (*Bacteroides fragilis*, *B. melanococcus* and *Streptococcus faecalis*) are the most common. **Staphylococcus aureus** *is a common skin commensal and potential pathogen, but is rarely found in appendiceal abscess or in other infections associated with enteric organisms.*

SU-C73   CORRECT RESPONSE B

Abdominal wound dehiscence ('burst abdomen') most usually represents a failure of surgical technique. Abdominal wound closure, particularly for long vertical wounds, must be designed to resist the potential disrupting force of postoperative increases in intra-abdominal pressure from coughing, straining, distension and ileus. Mass closure of the abdominal parietes taking large bites, with heavy gauge non-absorbable suture material (for example Gauge I nylon), tied with sufficient tension to coopt the wound snugly (but without excessive tension causing ischaemia) satisfies these aims and can almost eliminate the complication. Premature loss of tensile strength of suture material could occur with absorbable sutures such as catgut, which is derived from animal intestine. Modern synthetic non-absorbable (nylon, polyester, polypropylene etc.) and absorbable (polyglycolic acid, polydioxane etc.) sutures are more reliable and can maintain tensile strength over the days and weeks required for the wound to reach maximum intrinsic strength from formation and maturation of collagen. Premature giving way or breakage of knots is minimised by careful technique. General causes of failure of wound repair (vitamin C deficiency, major protein depletions, gross anaemia, renal failure) are less common causes.

SU-C74   CORRECT RESPONSE C

A patient aged 65 years with a history of altered bowel habit needs first to have a large bowel cancer excluded. *Sigmoidoscopy is the optimum first investigation to diagnose carcinoma of the rectum and lower sigmoid.* Barium enema is neither as sensitive nor as specific as endoscopy; small tumours can easily be missed by overlapping bowel shadows. Barium meal and follow-through is an investigation used for disorders of gastric and small bowel mobility. Abdominal CT scan is more helpful for imaging solid viscera than for picking up bowel pathology, but may be useful for imaging liver metastases after the primary diagnosis has been made. Pulmonary metastases are less common in relation to large bowel cancer than are liver metastases. In addition to sigmoidoscopy, colonoscopy will also be required to confirm or exclude associated polyps or second cancers.

SU-C75   CORRECT RESPONSE A

Defaecatory rectal bleeding from surface ulceration is the most common and most important symptom of rectal cancer. The rectum extends from the third piece of the sacrum to the dentate line. The rectum is a distensible large diameter tube and intestinal obstruction from carcinoma of the lower rectum is quite uncommon.

Anaemia requires prolonged chronic blood loss and is classically associated with right-sided colonic lesions. Alterations in bowel habit (constipation, diarrhoea) are less common and usually later symptoms of rectal lesions, although 'spurious' diarrhoea with unsatisfied defaecation and a sense of incomplete evacuation (tenesmus) are also important symptoms.

SU-C76 CORRECT RESPONSE E

A fistula between the sigmoid colon and upper vagina is most commonly due to diverticular disease of the sigmoid. Adherence occurs between the area of diverticulitis and vagina in the pouch of Douglas.

Each of the other responses (colon carcinoma, radiation therapy to the pelvis, extension of uterine or cervical cancer and foreign body perforation of the vagina or bowel) is also a possible cause, but each is less common overall.

SU-C77 CORRECT RESPONSE C

Paget disease of the nipple is a surface eczematous manifestation of an underlying ductal carcinoma, which is usually impalpable. The symptoms may be itching, crusting or erosion. Any persisting nipple abnormality with such symptoms requires nipple biopsy, which reveals the characteristic intraepithelial neoplastic pagetoid cells.

SU-C78 CORRECT RESPONSE A

Adjuvant chemotherapy is combined with local breast surgery in patients at HIGH risk of metastatic or recurrent cancer. Known factors contributing to high risk include advanced disease indicated by spread to axillary nodes, a large primary tumour and histological tumour type.

Although chemotherapeutic drugs are potentially mitogenic and carcinogenic to a variety of tissues, there is no statistical evidence that chemotherapy increases the risk or causes second tumours of the breast.

Chemotherapy is not standard therapy for all patients with breast cancer. Adjuvant hormone manipulation treatment with tamoxifen, an anti-oestrogen, is used as first-line adjuvant treatment in high-risk patients who are postmenopausal and have tumours that are oestrogen or progesterone receptor positive. Chemotherapy tends to be used in premenopausal women and those who are receptor negative. Adjuvant chemotherapy causes some morbidity in its own right and is accordingly reserved for patients at higher risk to avoid unnecessary morbidity of treatment in the lower risk group, where improvement in results from adjuvant therapy is less marked.

Chemotherapy increases survival in high risk patients by approximately 15–30% at 5 years, as well as prolonging the disease-free interval. Chemotherapy using several drugs in combination is more effective and less toxic than use of one drug alone. Commonly used combinations are CMF (cyclophosphamide, methotrexate and 5-fluorouracil), AC (adriamycin and cyclophosphamide) and EC (epirubicin, cyclophosphamide).

SU-C79 CORRECT RESPONSE B

A discrete or 'dominant' breast lump is the most significant clinical presentation of breast cancer, but many other conditions can cause a breast lump. Although all discrete lumps should be considered due to cancer until proven otherwise, the most probable diagnosis of a discrete breast lump will vary with patient age. *In a 25-year-old female the MOST likely diagnosis is a fibroadenoma, a benign lesion usually with a typical picture of a firm, discrete, mobile swelling.* Each of the other responses is a possible cause at this age, but none is as likely as fibroadenoma overall. Cancer is the most likely cause of a lump in patients over 50 years of age, while fibroadenosis (fibrocystic disease, benign mammary dysplasia) presents as a lump in the 30–50 years age group in particular. Fat necrosis can cause confusion at any age, particularly as a history of previous injury is often overlooked or absent.

Intraduct papillomas may present as palpable lumps, but more commonly are associated with bleeding from the nipple.

SU-C80   CORRECT RESPONSE B

A painless lump in the breast in a woman aged 67 years must be considered cancerous until this diagnosis is confirmed or excluded. The illustration shows 'peau d'orange' over a wide area associated with skin dimpling. Peau d'orange is due to dermal oedema, the oedematous skin is pock-marked like the surface of an orange with depressions at the site of attachment of the ligaments of Cooper. Although such a sign may be due to inflammatory oedema, it is far more likely in a woman of 67 with a painless breast lump to be due to malignant lymphatic obstruction. The extensive area of peau d'orange involving more than one quadrant and extending wide of the tumour indicates an *advanced adenocarcinoma of the breast,* rather than an early cancer.

Dermal oedema and peau d'orange may also be seen in mastitis with an associated abscess, but this condition would be far more usual in a lactating breast with other signs of acute inflammation.

Involvement of large mammary ducts with a breast cancer is more likely to cause a blood-stained nipple discharge than peau d'orange.

Fibrocystic breast disease (fibroadenosis) would not be expected to be associated with lymphoedema and would be an extremely rare cause of peau d'orange.

Extensive fat necrosis of the breast could cause the features illustrated, but would be much less common in this age group than breast cancer.

SU-C81   CORRECT RESPONSE A

A varicocele is a dilatation of the veins of the pampiniform plexus of the scrotum and spermatic cord and is clinically evident as a soft, compressible collection of tortuous swollen vessels in the subcutaneous tissues of the scrotum resembling a 'bag of worms'. The abnormality is more common on the left side of the scrotum. The patient is often not aware of the varicocele and symptoms other than minor heaviness are rare. Development of a varicocele for the first time in later life can be a harbinger of a renal carcinoma.

Varicoceles are often found in adult males during investigation of infertility, but whether the former is the cause of the latter problem is a moot point. There is *no known association of varicocele with inguinal hernia.*

SU-C82   CORRECT RESPONSE E

The picture demonstrates the right testis to be lying transversely in the scrotum, suggestive of an abnormally mobile testis with a long sagittal mesorchium (the 'bell clapper' testis), liable to torsion. Episodic scrotal pain, tending to radiate to groin and lower abdomen, often characterises self-resolving episodes of testicular torsion. Repeated minor attacks occur in approximately one-third of patients and can presage an episode leading to continuing ischaemia and gangrene. *Operation with fixation of both testes within the tunica vaginalis is the only reliable method of prevention.* Expectant treatment invites recurrence and gangrene. Mumps orchitis is not associated with recurrent episodic pain and is usually accompanied by parotitis. Bladder pathology or urinary infection are not suggested by the history.

SU-C83   CORRECT RESPONSE D

The clinical presentation is classical of a torsion of the testis. Young males (teenagers and younger) who present with a history of acute scrotal pain and swelling, with a tender swollen testis, represent an acute surgical emergency — the diagnosis must be presumed testicular torsion and operation should proceed forthwith. The testis will infarct if the blood supply is not restored within an hour or two of onset of total ischaemia. The most difficult differential diagnosis is acute epididymo-orchitis in older males, but exploring a patient with epididymo-orchitis or one of the other causes is preferable to missing an ischaemic testis.

SU-C84   CORRECT RESPONSE A

Iron-deficiency anaemia in adults in the cancer age group without overt blood loss should be considered due to an occult bleeding gastrointestinal carcinoma, classically of the caecum, until this diagnosis can be excluded. Barium enema may often miss small epithelial lesions.

Colonoscopy with a view of the whole colon is the essential investigation if the cancer is not to be missed. Angiography can be helpful in diagnosing acute lower gastrointestinal haemorrhage; it is not appropriate as the next step of management in the patient described. Discharging the patient after giving iron supplements with advice regarding nutritional causes of iron deficiency is a classical error that can seriously and significantly delay the diagnosis of colonic cancer because of the mistaken belief that the anaemia is likely to be of dietary deficiency origin. Treatment of the anaemia with replacement of iron stores is appropriate, but the colon (and if this proves negative, the stomach) MUST also and urgently be visualised fully by an experienced endoscopist. Carcinoma of the bladder usually presents with frank haematuria and would rarely be a cause of occult blood loss.

SU-C85   CORRECT RESPONSE C

Pulmonary emboli may arise from limb or pelvic veins. The upper limb is a rare source. Although deep venous thrombosis (DVT) usually commences in the deep calf veins, *symptomatic pulmonary emboli which are large enough to block major pulmonary vessels most usually arise from iliofemoral vein thrombi which are large enough to block the large pulmonary vessels.* Both calf vein DVT or iliofemoral DVT may be asymptomatic, which may make the clinical diagnosis of thrombo-embolic disease difficult.

Areas of localised superficial thrombophlebitis affecting superficial calf or thigh veins present as tender firm subcutaneous cords. These are less liable to embolise than DVT. Pulmonary embolism complicating superficial thrombophlebitis only occurs if thrombosis spreads to involve the deep veins.

SU-C86   CORRECT RESPONSE C

The most important diagnostic aid in a patient with a possible bleeding tendency who is being prepared for operation is the clinical history. If there is a bleeding tendency, it is important to know when the patient bleeds and whether it is spontaneous or follows trauma. Any medications the patient is on should be noted. Many patients take aspirin regularly and may not volunteer this fact, although most patients on anticoagulants will be fully aware of the risks of haemorrhage.

If the patient has been on aspirin, then platelet function might be impaired. Any elective surgery should be deferred and the patient should be asked to stop the drug for 1 week prior to the procedure. Restoration of normal platelet function can be checked by measuring the bleeding time and platelet aggregation studies.

For patients who have been on warfarin, it will be necessary to measure the international normalised ratio (INR) of the prothrombin time; and for those on heparin, the activated partial thromboplastin time (APTT) should be determined. More detailed clotting studies will be required if the patient is thought to have a coagulation defect.

SU-C87   CORRECT RESPONSE C

Overwhelming sepsis after operative removal of the spleen is an important potential sequel to loss of splenic immune functions.

The risk of overwhelming sepsis is increased by approximately 10-fold after splenectomy, compared with the risk in the general population. The risk is highest in the first 12 months after splenectomy.

Brief prodromal symptoms of headache, nausea and vomiting may be followed within a few hours by prostration and refractory shock, with confusion progressing to coma. The risk is higher in children than in adults, making splenic conservation surgery after splenic injury even more important in children. The infections are most likely to occur with bacteria such as pneumococcus, *Haemophilus influenza*, meningococcus. When elective or semi-elective splenectomy can be planned, preliminary vaccination against these organisms is advisable.

SU-C88   CORRECT RESPONSE E

This textbook description fits an injury to the urethra and its classic description perhaps dates from an era when everyone rode a bicycle. People no longer fall astride manhole covers. More common causes now include instrumentation, falling astride a beam during building construction or being kicked in the perineum during an assault. The bulbous urethra can be damaged by forces compressing that section of the urethra against the adjacent pubic symphysis, the so-called 'straddle injury'.

This patient has swelling in the perineum and a subsequent fever, both of which support a diagnosis of rupture of the bulbous urethra and extravasation of urine.

SU-C89   CORRECT RESPONSE D

Pneumaturia (air passed with urine) is almost always due to a vesicocolic fistula. Faecaluria is rare; intermittent attacks of urinary infection, with air causing frothing or whistling on micturition comprise the usual clinical picture. *Diverticular disease of the colon is the most usual cause.* Carcinoma of the colon is a much less common cause. Neither urachal cyst remnants nor a ruptured bladder cause pneumaturia. Pneumatosis intestinalis is a condition of gas cysts affecting mucosal and serosal aspects of the colon or small bowel and is an acquired condition associated with chronic emphysema.

SU-C90   CORRECT RESPONSE A

Oliguria following surgery may be due to primary renal failure (intrinsic acute renal failure, usually due to acute tubular necrosis (ATN)) or to reversible acute renal insufficiency (extrinsic renal failure, acute renal vascular insufficiency) due to volume depletion. Differentiation between the two causes is of great clinical importance and may be helped by examination of urine composition.

Established acute renal failure (primary renal failure with ATN) gives urine approximating the composition of a plasma ultrafiltrate with low osmolality and high sodium concentration. By contrast, *the urine in depletional oliguria is concentrated with high osmolality and is also associated with sodium reabsorption and a low urinary sodium content.*

SU-C91   CORRECT RESPONSE D

Of concern in this patient is that he has injured his lower urinary tract. *The presence of blood at the external urethral meatus suggests damage to the urethra and a likely rupture of the membranous component.*

Passage of a urethral catheter may be unsuccessful and could cause further injury.

Excretory urography will show the upper urinary tract (kidney and ureters) well, but the concern here is with the urethra.

Asking the patient to attempt to void runs the risk of extravasation of urine at the site of urethral injury.

Urethroscopy is not the best way to demonstrate recent urethral injury and it also runs the risk of causing further damage.

The urgent investigation required is an ascending urethrogram using water soluble contrast material injected with minimal pressure through a balloon catheter inserted just inside the urethral meatus. Films are taken in different planes to demonstrate the penile, membranous and prostatic urethra, looking for evidence of injury and extravasation. If the examination of the urethra is normal a sterile catheter is passed into the bladder and a cystogram is performed to check for bladder injury.

If the suspected urethral injury is confirmed, proximal urinary diversion by suprapubic cystostomy will be required, with or without primary urethral realignment and splintage.

SU-C92   CORRECT RESPONSE C

An intravenous pyelogram (IVP) is often diagnostic during an attack of ureteric colic, showing delayed excretion or dilated urinary passages proximal to a filling defect. The line of the ureter is lateral to the lumbar transverse processes, but an opacity along this line can also be due to other causes (tablets in the intestine, calcified lymph nodes).

Red cells in the urine suggest stone disease, white cells suggest infection. Medullary sponge kidney is commonly associated with stones.

Demonstration of contrast in the obstructed collecting system, confirming the presence and site of the obstruction, is often best seen in delayed films.

SU-C93   CORRECT RESPONSE C

The correct response is 55 mmol.

Potassium is an essential element in the diet and the healthy individual requires a daily intake of between 40 and 80 mmol. One gram of potassium chloride is the equivalent of 13 mmol of potassium. Potassium is contained in vegetables and fruits and in meat, being a major intracellular cation. Given intravenously, it is safest to give in concentrations that do not exceed 40 mmol/L, as the rapid delivery of a large bolus of potassium can cause cardiac irregularities or cardiac arrest.

SU-C 94   CORRECT RESPONSE C

The history strongly suggests gastric outlet obstruction ('pyloric stenosis'). Common causes are stricture and spasm of a chronic duodenal or prepyloric benign peptic ulcer; distal gastric carcinoma is another important cause. The illustration shows a scaphoid lower abdomen with abdominal upper distension consistent with a distended J-shaped stomach. A succussion splash would be expected to be demonstrable.

Loss of gastric content gives an isotonic loss of HCl, causing a subtractional metabolic alkalosis with diminished serum chloride, a high serum bicarbonate and an elevated pH with little change in P_aco_2. The renal response is of increased bicarbonate excretion and is accompanied by concomitant loss of sodium, and later potassium, in the urine. Sodium and potassium are also lost in the vomitus. The full-blown picture is of water, electrolyte and nutritional depletion. The clinical syndrome commonly described as 'dehydration' is actually one of combined salt and water loss ('saline' deficit). *The major depletion requiring initial correction in this patient, who has clinical signs of 'dehydration' with oliguria, is to replenish extracellular fluid depletion with isotonic (normal) saline. The amount required to replace the deficit, in the absence of circulatory collapse, is approximately 3–5% of bodyweight (approximately 2–3 L); and isotonic saline is the preferred replacement fluid.* Hypertonic solution is not appropriate; gastrointestinal losses are isosmolar with body fluids. None of the other replacement solutions adequately replenishes the combined losses in the vomitus and urine. Dextrose in water supplies only water; 4% dextrose in 1/5 isotonic saline does not provide enough sodium and chloride (only 30 rather than 155 mmol/L). Hartmann solution would adequately replace sodium and water losses and is an admirable replacement fluid for mixed extracellular fluid deficits such as occur from small bowel obstruction. It contains inadequate chloride to replace gastric losses and the small amounts of potassium (5 mmol) are not suitable for potassium replacement. Once initial resuscitation with saline has restored urine output towards normal, large amounts of potassium (up to 150 mmol in 24 h) will be required to replace potassium losses, but infusion of potassium is best delayed until renal function has been shown to be satisfactory.

SU-C95   CORRECT RESPONSE B

'Normal' saline is an isotonic solution of sodium chloride without any additives, suitable for peripheral intravenous drips as it is isosmolar with body fluids. The total osmolality of extracellular fluid (approximately 300 mOsmol/L) is made up predominantly by the electrolytes sodium and chloride, with minor contribution from other electrolytes, from non-electrolytes (glucose, creatinine) and protein. Total osmolality is usually approximately 2 x [Na^+] + 10 mmol/L.

An isosmolar (0.9 g%) sodium chloride solution has an osmolality of approximately 300 mmol /L, with approximately 155 mmol /L Na and 155 mmol /L Cl. It contains 9 g/L NaCl, so each gram of NaCl contains approximately 17 mmol Na. Saline is often used as a replacement fluid for extracellular fluid deficits or to provide basal sodium requirements, which in an adult amount to approximately 80 mmol Na daily (or approximately 0.5 L of saline).

Another commonly used isotonic intravenous solution is 4% dextrose in 1/5 isotonic saline containing approximately 30 mmol Na and Cl [1/5 x155] and 40 g/L dextrose (4/5 isotonic). Isotonic (5%) dextrose contains about 300 mmol/L (50 g) dextrose, so 4% dextrose is roughly equivalent to 240 mmol dextrose.

Sodium (135–145 mmol), potassium (5 mmol) and calcium (2 mmol) are the cation concentrations found in Hartmann solution (response A: compound sodium lactate or lactated Ringer solution), which is a solution with electrolyte composition (in mmol/L: Na 135–145; K 5; Ca 2; Mg 2; Cl 110; lactate 40) more akin to extracellular fluid than saline.

Daily requirements of potassium (60–80 mmol) are provided by none of the above solutions. Potassium is often added to intravenous solutions as KCl (1 g = 13 mmol K) in concentrations of about 26 mmol/L (e.g. as additions to 4% dextrose in 1/5 saline, as in response E). Potassium administration is only commenced when urine output is adequate.

SU-C96   CORRECT RESPONSE C

Of the responses, *vitamin B deficiency is the least likely to affect wound healing.* Wound healing is influenced markedly by local factors, such as infection, local blood supply and previous irradiation, but also by a number of general factors, of which diabetes mellitus, vitamin C deficiency and uraemia are examples that act by impairing collagen formation and maturation or by association with ischaemia, neuropathy and impaired resistance to infection. Patients with liver failure will also have potential complications of wound healing associated with a bleeding tendency due to vitamin K-linked haemostatic deficiencies.

SU-C97   CORRECT RESPONSE B

'Gas gangrene' is an overwhelming anaerobic infection (clostridial myonecrosis with systemic toxaemia) and may complicate wounds, such as compound limb fractures and amputations for ischaemic vascular disease, or injections of vasoconstrictive agents such as adrenaline. *Adequate and early wound debridement with removal of devitalised tissue is both the best preventive and the most important aspect of treatment.*

Gas gangrene antitoxin carries a moderately high risk of anaphylaxis and is not now generally used.

Systemic (not local) antibiotics, usually penicillin, are important adjuncts, secondary to removal of dead or suspect tissue. Hyperbaric oxygen treatment aims to increase local oxygen tensions and thus diminish the likelihood that colonisation will progress to infection. It is, like antibiotics, valuable as a follow-up to surgical removal of dead tissue and foreign bodies, but must not delay primary operative treatment.

SU-C98   CORRECT RESPONSE E

This puncture wound must be regarded as potentially contaminated with spores of *Clostridium tetani* and, thus, a tetanus-prone wound. Wound debridement is mandatory, but in these types of wounds it may not be possible to ensure adequate local wound toilet. In such cases it is prudent to complement local treatment with a single intramuscular dose of penicillin.

As this man has never been immunised against tetanus he must be given tetanus toxoid. In addition to correction of his non-immune status, the patient should be provided with transient protection through the administration of (human) tetanus immunoglobulin. He should be given the immunoglobulin intramuscularly, not intravenously, to reduce the risk of an anaphylactic reaction. Therefore, the correct management of this man should include the administration of *tetanus toxoid, tetanus immunoglobulin intramuscularly, and penicillin.*

SU-C99   CORRECT RESPONSE D

Acute rupture of a hepatic echinococcal (hydatid) cyst into the peritoneal cavity can occur spontaneously or after trauma. Escape of the contents (brood capsules, daughter cysts, scolices, hydatid fluid) can cause presentation as an acute abdomen. Haemorrhage, peritoneal seeding of daughter cysts, intraperitoneal sepsis and hepatorenal failure are all possible sequelae.

The most immediate serious risk to life, although it is rare, is an anaphylactic reaction (hypersensitivity) from sudden exposure to hydatid antigen. Anaphylactic reactions can be mild and manifested by fever and a skin rash; or, more severe reactions can occur, with anaphylactic shock, or even cardiac arrest. Such reactions can occur within minutes of cyst rupture.

SU-C100   CORRECT RESPONSE C

Each of the responses has the potential for malignant change *except the blue naevus, a bluish cutaneous nodule which is entirely benign.*

Leucoplakia is a descriptive term describing a white plaque on the oral mucous membrane. It is associated with squamous cell carcinoma. Hutchinson melanotic freckle is a pigmented skin lesion of long standing, often found on the face of elderly individuals, which ultimately progresses to invasive melanoma.

Thyroid irradiation in childhood for acne or other conditions, can lead to development of thyroid cancer.

Irradiation of skin can lead to radiation dermatitis and squamous skin cancers.

SU-C101   CORRECT RESPONSE C

Hamartoma (Greek: 'a swelling which has gone wrong') is a developmental malformation containing a variety of local tissues (an excessive focal overgrowth of mature normal cells and tissues indigenous to the region). A hamartoma is thus due to a developmental defect and is distinct from neoplasm or teratoma ('monster') which contain abnormal non-indigenous tissues.

Hamartoma should not be confused with malignant liver tumour (hepatoma), blood clot (haematoma), the hamstring muscles, or bone.

SU-C102   CORRECT RESPONSE D

The oral cavity is lined with squamous epithelium and squamous cell carcinoma is the most common malignant tumour occurring in the mouth. Risk factors and common associations include all the S's: Smoking, Spirits, Sepsis, Syphilis, Spices (betel nut), Stumps of teeth and Suppressed immune status. The other less common tumours listed involve bone, dental tissue or salivary glands.

SU-C103   CORRECT RESPONSE C

Radiation damage to surrounding tissues is unfortunately all too common after radiotherapy for cervical cancer. The gut is particularly radiosensitive and small and large bowel damage may occur. If the patient has had previous abdominal surgery, the risks to the small bowel are increased as adhesions may fix loops of bowel down in the pelvis, where they will be in the field of radiation. In the absence of adhesions, the small bowel is relatively mobile and the risk for any one section of intestine is less than that to *the rectum, a fixed structure lying immediately behind the cervix.* The sigmoid colon is more remote from the treatment field and *radiation proctitis is the most common complication of pelvic irradiation.*

SU-C104   CORRECT RESPONSE D

Severe pain on pressure over the thumbnail is characteristic of a glomus tumour of the nail bed. These benign lesions involve the glomus cells, which are myoepithelial cells associated with arteriovenous communications and are concentrated particularly in the finger pulp and nail bed. They are normally concerned with heat exchange and temperature regulation. A glomus tumour presents as a small vascular nodule in the subcutaneous tissues of the limb or nail bed. They are often so small as to be undetectable on clinical examination, but cause severe spasms of pain exacerbated by pressure. Occasionally nail growth is affected with ridging and deformity of the overlying nail. Excision is dramatically curative. Glomus tumours comprise the most striking member of a group of tumours exhibiting severe pain out of proportion to physical signs; leiomyomas can also be painful. Liposarcomas, giant cell tumours of bone, fibroadenomas and dermatofibromas are not usually painful.

SU-C105   CORRECT RESPONSE A

This man has a squamous cell cancer on his forearm which has been incompletely excised. He requires further excision with histological proof that there is no tumour in the resection margins. While squamous cell carcinomas do metastasise and may well spread to adjacent lymph nodes, there is no evidence at this stage that the tumour has spread in this man; treatment should be directed at the primary lesion and restricted to *wider local excision*. Follow-up will be required to monitor for local recurrence and regional lymph node status.

SU-C106   CORRECT RESPONSE D

Metastatic bony deposits are commonly found in many malignant tumours, particularly those with primary sites in the lung, breast, prostate, kidney and thyroid. While deposits may occur in any bone site, they go less frequently to the *bones below the knee or elbow,* probably relating to the lesser vascularity at these latter sites. Skull, vertebral column, long bones of femur and humerus and pelvis are all common sites of metastatic deposits.

SU-C107   CORRECT RESPONSE E

While it is a well accepted procedure for the determination of the presence of free blood within the abdominal cavity, diagnostic peritoneal lavage has now been supplanted by CT scanning (where available) as the preferred method of assessment in circumstances such as those described in the question.

From the stem it can be implied that the patient is haemodynamically unstable, as the presence of blood *per se* in the abdominal cavity is not an indication for surgery. For example, splenic rupture is normally managed conservatively in the first instance. In this case, the degree of continuing intra-abdominal haemorrhage may be such that the blood pressure cannot be restored to normal without surgical control of the bleeding vessel. Surgery in such circumstances is an integral part of resuscitation and must not be delayed. A central venous pressure line is very useful in the diagnosis and management of refractory shock when the cause of continuing hypotension is unclear.

A nasogastric tube may be inserted prior to induction of anaesthesia if it is thought the patient has a full stomach. However, this is an uncomfortable procedure and attempted insertion may induce vomiting — with the subsequent risk of inhalation. To avoid regurgitation and inhalation, judicious use of cricoid pressure during induction is a far more effective measure.

In this case, the patient has a small pneumothorax and pain from the fractured ribs may interfere with respiration. It would be helpful to know what has happened to oxygen saturation, but this patient will be given oxygen through a face mask, whether or not blood gas analysis is done.

An intercostal drain would normally be inserted only if the patient had a large initial haemopneumothorax, or if a pneumothorax was of sufficient size to cause respiratory embarrassment. However, this patient is about to be anaesthetised and ventilated and the *positive pressure ventilation during general anaesthesia may worsen the pneumothorax, so a chest drain must be inserted as a precautionary measure under local anaesthetic prior to induction of anaesthesia and laparotomy, even though the pneumothorax is, at present, small.*

SUMMARY OF CORRECT RESPONSES

CATEGORY & QUESTION NO.	CORRECT RESPONSE	CATEGORY & QUESTION NO.	CORRECT RESPONSE	CATEGORY & QUESTION NO.	CORRECT RESPONSE
SU-Q 1	A	SU-Q 32	B	SU-Q 63	A
SU-Q 2	C	SU-Q 33	D	SU-Q 64	E
SU-Q 3	A	SU-Q 34	C	SU-Q 65	D
SU-Q 4	A	SU-Q 35	C	SU-Q 66	A
SU-Q 5	E	SU-Q 36	A	SU-Q 67	B
SU-Q 6	E	SU-Q 37	A	SU-Q 68	A
SU-Q 7	B	SU-Q 38	D	SU-Q 69	C
SU-Q 8	E	SU-Q 39	C	SU-Q 70	C
SU-Q 9	D	SU-Q 40	C	SU-Q 71	E
SU-Q 10	B	SU-Q 41	D	SU-Q 72	E
SU-Q 11	B	SU-Q 42	B	SU-Q 73	B
SU-Q 12	E	SU-Q 43	D	SU-Q 74	C
SU-Q 13	C	SU-Q 44	D	SU-Q 75	A
SU-Q 14	B	SU-Q 45	C	SU-Q 76	E
SU-Q 15	E	SU-Q 46	E	SU-Q 77	C
SU-Q 16	A	SU-Q 47	D	SU-Q 78	A
SU-Q 17	E	SU-Q 48	B	SU-Q 79	B
SU-Q 18	C	SU-Q 49	A	SU-Q 80	B
SU-Q 19	C	SU-Q 50	A	SU-Q 81	A
SU-Q 20	C	SU-Q 51	C	SU-Q 82	E
SU-Q 21	C	SU-Q 52	E	SU-Q 83	D
SU-Q 22	C	SU-Q 53	A	SU-Q 84	A
SU-Q 23	E	SU-Q 54	D	SU-Q 85	C
SU-Q 24	B	SU-Q 55	A	SU-Q 86	C
SU-Q 25	D	SU-Q 56	B	SU-Q 87	C
SU-Q 26	D	SU-Q 57	D	SU-Q 88	E
SU-Q 27	E	SU-Q 58	D	SU-Q 89	D
SU-Q 28	C	SU-Q 59	B	SU-Q 90	A
SU-Q 29	D	SU-Q 60	B	SU-Q 91	D
SU-Q 30	B	SU-Q 61	B	SU-Q 92	C
SU-Q 31	D	SU-Q 62	A	SU-Q 93	C

CATEGORY & QUESTION NO.	CORRECT RESPONSE
SU-Q 94	C
SU-Q 95	B
SU-Q 96	C
SU-Q 97	B
SU-Q 98	E
SU-Q 99	D
SU-Q 100	C
SU-Q 101	C
SU-Q 102	D
SU-Q 103	C
SU-Q 104	D
SU-Q 105	A
SU-Q 106	D
SU-Q 107	E

Surgery
Commentaries
and Summary of Correct Responses
TYPE
J

Commentaries SU-C108 to SU-C187

Correct Responses SU-Q108 to SU-Q187

SURGERY COMMENTARIES AND CORRECT RESPONSES — TYPE J

SU-C108   CORRECT RESPONSE A,B,C,D

Basal cell carcinomas (BCC) occur *most commonly on the face* and *rarely if ever metastasise by lymphatic or by systemic spread.* *They spread deeply and extensively by local invasion* ('nothing burrows like a basal cell'). *They are associated with solar exposure,* as are squamous cell carcinomas (SCC). In Australia, both BCC and SCC are common, BCC being approximately 3–4-fold more common than SCC.

As distinct from SCC, which are almost confined to sun-exposed areas (face, head and neck, lower lip, back of hands), BCC also occur quite commonly on non-exposed areas.

SU-C109   CORRECT RESPONSE C,D,E

Pilonidal ('nest of hairs') sinus has its peak incidence in young hairy adult males. It is less common in older males aged 40–50 years unless a predisposing unstable operative scar exists.

It is an acquired disease not associated with congenital tracks; and is due to hair penetrating the skin. Penetration is more likely through sweaty and macerated skin, by freshly-cut sharp hairs and by the frictional force of opposing large buttocks drilling hairs into the subcutaneous tissues.

Thus, primary pits and sinuses usually lie in the midline in the depths of the natal cleft.

The hairs deviate laterally as they burrow in the subcutaneous tissues; **and *an abscess may rupture or be incised causing 'secondary' granulating sinuses lateral to the midline*.** Pilonidal infection and sinuses also occur at other predisposed sites where skin clefts and hair coexist: *at the umbilicus, in the groin or axilla and as 'barber's sinuses' between the fingers.*

SU-C 110   CORRECT RESPONSE B

This black macular lesion on the temple of an elderly patient looks typical of a Hutchinson melanotic freckle. These lesions are slowly progressive, superficial, spreading melanomas. Although they commonly have a long latent period of some years before invasive spread occurs, they have a high malignant potential and, if left long enough, malignant transformation is virtually inevitable. An intradermal naevus is a wholly benign melanocytic naevus and accounts for most raised benign papular congenital moles with negligible risk of malignancy. Pigmented BCC can be difficult to pick from melanoma, but are usually nodular or papular lesions with surface telangiectases. Seborrhoeic keratoses are also common on the face. They are papular, verrucous, greasy, pigmented lesions of characteristic appearance.

SU-C111   CORRECT RESPONSE E

The appearance of extensive patchy gangrene of the skin of scrotum and perineum is typical of Fournier gangrene. It presents as a necrotising infection of skin and subcutaneous tissues due to a mixed group of infecting organisms and is common in elderly and debilitated patients with diminished resistance to infection, *often with associated diabetes mellitus.*

The most immediately important and potentially life-saving aspect of treatment is radical excision of necrotic skin and subcutaneous tissue. Antibiotics are secondary to the requirement of early surgery. Metronidazole is not the preferred antibiotic, as it is only effective against anaerobes such as bacteroides species and the infection is usually a mixed one with Gram-positive and -negative bowel organisms as well as anaerobes. Triple therapy using a penicillin, an aminoglycoside and an anti-anaerobe may thus be required; alternatively to triple therapy, a late generation cephalosporin. Antibiotics are always only an adjunct to definitive surgery, which may need to be repeated more than once.

Surgery must be early and should NEVER be left until a local abscess presents.

Hyperbaric oxygen therapy to help combat anaerobic infection is, like antibiotics, useful as an adjunct and follow up to adequate excisional surgery with free drainage and must NOT delay surgery.

SU-C112   CORRECT RESPONSE A,B

Thyroglossal cysts form from remnants of the thyroglossal duct. This follows the course of thyroid descent *in utero* from the foramen caecum at the base of the tongue to its position at the root of the neck. The track and any cyst that may develop runs *in the midline* to the level of the hyoid bone, with which it is intimately related. Most cysts lie near the hyoid bone, although they may be found at any site along the line of the thyroglossal duct. The duct below the hyoid diverges slightly from the midline (usually to the left), leaving as vestigial remnant the levator glandulae thyroidae muscle running to the apex of the pyramidal lobe of the thyroid above the isthmus. A fibrous cord often joins the cyst to the hyoid and the *cyst moves upwards* with the hyoid on swallowing and *when the tongue is protruded.*

The cysts can present at any age, although most are seen in patients in their teens or in their twenties. Malignant change is much less common as a presenting symptom and there appears to be no more liability to malignant change than in the normal thyroid.

SU-C113   CORRECT RESPONSE A,B

Benign nodular goitre in Western communities can present as a multinodular enlargement affecting the whole gland or as a 'solitary' lump in the neck, which is subsequently found to be a prominent component of a multinodular goitre. These goitres can be of sufficient size to *cause tracheal or oesophageal or venous obstruction* and this often relates to retrosternal extension of the gland. Involvement of the recurrent laryngeal nerve would be very unusual and highly suggestive of malignant infiltration, as would the much rarer Horner syndrome. There is no connection between the development of malignancy in such a goitre and glandular overactivity.

SU-C114   CORRECT RESPONSE C,D,E

Lip cancer most commonly affects the sun-exposed lower lip and *is nearly always a squamous cell carcinoma.*

Risk factors include sun exposure and smoking and *the great majority of lip cancers occur in males.* Spread by local invasion and by lymphatic spread contributes to mortality and morbidity, but *the outlook is better than for tongue cancer, where the diagnosis is more often late or occult. Cervical lymph node metastases from lip cancer are best treated by surgery if resectable;* squamous cell carcinoma within lymph nodes is less amenable to radiotherapy than is the primary lesion.

SU-C115   CORRECT RESPONSE A,C,D,E

The photograph (Figure 29) shows a close-up view of the nose, the bridge of the nose and the upper lip. Accurate knowledge of local topography aids descriptions of lesions. This has particular medico–legal relevance. Several regions are labelled. Starting at the top, region *P is the glabella,* Q is the lower tarsal plate, *R is the columella, S is the philtrum and T is the vermilion border.* The lacrimal gland secretes tears by ducts which open into the conjunctival sac and drain medially through superior and inferior lacrimal canaliculi via the lacrimal sac and nasolacrimal duct, to an orifice within the inferior meatus of the lateral wall of the nose.

SU-C116   CORRECT RESPONSE A,B,D,E

Submandibular duct calculus causes an *acute and painful swelling of the blocked submandibular salivary gland. The stone is usually palpable on bimanual examination of the floor of the mouth* within the submandibular salivary duct (Wharton duct). *Submandibular calculi are virtually always radio-opaque* and are best picked up on plain X-ray using an intra-oral view. *They can pass spontaneously through the duct orifice* but often require surgical excision for recurring obstructive attacks. Operative removal is usually done via an intra-oral approach. Removal of the gland itself is reserved for intraglandular or persisting recurrent calculi.

The only investigation usually required is a plain X-ray, which invariably shows the calculus. Sialography can precipitate infection, is unnecessary in making the diagnosis, is contraindicated in the acute attack and is best avoided. Sialography is more appropriate for chronic non-calculous sialitis, which often shows 'sialectasis' and is associated with autoimmune disease.

SU-C117   CORRECT RESPONSE B,C

Pharyngo-oesophageal diverticula are acquired pulsion diverticula occurring through the posterior wall of the pharynx near the midline, between the oblique and transverse fibres of the inferior pharyngeal constrictor.

They are false diverticula consisting of mucosa and submucosa without a muscular covering. *They usually occur in elderly males. Dysphagia is the main symptom and oesophageal cancer is the main differential diagnosis.*

Diagnosis is usually made by barium swallow: endoscopy is required to exclude any mucosal lesions. Endoscopy without the prior evidence of a contrast swallow is potentially hazardous, particularly in inexperienced hands, as the endoscope tends to pass into the cul-de-sac of the diverticulum and oesophageal perforation is a possible complication. One-stage resection has replaced two-stage resection as preferred treatment.

The diverticulum, although commencing near the midline, diverges and presents laterally, more commonly on the left than on the right.

SU-C118   CORRECT RESPONSE D

A Horner syndrome results from paralysis of the cervical sympathetic nerve fibres and is characterised by enophthalmos, miosis, ptosis and a warm, dry skin on the affected side of the face. The loss of sympathetic tone causes vasodilatation of the cutaneous vessels of the cheek and nasal mucosa with absence of sweating and a feeling of nasal obstruction. There is also narrowing of the palpebral fissure *where the ptosis is due to weakness of the levator palpebrae superioris muscle*. There is also a contraction of the pupil due to the unopposed action of the autonomic parasympathetic inflow via the oculomotor nerve. The eyeball itself can maintain a full range of movement.

Conditions that can produce a Horner syndrome include anything that might destroy the cervical sympathetic chain. Examples include invading cancer at the apex of the lung, syringomyelia and deliberate obliteration of the inferior cervical ganglion to treat vasospastic vascular disease.

SU-C119   CORRECT RESPONSE B,D,E

This patient is likely to have divided his right ulnar nerve. In the forearm the ulnar nerve innervates the flexor carpi ulnaris and the medial half of the flexor digitorum profundus. The ulnar nerve supplies motor fibres to the short muscles of the hand (except the first two lumbricals and muscles of the thenar eminence, which are supplied by the median nerve) and sensory fibres to the little finger and medial aspect of the ring finger.

If he has damaged the ulnar nerve, the patient will be **unable to abduct and adduct the extended fingers**, but will be able to pinch thumb and index finger together, as this latter movement depends on median nerve function. There would also be some **reduced power on flexion of the wrist** and **anaesthesia of the little and ring fingers.**

SU-C120   CORRECT RESPONSE A,B,D

A neuropathic (Charcot) joint can occur in any condition in which the sensory pathways from the joint become impaired, allowing destructive processes to go unnoticed and not appreciated. The impairment of sensation of pain or position may be due to a lesion of the central spinal cord (**syringomyelia**), the posterior spinal columns (the tabes dorsalis of **syphilis**) or involve peripheral nerve fibres from the joint itself (**diabetes mellitus** and leprosy (Hansen disease)). In motor neuron disease and progressive muscular dystrophy, it is the motor component of the nervous system that is affected and joint sensation is preserved. Progressive muscular dystrophy affects muscles only, without sensory involvement.

SU-C121   CORRECT RESPONSE B,D

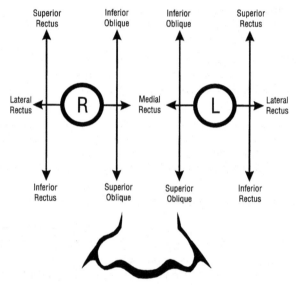

Actions of individual eye muscles
When the eye is turned out, SR & IR move eye up and down
When turned in, IO & SO move eye up and down

Figure 44a

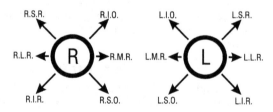

Muscles involved in Conjugate Eye Gaze
Figure 44b

Eye movements normally occur congruently and synchronously with control of individual eye movements as indicated (Figure 44a and Figure 44b). The external (lateral) rectus muscle moves the eye laterally and is supplied by the abducens (VIth) nerve. This nerve has a relatively long intracranial course before entering the cavernous sinus on its way to the orbit. Isolated VIth nerve palsies are accordingly quite common. The superior oblique muscle, moving the eye down and in, is supplied by the trochlear (IVth) nerve. Isolated IVth nerve palsies are rare; such lesions affect activities involving looking downwards (like descending a flight of steps).

The other muscles (internal rectus, superior and inferior recti, inferior oblique) are all supplied by the oculomotor (IIIrd) nerve, which also carries autonomic efferent pupilloconstrictor fibres from the Edinger–Westphal nucleus. Third nerve lesions thus cause ophthalmoplegia apart from outward lateral gaze, a divergent squint ('down and out eye') and a dilated pupil unresponsive to light (direct and consensual reflexes) or accommodation. The left oculomotor nerve is not involved, as the pupils are of equal size.

The patient's left eye is remaining central when attempting outward gaze. Inward gaze of the right eye appears normal. *The appearances suggest a lesion of the left abducens (VIth) nerve. This will cause diplopia*, the false image of the left eye being medial to the real image. The pupil size would not be expected to alter with a VIth nerve palsy. The corneal reflex, mediated by Vth and VIIth nerves, would be unaffected also. Direct and consensual light responses will also be unaffected. A blind eye due to injury of the optic nerve will lose the direct response of the affected pupil to light, but will maintain the consensual response.

SU-C122   CORRECT RESPONSE A,C

The patient is unable to close his right eye; the eye, instead, is rolling up under the upper lid with an open palpebral fissure and failure of action of orbicularis oculi (Bell Sign). The right side of the mouth also appears asymmetric and paralysed. These appearances are typical of *a right facial nerve palsy involving both upper and lower facial muscle groups.*

Facial nerve palsies may affect the upper motor neuron (supranuclear lesion) due to lesions such as cerebrovascular accidents or tumours, or may be lower motor neuron (nuclear and infranuclear) lesions due to basal skull fractures, acoustic nerve tumours, parotid lesions or brain stem pathology affecting the pons. The upper facial musculature (e.g. occipitofrontalis, orbicularis oculi) is bilaterally innervated from the upper motor neuron fibres, so the right upper facial muscles would be relatively spared in a right upper motor neuron lesion. Taste fibres to the anterior two-thirds of the tongue are carried via the lingual nerve to the chorda tympani, which joins the facial nerve within the facial canal of the petrous temporal bone on its way to the nucleus tractus solitarius in the pons. *Facial nerve lesions distal to the junction of chorda tympani with the facial nerve (extracranial lesions, such as those within the parotid gland) will thus spare taste fibres and taste to the anterior tongue will be retained.*

The corneal reflex (eye closure on corneal stimulation) depends on integrity of both afferent fibres via the Vth nerve and the efferent supply to orbicularis oculi by the VIIth nerve. In the case shown, it would be absent whatever the state of the Vth nerve and protection of the eye is a major concern in facial nerve palsies.

Collapse of the cheek on the affected side occurs due to paralysis of buccinator muscle, which is supplied by the facial nerve. The trigeminal nerve supplies muscles of mastication only (temporalis, masseter, pterygoids).

SU-C123   CORRECT RESPONSE A,C,E

'Stress' fractures are spontaneous fractures occurring, as their name suggests, in regions where a normal bone is subjected to forces of stress beyond what is normally expected in terms of support. In engineering terms stress is the measure of the amount of force per unit area and is that force which will produce a deformation on strain. In the biological sense, stress is that which goes beyond support and causes fracture of the *normal* bone. Stress fractures are thus to be distinguished from pathological fractures, which are also spontaneous, but occur in bones weakened by disease (osteoporosis, tumour, congenital deficiencies).

A classical site for stress fracture is the *neck of the second metatarsal.* This is the longest metatarsal. Its head projects forward beyond the others, leading to stress fractures across its narrow neck in individuals exposed to prolonged weight-bearing load ('march fracture' in army recruits). Another fracture from similar causes occurs *in athletes across the upper tibial shaft.*

The short and flat first rib is well protected from external trauma, but has the powerful scalene muscles attached to its upper surface. *The first rib is liable to spontaneous fracture across its neck in patients such as chronic asthmatics in whom accessory muscles of ventilation are in excessive and prolonged activity.*

Neither the femur nor the mandible is a common site of stress fracture.

SU-C124   CORRECT RESPONSE B,D,E

Dupuytren disease, usually presenting as palmar fasciitis (fibromatosis), is a condition of unknown aetiology, although there are several conditions which are associated with Dupuytren disease. It presents as a slowly progressive *painless* nodule or contracture of the palmar fascia (not the underlying flexor tendons) affecting particularly the ring and little fingers. The thumb is uncommonly involved. The condition is almost exclusively *confined to men* and it can *occasionally affect the foot.* In the foot, it presents as a subcutaneous nodule rather than a contracture.

SU-C125   CORRECT RESPONSE A,B,C,D

All of the fractures described involve the wrist or hand except the Monteggia fracture, which is a fracture–dislocation of the forearm and elbow. Fracture of the upper one-third of the ulna is associated with a dislocation at the elbow of the head of the radius, not of the wrist.

Colles fracture is a common fracture occurring in elderly women with osteoporotic bones after a fall on the hand. The fracture is through the distal radius and the ulnar styloid or collateral ligament. *The distal fracture segment is dorsally displaced and angulated, radially displaced and angulated and impacted.*

Smith fracture describes a lower radial fracture with displacements which are the reverse of Colles fracture.

Fractures of the scaphoid, without associated injuries, *usually have minimal or no displacement.*

Bennett fracture–dislocation of the thumb is an unstable fracture–dislocation of the base of the thumb–metacarpal *involving the carpo–metacarpal joint.*

SU-C126   CORRECT RESPONSE A,B,C,D,E

All of the responses are correct in relation to varicose veins. Varicose veins can primarily affect the superficial venous system. Superficial varices can also be *secondary to obstruction of the deep venous system by a previous deep venous thrombosis.* The deep venous obstruction or thrombosis can be the result of altered coagulation, diminished flow or direct trauma to the vein, such as might occur with a *previous tibial fracture.* In primary varicosities, the defect can be *incompetence at the sapheno–femoral junction* or at the site of incompetence of perforating veins in the leg or thigh. Occasionally, varicose veins develop as the result of *arterio–venous fistulae* in the leg. There can be a *familial predisposition* to the development of varicose veins.

SU-C127   CORRECT RESPONSE A,B,C

Until proven otherwise, this patient has developed a deep venous thrombosis of her right leg and thigh. The diagnosis can be confirmed by *Doppler studies and a Duplex scan and if any doubt still exists this can be followed by venography.*

An intravenous heparin infusion of 1000 units hourly (therapeutic dosage, not prophylactic) should be commenced and the patient should be given a loading dose of 10 mg warfarin. The leg should be elevated and a *compression stocking applied.*

A ventilation–perfusion scan would only be undertaken if it was thought that the patient had suffered a pulmonary embolism.

SU-C128   CORRECT RESPONSE D

A lumbar sympathectomy of the L2,3,4 sympathetic trunk segments interrupts sympathetic outflow to the lower limb. It can be performed by percutaneous chemical injection or by open operation.

Its major circulatory effect is to increase circulation to the skin of the foot in patients with vessels capable of dilating after interruption of vasoconstrictive sympathetic fibres. In established macrovascular or microvascular atherosclerotic arterial disease it is much less effective.

Sympathectomy does not influence claudication distance, recanalisation of vessels or establishment of collaterals. Afferent somatic pain fibres are not present in the sympathetic trunk. The risk of venous thrombosis is not affected significantly by sympathectomy.

SU-C129   CORRECT RESPONSE B,D,E

Micturition and defaecation are accompanied by Valsalva procedures and increased intra-abdominal and intra-thoracic pressures, contributing to syncope in patients at risk. *Micturition syncope in patients with bladder neck obstruction usually resolves without post-syncopal morbidity. Cerebral transient ischaemic attacks due to carotid artery stenosis or emboli can also resolve without residual neurological deficit, as can the syncope occurring with aortic stenosis.*

Syncope associated with gastrointestinal haemorrhage would have the associated haemorrhage as a dramatic symptom and would be expected to have persisting symptoms of faintness and shock requiring continuing medical attention. Myocardial infarct of sufficient degree to cause syncope would also be unlikely to result in the patient being able to return to bed without noticing additional subsequent symptoms.

SU-C130   CORRECT RESPONSE A,C,E

The patient's legs show incompetent and dilated varicose veins while standing. The left leg illustrates grossly tortuous veins of the greater saphenous system in both thigh and leg.

The most common site of incompetence and reflux between deep and superficial veins occurs at the sapheno–femoral junction. In the illustration, dilatation of the long saphenous system on the left leg extends up to mid-thigh and ***Trendelenburg test*** (emptying the veins on recumbency, occluding by finger or tourniquet the sapheno–femoral opening, standing the patient up, removing the compression and observing rapid reverse filling of long saphenous vein from above; a positive Trendelenburg test) ***would be expected to confirm sapheno–femoral incompetence.***

A doubly positive Trendelenburg test describes the additional finding of incompetence into the long saphenous system at some point below the sapheno–femoral junction (veins below the knee will fill on standing before release of the occluding tournique); ***such incompetence can be through a lower thigh perforator from the subsartorial canal (very common: Hunterian perforating vein).*** Incompetence of the sapheno–femoral valve itself is then demonstrated when the tourniquet is released by further filling from above via the sapheno–femoral junction incompetence. Signs of sapheno–femoral incompetence were actually described earlier by Benjamin Brodie.

The patient's legs show superficial varicosities of thigh and leg. However, evidence of long-standing deep venous insufficiency is not apparent from the photograph (Figure 32).

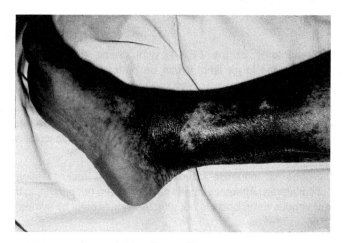

Figure 45

Chronic deep venous insufficiency often follows a previous deep venous thrombosis with perforating calf vein incompetence and sustained severe ambulatory superficial venous hypertension. Suggestive signs (Figure 45) are a glossy, shiny skin and a desquamatory venous eczema, brown discolouration due to extravasatory sclerosing periphlebitis with fibrous induration of subcutaneous tissues leading to 'inverted champagne bottle' deformity and a plantar flexion contracture, skin ulceration from minor trauma in the gaiter area above the ankle and venous cutaneous telangiectases and venous stars over the malleoli.

Haemorrhage from an eroded superficial varix is a serious complication but venous bleeding responds well to emergency treatment of elevation of the leg and local compression.

SU-C131   CORRECT RESPONSE A,B,E

Adult Respiratory Distress Syndrome ('shock lung') developing after femoral fracture, without associated chest injury, is strongly suggestive of fat embolism syndrome. The clinical onset is often delayed for 24–72 h after injury and the condition is associated with an interstitial pulmonary infiltrate.

Tachycardia, tachypnoea and hypoxia (decreased P_aO_2*)* are associated with loss of lung compliance. Tachypnoea is associated with hypocapnia (decreased P_aCO_2). The patient may become hypotensive and shocked; hypertension is not a feature.

SU-C132   CORRECT RESPONSE D,E

In Australia and other countries with similar lifestyles, this patient would almost certainly have Crohn disease. One-third of patients with Crohn enteritis have the disease limited to the terminal ileum, where a strictured segment may be identified on contrast studies. Some patients with ulcerative colitis may get ulceration of the terminal section of the ileum and the changes could rarely resemble Crohn disease, but with ulcerative colitis other radiological changes in the large bowel would be expected.

If the terminal ileum is severely diseased, re-absorption of bile salts may be affected. Any reduction in the bile salt pool will alter the dynamics of cholesterol saturation in the bile and *increase the risk of gallstone formation. Renal calculi are also more likely in patients with inflammatory bowel disease.*

Crohn disease can be complicated by fistula or abscess and these are definite indications for surgery. However, a small bowel stricture due to Crohn disease is also an indication for surgery, which should be as conservative as possible because of the high incidence of recurrence. Stricturoplasty or small bowel resection are each common operations for persistent stricturing. Medical management of Crohn disease includes steroids for acute exacerbations, and mesalazine and azathioprine are used for maintenance. Recurrence after surgery is a real risk and is in the order of 50%.

SU-C133   CORRECT RESPONSE B,C,D

Carcinoma of the colon is one of the important cancers of so-called developed societies and, after lung cancer, is the most common cause of cancer death. In some countries, such as Scotland, the lifetime risk for the disease is approximately 1 in 30. The disease is rare in Africa and it is likely that dietary factors, such as high fat and low fibre, contribute to the high incidence of the disease in Western communities.

Another factor which increases the risk is *a family history and if a first degree relative has had colorectal cancer, the risk is 1 in 10.* Patients with *ulcerative colitis and the rare hereditary condition of familial adenomatous polyposis are also at increased risk.* In the latter condition, malignant change is invariable. In patients with ulcerative colitis, the risk is approximately 10% at 10 years rising to 20% at 20 years after the onset of the disease. Amoebic colitis is not a risk factor.

SU-C134   CORRECT RESPONSE B,C

Gallstones are exceedingly common in Western countries and perhaps 30% of women in these communities will develop gallstones over their lifetimes. The risk is approximately 10% for men. Approximately 15% of patients with gallstones will also have stones in the biliary ductal system. Despite the high prevalence, only approximately one-third of patients with gallstones will develop symptoms that can be attributed to the stones and will require surgery.

Once gallstones have been detected, the question arises of how they should be managed.

If left untreated, it has been estimated that each year 2% of patients become symptomatic. This being the case, most clinicians would advise young patients with asymptomatic gallstones to have their gall-bladder removed. An additional reason for advocating surgery in young patients is that *carcinoma of the gall-bladder, although uncommon, is associated with gallstones in at least two-thirds of cases.*

If a patient with acute abdominal pain is thought to have underlying biliary disease, an ultrasound examination can confirm the presence of gallstones and a DIDA scan can be used to assess the function of the gall-bladder. *If isotope is not taken up by the gall-bladder in such a patient, this can be taken as an indication of absence of function of the gall-bladder, consistent with a diagnosis of acute cholecystitis.*

The most appropriate current treatment for gallstones is laparoscopic cholecystectomy. Other options include dissolution with chenodeoxycholic acid and shattering with focused shock waves of ultrasound (lithotripsy). These two modes of treatment are only suitable if the stones can be readily dissolved (not calcified) and are contained in a functioning gall-bladder.

SU-C135   CORRECT RESPONSE A

Pseudocysts occur in approximately 10% of patients who have an episode of acute pancreatitis and usually become evident *some weeks after the acute attack.* The mass may be visible and palpable in the epigastrium, but as the pancreas is a fixed retroperitoneal structure, the mass will not move with respiration. The development of a pseudocyst does not point to a particular cause for acute pancreatitis, although it will be remembered that the two most common causes of pancreatitis are gallstones and alcohol.

Pseudocysts often contain amylase and the concentration in the cyst fluid will far exceed that found in the serum.

Many pseudocysts, especially small ones discovered incidentally on imaging, will resolve spontaneously. But a large cyst measuring 15 cm in diameter in the body of the pancreas is more likely to require intervention and drainage percutaneously or by cystogastrostomy.

SU-C136   CORRECT RESPONSE A,B,C,D,E

The likely diagnosis in this man is *acute pancreatitis* secondary to an alcoholic binge. The photograph (Figure 33) shows discolouration at the umbilicus; this is typical of haemorrhagic extravasation from within the abdomen into the subcutaneous tissues around the umbilical cicatrix and is known as Cullen sign. This is a feature that can be associated with haemorrhagic pancreatitis; a condition with a *mortality rate approaching 50%.* Another sign which can indicate intraperitoneal and retroperitoneal haemorrhage in pancreatitis is Grey Turner sign, a discolouration of the skin of the loin or flanks. Haemorrhagic or necrotising pancreatitis accounts for less than 10% of all cases of pancreatitis, but is a particularly severe form of the disease. The patients are frequently shocked and oliguric on admission and *acute renal failure may develop.* Hypoxaemia is common and patients may require assisted ventilation. Liver function tests are deranged and hyperglycaemia and glycosuria develop. Serum *calcium levels may fall to such an extent that tetany becomes apparent.*

When there is a haemorrhagic process within the pancreas and adjacent tissues, **the bleeding may be of such a degree to require transfusion to replace blood loss.** The more severe the pancreatitis the more likely complications are to develop; and patients with haemorrhagic pancreatitis are prone to *pancreatic abscess formation.*

SU-C137   CORRECT RESPONSE A,C,E

The expression 'abdominal wound dehiscence' or 'burst abdomen' refers to a giving way of the deep layers of a (recent) surgically created wound involving the anterior abdominal wall. The skin and superficial layers may initially remain intact and the accompanying premonitory *serosanguineous discharge can give the false impression of underlying infection* or a haematoma. Eventually the whole wound gives way and intestine may spill outside the wound. *The complication typically occurs in the first 10 days after operation* and is a surgical emergency. The wounds that most commonly give way are those created vertically, those that become infected, those subjected to increased stress because of increased intra-abdominal pressure (coughing from postoperative chest infection) or *abdominal distension (ileus).*

The complication can be minimised by sound surgical techniques of wound closure.

A wound that suffers only partial dehiscence is very likely to be weakened and prone to later incisional hernia formation.

SU-C138   CORRECT RESPONSE A,C,E

Marked colonic dilatation with fluid levels on X-ray can be due to distal mechanical obstruction of the large bowel or colonic ileus (functional obstruction*). Carcinoma of sigmoid colon causing a ring stricture is a common cause of mechanical obstruction.* Carcinoma of the distal rectum occurs in a distensible and wide-lumen part of the bowel; and is unlikely to present with bowel obstruction. *Severe ulcerative colitis can present with acute toxic colonic dilatation heralding perforation ('toxic megacolon') and requires urgent surgery.*

Faecal impaction is usually a very slowly progressive loading affecting both rectum and more proximal colon. Plain X-ray usually shows a dilated colon stuffed with solid faeces, giving a 'ground glass' appearance, rather than air-fluid levels with dilatation.

Retroperitoneal inflammation or haemorrhage from a number of causes (acute pancreatitis, retroperitoneal trauma or abscess) is often associated with colonic ileus.

SU-C139   CORRECT RESPONSE A

Bile salts aid fat absorption in the duodenum and jejunum and are reabsorbed in the distal ileum as part of the enterohepatic circulation, so that usually only approximately 0.5 g bile salts are lost in the faeces daily. *Surgical resection of the distal ileum will significantly reduce the absorption of bile salts.*

Iron, folic acid, vitamin C and calcium are absorbed mainly in the proximal jejunum. The only vitamin absorbed in the distal ileum is vitamin B_{12}, whose absorption also requires intrinsic factor, a glycoprotein produced by gastric parietal cells.

SU-C140   CORRECT RESPONSE A,D

The photograph (Figure 34) shows a section of terminal ileum, caecum and ascending colon. The patient has undergone a right hemicolectomy. Adjacent to the ileocaecal valve there is an ulcerating tumour with a necrotic centre, typical of caecal adenocarcinoma. The dark patches may be areas of haemorrhage. Such patients classically present with the symptoms and signs of an iron-deficiency anaemia, which include *tiredness* and lethargy. The blood loss causing the anaemia is usually occult and chronic and not apparent as bright blood loss per rectum. This latter form of blood loss would be more typical of anorectal lesions. Back pain is not usually a symptom. The tumour may well have *been palpable on abdominal examination*, as these tumours can become quite large before they become clinically apparent. The proximity of the tumour to the ileocaecal valve also raises the possibility of a presentation with small bowel obstruction.

The tumour has not spread to the mesenteric lymph nodes, so it would be classified as Dukes A or B stage tumour. The 5 year survival for Dukes A is at least 80% and for Dukes B the figure is approximately 60%.

SU-C141   CORRECT RESPONSE A,B,D,E

Achalasia of the oesophagus is a motility disorder characterised by absence of coordinated peristaltic activity in the body of the oesophagus and a raised pressure in the lower oesophageal sphincter. The *lower oesophageal sphincter fails to relax on swallowing* and the patient may present with difficulty in swallowing and free regurgitation. Saliva and food accumulate in the oesophagus *and can show up as an air–fluid level in the oesophagus on an erect chest X-ray.* Because of the difficulty in getting any material through the lower oesophageal sphincter, the air that is normally swallowed with meals may not get into the stomach and the condition *is characterised by absence of a gastric air bubble on the erect chest X-ray.* These patients tend to have long histories and it is thought that the prolonged contact of the oesophageal mucosa with swallowed material may explain the *associated risk of late malignancy.*

Achalasia is usually an acquired degenerative condition of the myenteric nerve plexuses, whereas Hirschsprung disease, which can affect the same neuronal complexes at the other end of the digestive tract, is a congenital and unrelated condition.

SU-C142   CORRECT RESPONSE A,B,C,D,E

Ultrasound has now superseded oral cholecystography as the non-invasive imaging investigation of choice for biliary disease. However, an oral cholecystogram can usually give good definition of the gall-bladder and will also provide information on the function of the organ. *Patient non-compliance with ingestion of the oral contrast is an important cause of non-visualisation of the gall-bladder.* In addition to the oral contrast material, the patient is required to take a cathartic to empty the colon so that there is an unimpeded view of the gall bladder. Understandably, many patients do not take such medications.

If the patient has *intestinal hurry (e.g., due to gastroenteritis) the contrast will not be absorbed.* Even if the contrast is absorbed, poor liver function due to *hepatocellular failure* or secondary to *obstructive jaundice* will prevent the material from being excreted in the bile. Once in the bile, the contrast must be taken up and concentrated in the gall-bladder to a sufficient degree to permit radio-opacity. If the gall-bladder is obstructed, inflamed and non-functioning, with a blocked cystic duct (as occurs in *acute cholecystitis*) the contrast would not be concentrated and the gall-bladder is not visualised.

SU-C143   CORRECT RESPONSE B,C,D,E

Villous adenomas of the rectum can secrete large volumes of mucus leading to potassium deficiency.

Marfan syndrome is an inherited disorder of collagen and elastic tissue. Patients have characteristically long and narrow faces, a high palatal arch, arm span greater than height and arachnodactyly. Connective tissue deficits include double-jointedness, subluxation of the crystalline lens, aortic regurgitation and a tendency to aortic dissection.

Coeliac disease is an immune deficiency syndrome with steatorrhoea and other gastrointestinal symptoms and a tendency to develop intestinal lymphoma.

Immunosuppressive drugs such as azathioprine, 6-mercaptopurine, cyclo-

phosphamide, cyclosporine and antilymphocyte globulin are teratogenic and carcinogenic, often in synergistic association with oncogenic viruses. In Australia, the most common tumours induced are skin cancers, particularly squamous cell carcinoma.

Maternal hydramnios is an important indication of fetal abnormalities such as oesophageal atresia.

SU-C144 — CORRECT RESPONSE B

Ultrasound is the preferred non-invasive imaging investigation for the biliary tract. It is relatively cheap, easy to perform and has good diagnostic accuracy, although in difficult cases the interpretation is observer dependent. Interpretation is made more difficult in the obese and where there is a large amount of gas in the adjacent intestine. The *(common) bile duct, which lies anterior to the portal vein*, can be identified, particularly when it is dilated. Although not as accurate as a contrast examination, ultrasound can usually detect a dilated common bile duct, which is one more than 10 mm in diameter. A gallstone does not have to contain calcium to be detected ultrasonographically and ultrasound is the investigation of choice in pregnancy.

SU-C145 — CORRECT RESPONSE A,B,C,E

Intussusception may occur at any age. The aetiology will vary with the age of the patient. In children, the usual cause is enlargement of Peyer patches secondary to a viral infection.

An enlarged patch, *usually in the ileocolic region*, will form the apex of the intussusception. The child typically presents with screaming due to abdominal colic and passage of 'red currant jelly' stool, due to blood from ischaemic necrosis of the apex of the intussusceptum. If identified at an early stage these lesions can be *successfully treated without open operation* by instillation of barium into the colon and reduction under hydrostatic pressure.

Some of these patients are individuals who have Henoch–Schönlein purpura. Two-thirds of children with Henoch-Schönlein purpura develop gastrointestinal lesions and some will intussuscept a segment of intestine.

SU-C146 — CORRECT RESPONSE A,B,C,E

Hepatic encephalopathy is an important complication of chronic liver disease. While many patients with severe liver disease may not be troubled by encephalopathy, others will be easily tilted into trouble by a minor derangement of metabolic function, such as *hypokalaemic alkalosis from vomiting*, infections such as *pneumonia* or *bleeding into the gastrointestinal tract.* Many of these patients with liver disease have gastritis, peptic ulcer or varices and haemorrhage is common.

If blood is diverted away from the liver, either by a collateral circulation or a man-made *portosystemic shunt,* then toxins absorbed from the gut may pass directly to the brain and produce encephalopathy. Sterilisation of the gut with agents such as neomycin can be used to reduce the incidence and severity of encephalopathy.

SU-C147 — CORRECT RESPONSE A,C,E

There are various risk factors for cancers of the gastrointestinal tract. *Pernicious anaemia* is now uncommon, but sufferers are at increased risk of developing carcinoma of the stomach. Patients with *coeliac disease* are at increased risk for lymphoma of the proximal jejunum.

Melanosis coli is a consequence of chronic laxative abuse and neither the pigmentation of the colon nor excessive use of cathartics increases the risk of cancer.

Chronic gastritis associated with Helicobacter pylori is a risk factor for gastric ulceration and gastric cancer.

SU-C148   CORRECT RESPONSE C,E

Familial adenomatous polyposis (FAP) is a rare condition, which is inherited as an autosomal dominant, with males and females being equally affected and half the members of a family developing the disease. Polyps may occur at any site in the colon and rectum and *first appear between the ages of 10 and 15 years.* Symptoms commence usually in the second decade of life and consist of rectal bleeding, diarrhoea and mucorrhoea. *All patients with FAP will eventually develop malignant change* in one or more of the polyps, although this does not usually occur before the age of 20.

SU-C149   CORRECT RESPONSE A,B,C

The classical features of acute appendicitis in an otherwise fit young man are those of a short illness with gradual onset of worsening central abdominal pain which shifts after several hours and localises as a constant pain in the right iliac fossa. If the appendix is retrocaecal, the pain may radiate round to the loin or flank, but back pain is not usually a feature. The patient feels unwell, *loses interest in food* and may feel nauseated and vomit. He may be flushed with a *low grade fever of 37.5°C, as described.* Urinary symptoms may be present if the appendix is positioned in the pelvis, but macroscopic haematuria is rare and would suggest another cause for the pain. From the early stages the patient will have signs of *peritonitis with tenderness localised to the right iliac fossa,* although these may be less marked if the appendix is tucked in behind the caecum.

SU-C150   CORRECT RESPONSE B,C,E

A patient with a perforated ulcer of the anterior wall of the duodenum typically presents with severe unremitting epigastric pain of sudden onset. Depending on the degree of peritoneal soiling, the extent and magnitude of the pain will vary. Back pain is not a feature. *The patient usually lies supine with knees drawn up to diminish abdominal wall tension and the patient will be reluctant to move, because this exacerbates the pain.* The pain and peritonitis will also produce *pallor, sweating and a reluctance on the patient's part to make deep respiratory efforts.*

On examination, the abdomen will be rigid, particularly the upper abdomen, and the free gas in the abdomen may *diminish the area of liver dullness to percussion.*

SU-C151   CORRECT RESPONSE A,E

Eliciting local or general tenderness in the assessment of a patient with acute abdominal pain comprises a very important part of the assessment. Tenderness to palpation is an important sign of peritonitis and tenderness may be elicited on deep palpation before overlying reflex muscle guarding occurs. Thus, tenderness without guarding does not exclude peritonitis. Tenderness on rectal examination is a very important sign in pelvic appendicitis and is not, in such circumstances, indicative of pelvic abscess unless a boggy mass is also palpable. Muscle guarding and rigidity, when accompanying tenderness due to peritonitis, are often accompanied by release tenderness. *Release tenderness can be assessed most elegantly and most kindly by gentle finger percussion.* Colonic disease can cause tenderness over the site of the colonic pathology; this may be on either side or across the abdomen depending on whether the right or left colon is affected.

Local tenderness in the right iliac fossa is both a manifestation of peritonitis at the position of the appendix and also the most important single clinical sign of appendicitis.

SU-C152   CORRECT RESPONSE A,B,C,D,E

All of the responses can be typical of the clinical presentations of caecal carcinoma. Occult blood loss resulting in iron deficiency *anaemia* is a classical presentation. So is a *palpable mass* and so too is vague *dyspepsia* or indigestion. Alternatively, the presentation can be acute, with local pain *mimicking appendicitis* or as an *acute small bowel obstruction if the tumor involves the ileocaecal valve.* Change in bowel habit or overt bleeding are less common presentations for right colon cancer than they are for left colon cancer.

SU-C153   CORRECT RESPONSE A,E

A perianal fistula runs commonly from an orifice on the perianal skin to an internal opening in the anorectum, usually at the line of the anal valves. Anal glands open along this line; some penetrate deeply through submucosal layers into the muscular planes. Anal gland abscesses can burst onto the perianal skin, leading to chronic fistulae.

Most fistulae are low anal. *They can be associated with recurring abscesses, especially if the fistulous origin of perineal suppuration is not recognised and if recurring abscesses are treated just by drainage* rather than laying open the whole track. *A purulent discharge from the track*, marked by pouting granulation tissue, is common with chronic fistulae and is often painless.

Chronic fistulae are NOT typically or usually associated with persistent pain, diarrhoea or discharge of faecal material through the fistula track.

SU-C154   CORRECT RESPONSE A,C,D

Anal fissures typically present with a classical clinical picture of *anal pain on defaecation with associated bleeding. Pain is burning and severe and persists for some time after defaecation, which is inhibited by pain and sphincter spasm. Bleeding on defaecation* is bright but of small amount and is noted on the paper or on the surface of the stool. An episode of constipation often triggers the development of the initial mucosal tear. *An anal skin tag* and sentinel 'pile' are also usual in chronic fissures. Neither colicky abdominal pain nor faecal soiling are common, although self-administration of liquid paraffin or other stool-softening and liquefying agents may give a spurious diarrhoea.

SU-C155   CORRECT RESPONSE A,D

Gross generalised abdominal distension, as illustrated here, can be due to fluid (ascites), flatus (intestinal obstruction, pseudocyesis), faecal loading, the pregnant uterus, or *other masses filling the abdominal cavity, such as huge ovarian cysts*.

Percussion can help differentiate these causes. With ascites, fluid gravitates to the flanks and gas-containing bowel floats centrally in the recumbent position. *A central small area of resonance surrounded by dullness extending peripherally to the flanks suggests ascites.* Ovarian cysts tend to give reverse findings: a large area of central dullness over the cyst with the resonant gas-containing bowel displaced peripherally.

Pseudocyesis is accompanied by air swallowing and gaseous distension, with hyperresonance to percussion over a large area.

Physical examination will not detect the presence of ascites until sufficient fluid has accumulated to give signs of distension and shifting dullness. A minimum of approximately 250 mL fluid is required. A volume of 2.5 L would be expected to give very obvious signs.

Ascites due to cirrhosis may be associated with gross hepatomegaly, but may alternatively be accompanied by a contracted cirrhotic liver of less than normal size.

SU-C156   CORRECT RESPONSE A,B,C,E

The specimen shows an infarcted loop of small bowel with a constriction furrow across the base of the mesentery.

The clinical features would be those of *strangulated intestinal obstruction including central abdominal pain* in association with primary causes, such as *postoperative adhesions due to previous pelvic surgery* or *a strangulated femoral hernia* or *strangulated inguinal hernia.* Back pain is not a feature of intestinal obstruction.

SU-C157   CORRECT RESPONSE A,C,D

Primary hyperparathyroidism *is most often due to a solitary parathyroid adenoma* and the condition can quite commonly be an incidental finding in asymptomatic patients, coming to light when the patient is undergoing biochemical investigation for another reason. *It is essentially a disease of adults.* Typically, the serum calcium is elevated and the phosphate is depressed. The elevation of serum calcium is usually relatively minor, but it can be raised to such an extent that the patient may present with one of the complications of hypercalcaemia, such as a florid *psychiatric disorder* or urinary calculi. Other symptoms of hypercalcaemia with which patients commonly present include constipation, polyuria and polydypsia, loss of energy and abdominal pain.

SU-C158   CORRECT RESPONSE A,B,C

The Zollinger–Ellison syndrome is a rare condition, which has given additional insight into mechanisms of control of gastric secretion, in which a gastrin-producing tumour (gastrinoma) leads to *hypersecretion of gastric acid.* The patient can present with diarrhoea or intractable peptic ulceration. The *tumours can be multiple* and are situated within and often outside the pancreas, usually in the duodenum or peripancreatic tissue. Although these tumours secrete gastrin, they do not arise from the G cell population in the antrum, but appear to develop from cell rests at other sites or dedifferentiated pancreatic islet cells. *Approximately two-thirds of these tumours are malignant*, although the malignancy is extremely low grade and the tumours are slow-growing. There is no association with hypoglycaemia.

Treatment used to be by removal of the target organ, with performance of a total gastrectomy. Vagotomy does not control the hyperacidity. Current treatment is directed at tumour localisation and excision. If this is not possible, the patient is treated with an anti-secretory agent, such as one of the proton pump inhibitors.

SU-C159   CORRECT RESPONSE A,B,C,E,

Goitres have several causes and, worldwide, the most common is a *dietary deficiency of iodine.* Other causes include the presence of goitrogens in the diet, thyrotoxicosis and thyroiditis. The formation of antibodies to thyroid tissue occurs in several forms of thyroiditis, but not in the simple colloid goitre associated with iodine deficiency. Where the aetiology is a deficiency in iodine, there is initially a diffuse enlargement of the gland with engorgement of the follicles with colloid, the so-called 'simple colloid goitre'. Because most goitres are deficient in iodine, there will be an *increased uptake of iodine-131 on scanning. Goitre is more common in women.* While the goitrous enlargement may be diffusely uniform and smooth, **nodules often develop at a later stage** and, from a clinical perspective, the most common cause of an apparently isolated lump in the thyroid is a prominent component of a multinodular goitre.

SU-C160 CORRECT RESPONSE A,B,C

Mastectomy would be favoured over conservative surgery for **multifocal breast cancer, for large tumours over 5 cm in diameter and for peau d'orange wide of the tumour.** Both premenopausal and postmenopausal women are appropriately treated by conservative surgery; age is not, in itself, an indication for more radical surgery. Axillary node involvement in association with an infiltrating breast cancer is best treated by complete axillary clearance. This can be done in combination with either a total mastectomy or conservative breast surgery.

SU-C161 CORRECT RESPONSE A,D

This 64-year-old postmenopausal woman has had a mastectomy for carcinoma of the breast and now has the clinical picture of uncontrolled chest wall recurrence and ulceration. Adjuvant treatment at the time of surgery was not mentioned in the stem and there are no signs of previous radiotherapy in the form of skin pigmentation or telangiectases. **Local control after confirmation of the diagnosis by fine needle aspiration cytology (FNAC) or core biopsy would be preferably by local chest wall radiotherapy and the anti-oestrogen tamoxifen**, which is most effective in postmenopausal patients. Testosterone is not appropriate in such patients. Local conservative surgery is more likely to spread disease than to give control. Radical excisional surgery and reconstruction is best reserved for persisting, uncontrolled local recurrence despite radiotherapy and would not be the initial choice of treatment.

SU-C162 CORRECT RESPONSE E

Carcinoma of the prostate is one of the most common cancers of men and is the second most common cause of cancer deaths in Australian men. There appears to have been a rise in the incidence of the disease over the past decade, although this may be due to increased awareness of the condition, screening and more frequent diagnosis rather than any real change in the incidence.

Screening can be undertaken by the measurement of serum prostate-specific antigen, although the exact place of this screening tool is still debated. Prostate-specific antigen is a more reliable indicator of bony disease than serum acid phosphatase, which is frequently normal in patients with established metastatic disease.

Lymphangiography has been replaced by CT scanning as the imaging procedure of choice to assess lymph node involvement. **Radioisotope examination is used to look for skeletal metastatic disease, although areas of Paget disease can be mistaken for deposits of prostatic cancer.**

Although evidence of the disease only comes to light in many patients through histological analysis of prostatic tissue resected for urinary obstruction, almost 50% of patients with carcinoma of the prostate have established metastatic disease at the time of presentation. Metastatic disease occurs to pelvic nodes, the lumbar spine, pelvis and adjacent tissues.

SU-C163 CORRECT RESPONSE A,C,D,E

Testicular cancer is one of the most common cancers to affect young men. The disease usually presents with painless enlargement of a testicle and, by the time of presentation, **may have spread to para-aortic lymph nodes.**

Testicular tumours do not spread to inguinal lymph nodes unless the disease involves the scrotal skin, a rare event unless the illness has been complicated by an unwise scrotal incision in the mistaken belief that the condition was a hydrocele or some other benign lesion.

Pulmonary metastases can occur by blood spread and may be the first manifestation of an occult primary testicular neoplasm. The tumour markers *serum beta-human chorionic gonadotrophin* and *alpha-fetoprotein* are elevated in most non-seminomatous germ cell tumours and in a large proportion of seminomas. Serial measurement of these two markers, provided they were elevated in the first place, can provide a useful guide of response to treatment or re-activity of the disease.

SU-C164   CORRECT RESPONSE A,C,E

Risk factors for venous thrombosis relate to the Virchow triad: hypercoagulable states, endothelial injury and stasis. The medical therapy of peptic ulcer is usually done on an ambulatory basis and this is not associated with increased liability to deep venous thrombosis.

Pelvic surgery may be associated with damage to or pressure exerted on the iliac veins during surgery. In addition, patients undergoing pelvic surgery are often in the lithotomy position, whereby venous return from the legs may be impeded leading to stasis in calf veins.

Patients with complicated varicose veins have an increased risk of deep venous thrombosis, mainly because of increased venous stasis. Surgery for uncomplicated varicose veins is not in itself a risk factor. After surgery for varicose veins, early ambulation is encouraged and support stockings are used to compress the superficial veins and promote deep venous flow.

Any form of malignancy increases the risk of venous thrombo-embolism, perhaps due to increased hypercoagulability. *Polycythaemia rubra vera* is a primary hypercoagulable state associated with increased risk of venous thrombosis.

SU-C165   CORRECT RESPONSE A,B,C,E

Massive blood transfusions can cause problems with bleeding for several reasons. The anticoagulant used for blood storage contains excess citrate, which chelates calcium. *Thus, massive transfusion causes calcium deficiency.* Calcium is a co-factor in many of the steps of coagulation.

Factors V, VIII and XI degrade in stored blood and deficiencies of these factors may be induced. Platelets are lost when blood is stored under normal conditions at 4°C. Massive blood transfusion is often seen alongside major trauma, shock, hypoxia and surgery, *conditions in which fibrinolysis can occur secondary to release of excessive plasminogen activators.* Prostaglandins are involved in opposing ways in platelet aggregation, but there is no evidence that prostaglandin deficiency occurs as a result of massive blood transfusion.

SU-C166   CORRECT RESPONSE A,C,E

Bleeding that follows surgery is usually secondary to a problem with local haemostasis and, as often as not, reflects a defect in surgical technique. However, if the surgery has been major and complex, if the patient has underlying problems, such as liver disease, or has required massive blood transfusion, then there can be problems with general haemostatic mechanisms.

This would be suspected if blood was seen coming from many areas, including *venipuncture sites, if the platelet count was less than 30 x 10⁹ /L (30 000 /µL), if the INR was three-fold normal* or the fibrinogen level was low.

SU-C167   CORRECT RESPONSE A,C

Splenic enlargement can be the result of infection (bacterial septicaemia, malaria), disordered immunoregulation (systemic lupus erythematosus, Felty syndrome), disordered splenic blood flow (any cause of portal hypertension), diseases associated with abnormal erythrocytes (spherocytosis, thalassaemia) infiltration by malignancy (Hodgkin or non-Hodgkin lymphoma), benign infiltrations (amyloidosis) or one of several miscellaneous processes (sarcoidosis).

However, few of these conditions produce massive splenomegaly. *Malaria does, as may chronic myeloid leukaemia* (not chronic lymphatic leukaemia) and myelofibrosis, but the splenic enlargement associated with Hodgkin disease and portal hypertension is usually only moderate.

SU-C168   CORRECT RESPONSE A,B,D,E

Macrocytic anaemias are associated with a megaloblastic bone marrow picture and develop as the result of vitamin B_{12} or folate deficiency. The failure of cell maturation is brought about by impaired replication of DNA, particularly in cells with a high rate of turnover. Thus, this type of anaemia may develop either in conditions where there is malabsorption or where requirements are increased.

Intrinsic factor is required to facilitate the absorption of vitamin B_{12} and is produced in the stomach. *Gastric resection* may interfere with the production of intrinsic factor and thus lead to a macrocytic anaemia. Vitamin B_{12} is absorbed in the terminal ileum and disease processes affecting this region, for example *Crohn disease or tropical sprue*, are likely to impair absorption. Absorption of vitamin B_{12} may also be reduced if there is increased competition for the vitamin. This can happen in *blind loop syndromes, where stasis can lead to bacterial overgrowth* and increased demand for vitamin B_{12}.

Other conditions where macrocytic anaemias often occur include the poor intake of folate associated with alcoholism and the increased demands in pregnancy and malignancy.

An oesophageal hiatus hernia is not associated with macrocytic anaemia, but if there is an element of gastro-oesophageal reflux and oesophagitis with occult bleeding, an iron-deficiency microcytic anaemia can develop.

SU-C169   CORRECT RESPONSE A,D

Classic haemophilia due to deficiency of factor VIII *has an incidence of approximately 1:10 000.* Haemophilia is inherited as a sex-linked recessive character.

Recurrent bleeding into joints (haemarthroses) is the most common orthopaedic problem.

Factor VIII component therapy is required before elective surgery.

Cryoprecipitate, containing factor VIII and fibrinogen, has risks of transmission of hepatitis and HIV. Factor VIII is now given as a freeze-dried, heat-treated concentrate free of such risk.

SU-C170   CORRECT RESPONSE B,C,D

The right ureter starts its descent from the urinary pelvis at the level of the second lumbar vertebra. Through the *25 cm of its length,* the ureter is closely applied in its upper reaches to the peritoneum, in its middle section to the psoas fascia and in its lower reaches to the lateral wall of the pelvis.

The ureter receives a *blood supply from the renal artery at its upper end and the vesical artery at the lower extremity.* Branches from the aorta, common iliac or gonadal vessels supply the mid-section of the ureter. The inferior mesenteric artery does not supply the ureter.

SU-C171   CORRECT RESPONSE B,D

The aim of dehydration in intravenous urography is to ensure good concentration of the contrast material as it is excreted by the kidneys. Most patients, including those with leukaemia, raised intracranial pressure and renovascular hypertension can tolerate several hours (6–12 h) of dehydration; but this would be ill-advised in patients with *myelomatosis* and *chronic renal failure.* In myelomatosis, dehydration can significantly worsen renal function and is contraindicated prior to intravenous pyelography. Chronic renal failure is usually associated with lack of renal concentrating power and polyuria: dehydration is a common precipitant of increasing azotaemia and worsening renal function. Leukaemia has no special associations with renal insufficiency and patients with raised intracranial pressure (ICP) are often treated by dehydration to reduce ICP. Patients with renovascular hypertension may show increased density of contrast excretion by the affected ischaemic kidney, a finding enhanced by previous dehydration.

SU-C172   CORRECT RESPONSE B,C

Over 80% of renal calculi are radio-opaque and these stones contain calcium salts of oxalate, phosphate and carbonate. A smaller percentage of stones are based on uric acid. Stones composed of cystine and xanthine are rare and are associated with metabolic disorders. Stones that contain *uric acid* and *xanthine* are radiolucent.

SU-C173   CORRECT RESPONSE A,B,C,E

While solitary cysts of the kidney are common and usually silent, polycystic kidney disease is a serious, but less common, abnormality. It is a congenital disorder and affects both kidneys and *cysts are often found in the liver and sometimes in the pancreas.* The condition can be associated with *cerebral arterial aneurysms.* The patient can present with renal failure (usually in the fourth or fifth decade), with pain due to a bleed into a cyst, or with *haematuria* when a cyst ruptures into the pelvi–calyceal system.

SU-C174   CORRECT RESPONSE A,B,D,E

Analgesic nephropathy remains an important cause of chronic renal failure in communities that consume large quantities of phenacetin and aspirin. Australia has been one such community. The condition is characterised by papillary necrosis and the necrotic fragments may cause *ureteric obstruction* and colic. Over 50% of these patients have a pyuria, which may be sterile, but is *often associated with a urinary infection and pyelonephritis.* Long-term chronic changes within the kidney include *calcification of the papillae* and shrunken kidneys with deformed calyces. The incidence of *transitional cell carcinoma* is increased. These can develop in the renal pelvis or ureters as a late complication.

SU-C175   CORRECT RESPONSE B,C,D

Haematuria is not a common symptom of benign prostatomegaly, nor of hydronephrosis.

Haematuria is common *in urinary calculus disease and in urothelial cancer and renal cell carcinoma (hypernephroma).*

SU-C176   CORRECT RESPONSE A,B,C,E

It can be of value to identify before operation patients with factors that might increase their risk of developing problems postoperatively. This is particularly true for venous thrombo-embolism and is also applicable for patients with poor nutrition. These latter patients are at increased risk of problems related to the healing of tissues and wounds. It has been estimated that up to 25% of patients on general surgical wards may be malnourished. Measurement of weight alone is not an index of nutrition and obese individuals may suffer from malnutrition. Objective measurements of the nutritional status of a patient include the anthropomorphic measurements of **mid-arm muscle circumference, hand grip strength**, the **serum albumin concentration** and the state of anergy (**delayed cutaneous hypersensitivity** and total lymphocyte count). The haemoglobin level is not a helpful index of nutritional status.

A recent unintentional loss of more than 10% of bodyweight and a weight of less than 80% of ideal bodyweight are indices of poor nutrition. A serum albumin of less than 30 g/L and a total lymphocyte count of 1.2 /μL and a reduction of mid-arm muscle circumference to less than 80% (for a comparable population) are all indices of poor nutritional status.

SU-C177   CORRECT RESPONSE A,B,C,D,E

There are many factors that can lead to the breakdown of a wound. The condition can be a reflection of deficient surgical skills. The deficiency may be **inappropriate selection of suture material**, too tight or loose application of sutures, wrong placement of sutures or attempted wound closure when the wound should be left open.

Other factors which will influence the healing of a wound include local issues, such as the presence of foreign material, **infection**, malignancy and, where a hollow viscus is concerned, distal obstruction. A poor blood supply to the area, such as might follow **radiotherapy,** will reduce the ability of a wound to heal. The general state of health of the body is important and individuals with diabetes, **jaundice**, AIDS or **uraemia** tend to have increased problems with wound healing.

SU-C178   CORRECT RESPONSE A,B,C

The normal hydrogen ion content of arterial blood is held constant by respiratory and renal balancing control mechanisms between 36 and 44 nmol/L (serendipitously corresponding to a pH of 7.44–7.36).

Acidaemia is an absolute increase in the level (pH < 7.36), alkalaemia a decrease in the level (pH > 7.44) of hydrogen ion concentration. Acidosis and alkalosis are often used as synonyms for acidaemia and alkalaemia or can describe a tendency to acidaemia and alkalaemia without necessarily a change in pH, as secondary and compensatory mechanisms act to oppose and minimise change.

Acidosis and alkalosis may be due to gaseous (respiratory) causes or to non-gaseous (metabolic) causes. Metabolic causes relate to addition or subtraction of acidic or alkaline agents.

The relationship between the major types is given by the Henderson–Hasselbach equation, derived from the reversible reaction:

$$H^+ + HCO_3 \rightleftharpoons H_2CO_3 \rightleftharpoons H_2O + CO_2$$

The left side of the equation is governed by the balance between production of hydrogen ion by tissue perfusion and metabolism and its excretion by the kidney; the right side is governed by the balanced excretion of CO_2 via the lungs under the influence of the respiratory centre.

Respiratory acidosis is caused by underventilation. Decreased alveolar ventilation results in an elevated arterial P_aCO_2 (normal P_aCO_2 range is 35–45 mmHg).

Respiratory alkalosis is the reverse situation, caused by overventilation, which blows off CO_2 and lowers arterial P_aCO_2, with a rise in pH.

Respiratory alkalosis (and also metabolic alkalosis) will lower the arterial hydrogen ion concentration and will reciprocally increase renal tubular cell potassium excretion at the expense of hydrogen ion; the latter being retained. Alkalosis of either respiratory or metabolic type is commonly associated with increased potassium loss and potassium deficiency, frequently with hypokalaemia requiring potassium supplementation, not restriction.

SU-C179   CORRECT RESPONSE A,B,C,D,E

All the factors listed can contribute to an increased risk of wound infection.

Alcoholism is associated with nutritional deficiencies, a bleeding tendency and cirrhosis; and with a dishevelled and neglected general status predisposing to infection.

Diabetes mellitus is associated with increased risk both of wound infection and of general infections.

A urinary infection provides a further source of potential bacteraemia and colonisation.

Prolonged preoperative hospital stay allows skin colonisation by resistant organisms.

Shock is associated with decreased general tissue perfusion, thus increasing the risk of infection.

SU-C180   CORRECT RESPONSE A,C

Pre-operative use of antibiotics should always be considered in surgical procedures in contaminated fields. Another indication is when the surgery is clean, but any infection would have catastrophic consequences for the patients: for example, aortic valve replacement or *aortic aneurysm graft replacement* surgery or any sort of surgery in patients with prosthetic materials already *in situ.* Another instance is when the risk of infection is low, but the patient's resistance is diminished, such as surgery in diabetics or immunosuppressed patients. Yet another situation is the use of antibiotics to reduce the risk of infection in clean areas of incisional access (the wound and peritoneal cavity) when the large bowel is opened for an *appendicectomy for acute appendicitis.*

If the surgery is 'clean' and no contaminated or colonised cavity or viscus is to be opened, then use of antibiotics is not appropriate. Examples include highly selective vagotomy or elective repair of a femoral hernia. However, if the site to be operated on is already infected or extensively colonised and no clean area is to be broached, then antibiotics are of little value. Examples would include drainage of a superficial skin abscess or a haemorrhoidectomy.

SU-C181   CORRECT RESPONSE C,E

Hydatid infestation is an important disease in certain areas of the world, particularly Australia and Greece. The tapeworm *Echinococcus granulosa* lives in the intestine of its primary or definitive host, the dog. *Ova are shed in the stools* and are ingested by the secondary host, which is usually the sheep. Where people, sheep and dogs live in close proximity, human infestation occurs. Humans replace sheep or cattle as the secondary host. *Faecal ova contaminate the dog's fur and stroking or handling the dog results in ova being transferred to fingers and thus ingested.*

The ova hatch in the proximal small bowel and the embryos pass via the portal circulation to the liver where they grow into cysts. Cysts may occur anywhere in the body, the liver being by far the most common site, while the lungs are also a favoured area. Hydatid cysts in the bone are an unusual but *serious cause of pathological fracture.* Hydatid cysts may remain symptomless or may produce symptoms because of their size or from rupture and spillage of contents. The hydatid cyst is made of three layers: an outer fibrous host layer, a middle laminated membrane and an inner germinal epithelium from which daughter cysts can develop.

SU-C182   CORRECT RESPONSE D,E

Hydatid disease in humans is due to the cystic form of *Echinococcus granulosa,* a small (6 mm) tapeworm resident in the dog's intestinal tract. The sheep is the normal intermediate host with cysts developing in liver, lungs and other organs. Normally, the life cycle is completed by dogs ingesting infested sheep offal containing cysts.

Humans usually are infected in childhood by playing with dogs and ingesting ova: the ova reach the fingers and mouth from contaminated dog fur. Humans cannot contract the disease from eating sheep meat.

Liver cysts commonly calcify, but this does not necessarily imply death of the parasite. Surgery is the only reliably curative treatment of hydatid disease in humans. Scolicidals, such as albendazole and mebendazole, have some clinical activity; metronidazole is ineffective. *Liver cysts are often multiloculated and ultrasound can be virtually diagnostic of such multilocular cysts.*

Surgery for hydatid cyst involves removal of the endocyst component from within the host ectocyst, the endocyst comprises the chitinous laminated membrane produced by the parasite and the lining germinal epithelium and contained hydatid fluid, including daughter cysts and hydatid sand. Spillage of hydatid material containing scolices into serosal cavities can result in further transcoelomic spread. Special measures are taken to avoid spillage and to inject scolicidal agents (hypertonic saline, formalin, silver nitrate) into the cyst before aspiration.

SU-C183   CORRECT RESPONSE D,E

Antibiotic therapy is frequently abused and overused. If a patient has a localised purulent infection and is otherwise well, the most appropriate treatment is drainage. This is especially true of staphylococcal infections which, when forming abscesses in the skin and subcutaneous tissues, can be incised and drained. Many staphylococcal infections present as an abscess requiring drainage only. When the patient is not well and where there is evidence of spreading or systemic infection, then additional antimicrobial therapy may be indicated.

A young man with a furuncle or boil in the beard area is treated just by removing the appropriate hair, which provides free drainage and early resolution.

A wound infection after an antireflux procedure in a fit patient is usually a stitch abscess or subcutaneous collection. Both are treated best by adequate wound drainage alone.

A 40-year-old man with a peri-anal abscess needs incision and drainage, not antibiotics.

However, *a diabetic patient with a carbuncle (a more serious necrotising subcutaneous infection) requires both adequate drainage and administration of a systemic antibiotic.*

Similarly, a patient with a prosthetic mitral valve developing wound infection is at risk of systemic colonisation of the valve and needs both drainage and antibiotics.

SU-C184   CORRECT RESPONSE A,C

Medications that have peptic ulceration as a side effect include aspirin and prednisolone.

Aspirin acts on the gastric mucous membrane to decrease mucosal resistance to autodigestion.

Steroids (prednisone, prednisolone) are also associated with peptic ulceration as a side effect of prolonged immunosuppression.

Paracetamol, penicillin and erythromycin are not associated with peptic ulceration.

SU-C185   CORRECT RESPONSE D,E

Testicular malignant tumours are most commonly germ cell tumours (seminoma or teratoma).

Lymph node metastasis is to para-aortic, not inguinal nodes. Pain is not a common symptom, nor is haematuria. *An associated secondary hydrocele, which may obscure the primary tumour, is common.*

Testicular germ cell tumour is one of the few neoplasms that can sometimes be cured by combined chemoradiotherapy, even when metastatic.

SU-C186   CORRECT RESPONSE A,B,D

Patients who are immunosuppressed for any reason are at increased risk of developing malignancies. Perhaps the best known examples are Kaposi tumours in patients with AIDS. Patients who have renal allografts often *develop basal and squamous cell tumours* of the skin, where the *tumours develop as a result of the long-term immunosuppression* rather than the transplant itself. *The normal ratio of basal cell cancer to squamous cell cancer is approximately 4:1, but in immunosuppressed patients the ratio is reversed.*

SU-C187   CORRECT RESPONSE D,E

In the 1990s there has been a major shift from in-patient to out-patient care. In our hospitals a greater share of the work is being undertaken on a day case, short-stay or day of admission basis. While the move has been largely dollar-driven, health professionals must ensure that such moves are not to the detriment of the patients and the same high standards of medical care are delivered.

In day care surgery, the same standards must be maintained as exist for conventional in-patient surgery. If the procedure is to be done under a general anaesthetic the same rules of pre- and postoperative management must apply, including a period of pre-operative and postoperative fasting, and the patient should certainly not be permitted to drive to and from the day centre. All the facilities must exist in the day surgery centre that exist in any centre where surgery under general anaesthesia is to be performed. *These facilities must include oxygen, suction and equipment for cardiac resuscitation.*

SUMMARY OF CORRECT RESPONSES

CATEGORY & QUESTION NO.	CORRECT RESPONSE	CATEGORY & QUESTION NO.	CORRECT RESPONSE	CATEGORY & QUESTION NO.	CORRECT RESPONSE
SU-Q 108	A,B,C,D	SU-Q 139	A	SU-Q 170	B,C,D
SU-Q 109	C,D,E	SU-Q 140	A,D	SU-Q 171	B,D
SU-Q 110	B	SU-Q 141	A,B,D,E	SU-Q 172	B,C
SU-Q 111	E	SU-Q 142	A,B,C,D,E	SU-Q 173	A,B,C,E
SU-Q 112	A,B	SU-Q 143	B,C,D,E	SU-Q 174	A,B,D,E
SU-Q 113	A,B	SU-Q 144	B	SU-Q 175	B,C,D
SU-Q 114	C,D,E	SU-Q 145	A,B,C,E	SU-Q 176	A,B,C,E
SU-Q 115	A,C,D,E	SU-Q 146	A,B,C,E	SU-Q 177	A,B,C,D,E
SU-Q 116	A,B,D,E	SU-Q 147	A,C,E	SU-Q 178	A,B,C
SU-Q 117	B,C	SU-Q 148	C,E	SU-Q 179	A,B,C,D,E
SU-Q 118	D	SU-Q 149	A,B,C	SU-Q 180	A,C
SU-Q 119	B,D,E	SU-Q 150	B,C,E	SU-Q 181	C,E
SU-Q 120	A,B,D	SU-Q 151	A,E	SU-Q 182	D,E
SU-Q 121	B,D	SU-Q 152	A,B,C,D,E	SU-Q 183	D,E
SU-Q 122	A,C	SU-Q 153	A,E	SU-Q 184	A,C
SU-Q 123	A,C,E	SU-Q 154	A,C,D	SU-Q 185	D,E
SU-Q 124	B,D,E	SU-Q 155	A,D	SU-Q 186	A,B,D
SU-Q 125	A,B,C,D	SU-Q 156	A,B,C,E	SU-Q 187	D,E
SU-Q 126	A,B,C,D,E	SU-Q 157	A,C,D		
SU-Q 127	A,B,C	SU-Q 158	A,B,C		
SU-Q 128	D	SU-Q 159	A,B,C,E		
SU-Q 129	B,D,E	SU-Q 160	A,B,C		
SU-Q 130	A,C,E	SU-Q 161	A,D		
SU-Q 131	A,B,E	SU-Q 162	E		
SU-Q 132	D,E	SU-Q 163	A,C,D,E		
SU-Q 133	B,C,D	SU-Q 164	A,C,E		
SU-Q 134	B,C	SU-Q 165	A,B,C,E		
SU-Q 135	A	SU-Q 166	A,C,E		
SU-Q 136	A,B,C,D,E	SU-Q 167	A,C		
SU-Q 137	A,C,E	SU-Q 168	A,B,D,E		
SU-Q 138	A,C,E	SU-Q 169	A,D		

Paediatrics
Commentaries
and Summary of Correct Responses
TYPE
A

Commentaries PA-C1 to PA-C86

Correct Responses PA-Q1 to PA-Q86

PA-C1 CORRECT RESPONSE A

A mild keratolytic (salicylic acid) with sulphur is a long established and effective treatment for seborrhoeic dermatitis.

Vitamin E has no specific effect in this condition.

Seborrhoeic dermatitis is unrelated to diet, in contrast to some cases of atopic dermatitis.

Hydrocortisone cream may be used for its topical anti-inflammatory effect in severe cases, but increases the risk of infection, particularly with candida.

Gentian violet is messy. It has been used in the past for the complication of candida infection, but even in that condition it has been supplanted by other more effective topical anti-fungal preparations.

PA-C2 CORRECT RESPONSE E

All of the conditions listed may cause a white pupil. Such a finding is an indication for urgent referral to an ophthalmologist. *Retinoblastoma*, although uncommon, is highly malignant but responsive to appropriate treatment. *A cataract* also requires early treatment to maximise the chances of effective vision. *Retrolental fibroplasia* and *toxoplasmosis* of the retina, if severe enough to present with a white pupil, are not likely to respond to treatment, but require differentiation from treatable conditions.

PA-C3 CORRECT RESPONSE B

The significance of this question concerns the early diagnosis of deafness in children. Even if clinical tests of hearing appear normal, *a parental concern that a child does not seem to hear properly is an indication for prompt audiometric assessment.*

Tympanometry may be useful to determine the cause of deafness if present, but will be normal in sensorineural deafness. Similarly, tuning fork tests may help to distinguish conductive deafness from other forms. They are also impossible to perform in a child of 18 months who could not understand instructions.

PA-C4 CORRECT RESPONSE D

Research in the past decade has shown that a much smaller proportion of cerebral palsy is caused by perinatal hypoxia than was previously thought. Most cases have their origin earlier in pregnancy.

Spastic diplegia is the most common variety of cerebral palsy in Australia and elsewhere; choreoathetosis is much less common and is probably diminishing with the prevention of kernicterus, previously a significant cause.

Diazepam is ineffective as a treatment for spasticity.

Feeding difficulties are common in cerebral palsy, especially in the most severely affected, such as those with spastic quadriplegia. This group are also almost always significantly intellectually impaired, in contrast with those with spastic diplegia, in whom intelligence is usually within the normal range.

PA-C5 CORRECT RESPONSE E

There is evidence that long-term oral phenobarbitone can reduce the frequency of febrile convulsions, but it is relatively slowly absorbed and has a long half-life in plasma, making it unsuitable for oral use in an acute situation.

There is controversy about the value of gentle cooling in the management of febrile convulsions, but immersion in a bath of cold water is contraindicated because of the cutaneous vasoconstriction induced and the discomfort to the child.

Antipyretic therapy with paracetamol is also controversial, but aspirin is contraindicated in the febrile child because of a possible association with Reye syndrome. The dose is also excessive.

Antibiotic therapy is not generally indicated in upper respiratory infections, most of which are due to viruses. The previous history of febrile convulsion is not relevant.

Approximately 30% of children who have a single febrile convulsion can be expected to have a recurrence. The majority do not.

PA-C6   CORRECT RESPONSE C

Petit mal epilepsy characteristically has its onset between 5 and 10 years of age.

Intellectual development is usually normal.

Attacks can usually be brought on by hyperventilation and this is a useful step in diagnosis.

The drugs of first choice are ethosuximide or sodium valproate. More than 50% of children with Petit-mal also have a Grand-mal (generalised tonic-clonic) seizure at some time.

PA-C7   CORRECT RESPONSE A

Cerebral palsy (CP) is correctly defined as a disorder of posture and locomotion. It has a number of associations which are believed to result from non-progressive lesions of the central nervous system (CNS), generally occurring prior to birth.

Cerebral palsy does not cause intellectual disability (ID). It may be associated with ID, but other conditions, such as Down syndrome, are much more common with ID than CP.

Some types of CP are frequently associated with epilepsy, but overall epilepsy occurs in fewer than half the people with CP.

The traditional attribution of CP to birth trauma is now known to be incorrect, the majority of cases being due to insults to the CNS before birth.

Some cases of CP are due to malformations of the CNS. Such malformations are familial in a minority of cases only.

PA-C8   CORRECT RESPONSE D

Acute polymyositis is uncommon at any age, especially in childhood and would be unlikely to result in this clinical picture.

Myasthenia gravis is characterised by fatigability, although this may not always be present. It is a possible cause of the condition described. Myasthenia gravis, however, is much less common than *Guillain–Barré syndrome, which is the most likely diagnosis.* Guillain–Barré syndrome (acute postinfective neuropathy) is a disease of unknown cause, beginning 7–10 days after an infective illness, causing flaccid ascending muscle paralysis, usually without sensory loss. The cranial nerves may be affected and respiratory muscle paralysis can be fatal.

The disease presents as an acute symmetrical ascending lower motor neuron paralysis that can cause diaphragmatic and bulbar paralysis as it spreads proximally from its distal origins; usually it is self-limiting with complete recovery.

The more acute form of spinal muscular atrophy presents before 6 months of age and progresses rapidly to death before the second birthday. It is usually recessively inherited.

Botulism due to ingestion of toxin or wound infection is now rare and more acute in its progression, while infant botulism, which is due to colonisation of the gut with *Clostridium botulinus*, occurs in infants under 6 months of age.

PA-C9 CORRECT RESPONSE A

This infant clearly had an abnormally rapid growth of the head in the postnatal period. This would not occur in familial macrocephaly or as a variant of normal, in both of which the head would be expected to be large from birth.

The rapid head growth is highly suggestive of hydrocephalus due to partial obstruction of the flow of cerebrospinal fluid. Of the causes listed, aqueduct stenosis is more common than posterior fossa brain tumour.

A porencephalic cyst may be associated with hydrocephalus, but is also much less common than aqueduct stenosis.

PA-C10 CORRECT RESPONSE D

The development of pes cavus in an adolescent boy should alert one to the possibility of the neurological disorder known as Friedrich ataxia. This is a form of spinocerebellar degeneration presenting in late childhood or adolescence. The clumsy gait is generally due to cerebellar ataxia, but is sometimes incorrectly attributed to the high plantar arch foot deformity, pes cavus, which results from spastic contracture of the intrinsic muscles of the foot.

The disease runs a progressive course and no effective treatment is available. A most difficult aspect is the psychological impact of the disorder, which is likely to be made worse by misdiagnosis or inappropriate management. Surgical release of contractures sometimes provides temporary benefit, but would not be appropriate management at presentation.

PA-C11 CORRECT RESPONSE E

Inflammatory changes of the eye are a very important association with juvenile chronic arthritis (JCA). Although they are found in fewer than 25% of children with JCA, early diagnosis and treatment can avert severe loss of vision.

High, spiking fever is characteristic of the systemic onset form of JCA (Still disease), which may occur at any age in childhood.

Monoarticular arthritis most commonly affects the knee. Rheumatoid factor is rarely present in JCA, except in the late onset polyarticular form, which is relatively uncommon (approximately 10% of JCA).

Radiological changes occur late in the course of the disease and in most children with JCA little will be seen in the X-ray other than some non-specific bone demineralisation.

PA-C12 CORRECT RESPONSE D

The key to this question is the understanding of normal foot posture in the growing child. The relative flattening of the medial longitudinal arch, together with a fat pad filling the arch, accounts for the finding that most 2-year-olds have flat feet, which persist into adult life in approximately 15% of individuals. Such flat feet in 2-year-olds are not influenced by physiotherapy, metatarsal bars or plates in the shoes. *Reassurance of the parents that this is a normal developmental stage is appropriate.*

PA-C13　　　　　　　　　　　　　　CORRECT RESPONSE A

'In-toeing' in young children is usually due to one or more of three conditions: internal rotation of the hips, internal torsion of the tibia, or metatarsus adductus. All are common normal phenomena before the age of 5 years which correct themselves with growth. Only in rare extreme cases are splints or plasters considered and surgery is not required. *Thus the correct answer is to reassure the parents.*

PA-C14　　　　　　　　　　　　　　CORRECT RESPONSE A

Most small ventricular septal defects in infancy resolve spontaneously. Atrial septal defects, even if small, do not. Patent ductus commonly closes in infancy; should it persist to the toddler age group, spontaneous resolution is not anticipated. Aortic coarctation and congenital heart block are persisting disorders.

PA-C15　　　　　　　　　　　　　　CORRECT RESPONSE D

Ventricular septal defect in childhood commonly closes spontaneously. It is associated with frequent lower respiratory infections. Down syndrome is frequently complicated by cardiac anomaly, often complex defects of the ventricular septum. Approximately one-third of patients with oesophageal atresia have other congenital anomalies, of which cardiac malformations, including ventricular septal defect, are commonest. *Smoking in pregnancy has not been shown to be associated with the disorder.*

PA-C16　　　　　　　　　　　　　　CORRECT RESPONSE B

A diastolic blood pressure of 95 mmHg in a 15-year-old girl must be regarded as significant. Before embarking on any investigation or treatment, *the reading should be checked after a period of rest*, even though emotional factors have greater effect on the systolic, rather than diastolic, blood pressure.

PA-C17　　　　　　　　　　　　　　CORRECT RESPONSE D

Diagnosis of congestive cardiac failure in infancy can be difficult, as it lacks the typical features of the adult syndrome, such as ankle oedema. Tachycardia is common with minor febrile illnesses and is not suggestive of cardiac failure. Raised respiratory rate is more likely to occur with respiratory illness than in cardiac disease in infancy. Observation of jugular venous distension is unreliable. *The most useful feature is liver enlargement.*

PA-C18　　　　　　　　　　　　　　CORRECT RESPONSE E

The combination of colicky abdominal pain with an urticarial rash over the buttocks and lower extremities, together with arthritis and localised oedema is very suggestive of Henoch-Schönlein (anaphylactoid) purpura. The skin lesions characteristically progress from urticaria to purpura. Laboratory tests are generally unhelpful, but *up to 50% of children have haematuria on microscopy of urine.* Nephritis, when it occurs, is usually mild, but is an important manifestation of the disease as it may occasionally progress to renal failure.

Intussusception is a very rare complication and, when it occurs, generally involves the small bowel. Plain X-ray of the abdomen is not diagnostic.

PA-C19　　　　　　　　　　　　　　CORRECT RESPONSE B

The use of short courses of oral corticosteroids in acute attacks of asthma has been clearly demonstrated to reduce the duration of attacks and the requirement for admission to hospital. Systemic corticosteroids were under-utilised for many years because of unwarranted fears of complications, which are rarely seen with courses of 5 days or less.

Theophylline is less effective and has a high incidence of unwanted effects. The efficacy of added ipratropium bromide is less well established than that of steroids. Inhaled steroids are valuable for long-term preventive therapy, but are ineffective in the acute attack.

Antibiotics are frequently prescribed in asthma, but are of no value unless there is concurrent infection which itself justifies the use of antibiotics, an uncommon situation.

PA-C20   CORRECT RESPONSE E

Asthma is a common condition in childhood and is characterised by recurrent wheeze. There is underlying bronchial hyperreactivity, which often produces *a chronic unproductive cough in otherwise healthy children. Asthma is thus the most likely cause of the symptom described;* however, a definitive diagnosis of asthma should not be made on the basis of this symptom alone.

Bronchitis in childhood is usually an acute febrile illness of viral origin and is often associated with asthmatic symptoms. Whooping cough is relatively uncommon in the community, although the unimmunised child is at greater risk. It usually produces an acute spasmodic cough which lasts several weeks. Bronchiectasis and cystic fibrosis are associated with productive cough. Both are marked by acute exacerbations and a variable degree of ongoing debility.

PA-C21   CORRECT RESPONSE C

The description of the child provides some indication that the episode of asthma is of no more than moderate severity. *The most appropriate therapy would be repeated inhalations of salbutamol* with assessment of response. In this case the child has shown some improvement. Were this not so, a short course of systemic corticosteroid might be considered, but the oral route would be preferred. Oral aminophylline elixir, commonly prescribed in the past, is slow acting and associated with significant side effects and would not be helpful in this situation. Antibiotics are of no value in the treatment of asthma, even when the attack is associated with upper respiratory infection. Antibiotics should be restricted to those cases in which the infection itself justifies their use. Few upper respiratory infections meet this criterion.

Inhalation of beclomethasone is ineffective treatment for an acute attack of asthma. Its role is confined to preventive therapy.

PA-C22   CORRECT RESPONSE C

Facial suffusion followed by vomiting during a paroxysm of coughing is highly suggestive of pertussis, whether or not the typical inspiratory whoop is heard.

Erythromycin estolate has been shown to reduce the shedding of organisms and hence the infectivity of the patient, but it does not shorten the course of the disease. Cough frequently lasts longer than 6 weeks and often recurs with subsequent respiratory infections, but permanent lung damage is not a feature and bronchiectasis is rare unless other factors associated with chronic suppurative lung disease are present.

Unfortunately, currently available vaccines do not completely protect against infection, but they do greatly reduce its morbidity and mortality and are strongly recommended.

PA-C23   CORRECT RESPONSE D

Asymmetry of breath sounds and wheezes in a toddler with cough must raise the possibility of inhaled foreign body. *Inspiratory and expiratory chest X-rays may reveal partial lobar collapse on inspiration and lobar emphysema on expiration, due to partial obstruction of a major bronchus (ball-valve effect).*

Management of this condition requires early bronchoscopy and removal of the foreign body. Subsequently bronchodilators, antibiotics and physiotherapy could all have a place in certain circumstances. Oxygen would not be required in this 'generally well' boy.

PA-C24   CORRECT RESPONSE E

The chest X-ray findings are very suggestive of primary tuberculosis and the history is compatible with that diagnosis. There is a significant pool of people with active tuberculosis in Australia and the diagnosis must be considered in such cases. *Tuberculin testing by intradermal injection should be undertaken at presentation.*

Although both asthma and pneumonia are causes of segmental or lobar collapse, neither is associated with significant hilar lymphadenopathy. Skin prick tests with dust mite antigen are frequently positive in allergic children, but would not be helpful in clarifying the diagnosis in this patient. Both therapeutic trial of antibiotics and needle biopsy might be considered in certain circumstances, but not without excluding tuberculosis.

PA-C25   CORRECT RESPONSE D

The differentiation between 'croup' (laryngo-tracheo-bronchitis (LTB)) and acute epiglottitis may sometimes be difficult, but is important because of the potentially fatal consequence of failure to treat epiglottitis appropriately. *The distinctive barking cough in LTB, which reflects the involvement of the trachea and major bronchi, is most helpful in making the distinction.* Cough is not usually a feature of acute epiglottitis, in which the inflammatory swelling is confined to the supraglottic region.

Expiratory as well as inspiratory stridor occurs in both conditions as the airway narrows, as does subcostal retraction on inspiration. Both may be preceded by symptoms suggestive of upper respiratory infection. Although high fever is more suggestive of epiglottitis than of LTB, it may occur in both conditions.

The decline in frequency of epiglottitis since this question was written, which followed the introduction of *Haemophilus influenzae* B immunisation, does not negate the need for prompt recognition and treatment at presentation.

PA-C26   CORRECT RESPONSE B

You should explain that the baby probably has gastro-oesophageal reflux. If the mother and maternal grandmother continue to believe the baby is otherwise ill, then reassurance will not be effective. Investigation is not indicated in this common situation, but would be considered if the infant was not thriving. Although urinary tract infection is a common cause of vomiting in the new-born period, the otherwise normal progress makes this diagnosis very unlikely. Dilution of formula, by increasing the volume of gastric contents, is likely to lead to exacerbation of the vomiting.

PA-C27   CORRECT RESPONSE D

Childhood threadworm (*Enterobius vermicularis*) infestation is worldwide, is spread within families and, therefore, it is appropriate *to treat all members of the family with antihelminthics, such as mebendazole, when treatment is required.*

Most infested children are asymptomatic. Many have pruritus ani and occasionally vaginitis may occur. Threadworms are not, however, a common cause of enuresis. Constitutional features, such as anorexia, weight loss and abdominal pain, cannot be attributed to threadworms.

Because of its wide distribution and the ease with which it is transmitted from child to child, recurrence after treatment is quite common, but it would be impractical and inappropriate to isolate the infested child.

PA-C28   CORRECT RESPONSE C

This is a common event; it is appropriate to **await further developments,** after a solitary vomit by an otherwise normal infant. Should vomiting persist, different alternatives would be appropriate, depending on clinical features. Urinary microscopy may be appropriate. Changing milk formula is unlikely to be useful; it would not be appropriate if the infant were breast fed. Thickening of the feed is advised for gastro-oesophageal reflux, which usually produces symptoms from birth. Barium meal is occasionally used for investigation for possible pyloric stenosis, but would only be considered in cases of persistent vomiting, associated with weight loss, where other clinical signs are absent. It has largely been replaced by ultrasound of the pylorus.

PA-C29   CORRECT RESPONSE A

Intussusception is most common under the age of 2 years. The underlying cause is often not determined, but there is an association with adenovirus causing enlargement of intestinal lymphoid tissue. Henoch–Schönlein purpura is another less common precipitant, causing ileo–ileal intussusception from mucosal haemorrhage and oedema. Passage of a bloody stool is a late feature of intussusception. *If diagnosed early, over 75% of cases can be reduced by hydrostatic pressure under fluoroscopic control, without the need for laparotomy.*

PA-C30   CORRECT RESPONSE E

The volume of fluid required in the first 24 h in this moderately depleted infant will be about 100 mL/kg expected weight (400 mL) for maintenance of intravenous fluid requirements, plus approximately 5% of expected bodyweight (200 mL): *total 600 mL*. There is no need for a component for continuing losses, as vomiting should cease when oral intake is discontinued.

Hydrogen ion and chloride loss predominate, with alkalosis (pH 7.50), hypochloraemia and hypokalaemia. The appropriate electrolyte solution is therefore one containing adequate potassium, sodium and chloride, with dextrose to provide some energy requirement.

Half isotonic (N/2) saline with 5% dextrose and 40 mmol/L potassium chloride would be a good choice. Potassium should not generally be infused in concentrations above 40 mmol/L and urine output should be observed to be adequate. Hartmann solution, which is often chosen to correct 'dehydration' with acidosis because of its lactate content, is inappropriate as a replacement for gastric acid. Adequate potassium chloride with saline rehydration will correct the alkalosis and ammonium chloride is not required.

PA-C31   CORRECT RESPONSE A

Anal fissure is common in infancy, usually due to the passage of a hard constipated stool and causes blood staining on the surface of the stool or on the nappy. Anal fistula is much less common and does not cause rectal bleeding. Haemorrhoids are rare in infancy.

Meckel diverticulitis may be the source of passage of blood per rectum when ectopic gastric mucosa leads to peptic ulceration and intussusception is characterised by the passage of blood and mucus ('red currant jelly') late in the evolution of the condition. Neither of these conditions approaches anal fissure in frequency as causes of blood in the stools.

PA-C32   CORRECT RESPONSE E

Over 10% of primary school-aged children have recurrent attacks of abdominal pain for which no recognisable organic cause can be found. In the past, some such children have been subjected to appendicectomy for a diagnosis of 'chronic appendicitis', but pathological examination has not identified such a condition.

Meckel diverticulitis is uncommon and when it does occur it mimics acute appendicitis. Both hydronephrosis and urinary tract infections may cause acute attacks of pain, not usually periumbilical.

PA-C33   CORRECT RESPONSE D

Not much information is provided about this infant, beyond the observations that jaundice commenced on the second day of life and persists for 2 weeks and that the infant is thriving.

Physiological jaundice is the most common cause of jaundice in infancy, but does not persist for 2 weeks. Prolonged neonatal jaundice is usually due to unconjugated bilirubin, most often associated with breast feeding. *Breast milk jaundice occurs in approximately 5% of breast fed infants and can be cured by weaning, but this is not necessary if adequate explanation and support are provided.*

Blood group incompatibility is characterised by the early (first day) onset of jaundice and is unlikely to persist for 2 weeks without other signs of illness. Hypothyroidism is a rare cause of prolonged jaundice, but should be considered. It should be identified by neonatal screening programmes.

Conjugated bilirubinaemia is much less common in prolonged neonatal jaundice and is seen particularly in neonatal hepatitis and biliary atresia. Among the rarer causes is galactosaemia, prompting a test for reducing substances (galactose, not glucose) in the urine.

PA-C34   CORRECT RESPONSE E

The description is of *faecal retention with overflow. In this 5-year-old, this is probably due to chronic constipation.* Hirschsprung disease and volvulus usually present with symptoms of acute obstruction. Giardiasis is not associated with constipation. Neurological defects are uncommon in spina bifida occulta, in contrast with spina bifida with myelomeningocele.

PA-C35   CORRECT RESPONSE B

Hepatomegaly is expected in neonatal jaundice associated with galactosaemia, hepatitis and haemolytic disease, as well as being a feature of cardiac failure in infancy. *Hepatomegaly is not found in breast milk jaundice.*

PA-C36   CORRECT RESPONSE C

Strangulation is rare in infantile umbilical hernia. Strapping does not assist resolution, which occurs spontaneously in most cases, even if the defect is large. Surgery is not advised unless the hernia persists over the age of approximately 3 years. There is no familial incidence. Umbilical hernia is a feature of classical cretinism, but does not suggest hypothyroidism in the absence of other clinical features of that disorder.

PA-C37   CORRECT RESPONSE A

An inguinal hernia in an infant can be diagnosed on the history of swelling. Thickening of the spermatic cord on the side involved is further evidence, even if the doctor consulted is unable to demonstrate the hernia itself. In the absence of current swelling, operation is not urgent, but *surgical consultation should be arranged at an early time with a view to inguinal herniotomy* to remove the risk of strangulation.

PA-C38   CORRECT RESPONSE C

Intussusception must be considered as a possible cause of the sudden onset of intermittent crying and pallor in infancy. Pallor is unusual in crying spells in infancy, but is characteristic of intussusception. A mass may be found on abdominal examination, but its absence does not allow the diagnosis to be excluded. Early diagnosis is essential to avoid significant morbidity; reassurance is inappropriate. Urinary tract infections and gastroenteritis are less likely to present in this way; investigation for possible infection may delay the diagnosis, which should be established by radio-opaque enema without delay.

PA-C39   CORRECT RESPONSE A

Hirschsprung disease *presents most commonly as neonatal intestinal obstruction.* Where the abnormal segment of bowel is short, the diagnosis may not be made by contrast enema. Biopsy of the aganglionic bowel wall is the most reliable way of making the diagnosis. Surgical excision of most or all of the aganglionic segment remains the definitive treatment.

PA-C40   CORRECT RESPONSE A

Absorption of highly potent corticosteroids from the skin has been shown to cause suppression of adrenal function and growth suppression in children. Local effects include atrophy of the skin and susceptibility to local candida infection.

Although purpura may be seen in atrophic skin, this is due to local effects on small vessels, not to thrombocytopenia.

PA-C41   CORRECT RESPONSE E

The correct response is non-specific vulvovaginitis.

The vagina, before the onset of puberty, lacks the resistance to infection conferred by oestrogen-induced changes in the epithelium, so that almost any infection or irritating agent may cause inflammation. Colonisation by flora from the gastrointestinal tract occurs mainly when there is trauma from scratching or friction.

Trichomonal infection is rare before puberty. Gonorrhoea is characterised by a profuse purulent discharge. A foreign body could account for the symptoms, but the discharge is usually profuse and may be haemorrhagic.

Cystitis may cause the symptoms described, but is unlikely to have persisted for 3 months and would not account for inflammation of the vulva, whereas *non-specific vulvovaginitis* is common, low grade and difficult to eradicate.

PA-C42   CORRECT RESPONSE A

The key to this question is the recognition that *cutaneous petechiae result either from platelet deficiency or from microvascular haemorrhage and not from coagulation defects.* Although skin bleeding does occur in haemophilia, it is in the form of ecchymoses and is usually the result of direct trauma, even though the trauma may be trivial and unnoticed. *Spontaneous petechiae are not characteristic of haemophilia.*

Both idiopathic thrombocytopenia and aplastic anaemia are associated with a reduced platelet count and with spontaneous petechiae.

The rash in Henoch–Schönlein syndrome is typically papular or urticarial at first, with petechiae developing later, the result of vasculitis of small vessels. The characteristic petechial rash of meningococcal septicaemia is thought to be due to micro-emboli and vasculitis.

PA-C43   CORRECT RESPONSE B

The infant described has severe hypochromic microcytic anaemia, which at this age is most often nutritional in origin and is associated with a high intake of cow milk. Such infants are generally well nourished in other respects, but *iron absorption from cow milk is poor, leading to iron deficiency.*

In adults, iron deficiency is more commonly due to chronic blood loss; however, even though this may be a factor in infants, it would not be the most likely cause.

Thalassaemia major is a cause of hypochromic anaemia, but the blood film would be expected to show macrocytes, anisocytosis, target cells and nucleated red cells and an elevated reticulocyte count. Anaemia of the severity described would generally be associated with hepatosplenomegaly.

Megaloblastic anaemia of infancy is now rare in developed countries. It is occasionally seen when a folate-deficient diet is accompanied by increased folate consumption, as in chronic enteric infection. The blood picture in this case does not suggest megaloblastic anaemia.

Although anaemia of infection is common in childhood, it is usually of a mild degree and the blood picture is normocytic.

PA-C44   CORRECT RESPONSE B

The combination of lethargy and development of jaundice towards the end of the first week of life should give rise to a suspicion of sepsis, whatever the racial origin of the infant. In particular, jaundice due to a rise in both conjugated and unconjugated bilirubin is typical of sepsis, whereas both haemolysis and defective conjugation of bilirubin, such as occurs in hypothyroidism, would lead to a rise in unconjugated bilirubin predominantly. Accordingly, *blood culture is the most likely of the listed tests to indicate the cause of the jaundice.*

Tests directed to possible causes of haemolysis, such as glucose-6-phosphate dehydrogenase activity or osmotic fragility of erythrocytes, are much less likely to indicate the cause of jaundice in this infant and haemoglobin electrophoresis would rarely be helpful at this age, even if haemolysis were suspected.

PA-C45   CORRECT RESPONSE C

The key to this question is in the recognition that the gene for haemophilia is X chromosome-linked. The affected man has only one X chromosome, which must have the defective gene. *Any sons he may have will receive his normal Y chromosome and be free of disease. Any daughters he may have must have received his defective X-linked gene and be carriers. Thus, the possible offspring are female carriers or normal males.*

PA-C46   CORRECT RESPONSE E

Regular bed wetting occurs in approximately 10% of children, but is not usual at the age of 4 years. The majority of children (75%) are dry at night by 3 years of age.

Disorders of the upper urinary tract do not cause enuresis. Intravenous pyelogram is not indicated.

A positive family history is very common, especially in boys, but is found in over 50% of both sexes.

Psychological factors may lead to secondary enuresis, usually transient, but if relevant at all are certainly not predominant in the aetiology of primary enuresis.

Tricyclic antidepressants, vasopressin analogues and conditioning apparatus have all been shown to be effective in the treatment of enuresis. *Safety considerations favour a conditioning apparatus, which is also least often associated with relapse in children old enough to understand the treatment objective. A conditioning apparatus is thus the most effective treatment for children who are over 8 years old.*

PA-C47   CORRECT RESPONSE B

The clinical picture described is that of nephrotic syndrome, which in early childhood is associated with the minimal change lesion in over 80% of cases.

Serum albumin is low, due to selective clearance of lower molecular weight proteins. While some low molecular weight globulins are also lost there is some compensatory increase in higher molecular weight globulins in the serum resulting in hyperlipidaemia, including raised cholesterol, but total globulin is normal. Microscopic haematuria is seen in approximately 30% of cases, but macroscopic haematuria is rare and, if present, requires review of the diagnosis.

The prognosis for minimal change nephrotic syndrome appropriately treated is ultimately good, although some 70% have relapses during childhood.

PA-C48   CORRECT RESPONSE A

Acute scrotal pain and swelling in childhood suggests torsion of the testis. *This diagnosis must be made by surgical exploration.* Confirmation of the diagnosis of torsion requires fixation of both testes because it is due to a bilateral congenital defect. Alternative investigations are contraindicated as this delays diagnosis. Observation will increase morbidity and antibiotic treatment is ineffective for torsion and of little use for epididymo-orchitis which is usually viral in origin in childhood.

PA-C49   CORRECT RESPONSE A

Meatal ulceration is one of the most common complications of circumcision. Neonatal circumcision is not painless and may be catastrophic in haemophilia. It is contraindicated in hypospadias, as the skin may be used in the surgical repair. The prepuce becomes retractile in the first years, but in the majority of uncircumcised boys of 6 months, it is still not fully retractile.

PA-C50   CORRECT RESPONSE A

There is a wide range of normality in many of the developmental milestones, but only one of those listed is clearly outside the normal range. *An infant at 2 weeks has a grasp reflex and will grasp an object placed in the palm of the hand, but the voluntary grasp associated with reaching for an object is not seen before 12–14 weeks.*

All the other activities listed are within the normal range.

PA-C51   CORRECT RESPONSE E

All of the activities listed are among those for which normal ranges are documented in the Denver Developmental Screening Test.

At 11 months, fewer than 25% of children can walk independently.

Mean age for building a tower of four blocks is 18 months, pointing to a named body part is 17 months and feeding with a spoon is 14–15 months.

Pincer grasp between thumb and finger is seen in some infants at 9 months and most have achieved it before 11 months. The ability to pick up a raisin between thumb and finger is, thus, the only one of the responses listed expected to be present in an 11-month-old child.

PA-C52   CORRECT RESPONSE C

All of the activities listed are among those for which normal ranges are documented in the Denver Developmental Screening Test.

The mean age at which children give their first and last names is between 2½ and 3 years.

Children can undress during the 2nd year and dress with supervision around 3 years.

The mean age for drawing a man of three parts is around 4 years, but for six parts is closer to 5 years.

The mean age for hopping on one foot is about 3½ years.

The age at which children separate easily from mother varies widely, but most 3-year-olds can achieve this so that kindergarten activities are enjoyed. The mean age in a test population was just over 3 years and, at 4 years, approximately 80% were able to separate easily.

PA-C53   CORRECT RESPONSE C

Social deprivation, especially lack of a mother, is a potent cause of delayed speech development. Hypothyroidism, although not often seen in Australian children because of population screening and treatment from the newborn period, is an important cause of global developmental delay, including speech development.

Contrary to popular belief, tongue-tie does not cause delayed speech development. Some believe that severe tongue-tie can cause dysarthria, but if so, it is very rare.

Infantile autism is strongly associated with delayed speech development and this is often the presenting symptom.

Sensorineural deafness most often affects the higher frequency responses, leading to high-tone deafness. If mild, this leads to difficulty in articulation of high-pitched sounds, but if more severe is a cause of delayed speech development.

PA-C54   CORRECT RESPONSE D

Anorexia nervosa is more common in adolescent girls than in boys. It is associated with marked weight loss, preoccupation with food and amenorrhoea. All these features are descriptive of anorexia nervosa in adolescents. *Patients usually remain remarkably active physically.*

PA-C55   CORRECT RESPONSE D

Failure to thrive in infancy is most often attributable to a disordered relationship between child and parent and is commonly part of the child maltreatment syndrome.

Laceration of the frenulum of the lower lip often occurs during forceful attempts at feeding a distressed child and should lead to consideration of maltreatment by the carer.

Scalds of the feet or buttocks may result from the carer, usually a parent, placing the child in very hot water, whereas scalds of the head, upper trunk and hands more often result from domestic accidents.

Epistaxes are uncommon in infants, but very common in older children, when they are usually spontaneous or associated with nose-picking or other minor trauma. *Of the conditions listed, epistaxes are the least suggestive of child maltreatment.*

PA-C56   CORRECT RESPONSE B

Intellectual disability is characterised by delay in all aspects of development, although some may be affected more than others. The absence of delay other than in speech development rules out this cause.

Deafness is the most likely cause. Deafness frequently escapes detection unless specifically sought by audiography. Severe deafness may lead to speech delay and to poor articulation.

Manipulative behaviour may lead to mutism, usually transient and associated with other evidence of behaviour disorder. This would occur most commonly in older children and adolescents and would be very rare at this age.

Dysarthria has many causes, but is not associated with failure to develop a vocabulary unless due to profound deafness.

Autism is often associated with delayed speech development, but is unlikely to be associated with development of gestures for communication. Other aspects of development are likely to be atypical.

PA-C57   CORRECT RESPONSE C

Brachycephaly, epicanthic folds, muscular hypotonia and duodenal atresia are all associated with Down syndrome, *but cleft palate is not.*

PA-C58   CORRECT RESPONSE D

The situation described is not rare and is a difficult one to manage well. The final decision by the parents of the child with Down syndrome regarding their ability and wish to care for the child at home may not be reached for some weeks after the birth, especially if the diagnosis is unexpected. During this time all options should be kept open. It is inappropriate to keep the baby in hospital, which is an unsuitable environment for optimal development. *A better course is to arrange temporary foster care, where the child can be cared for by a mother-substitute while the parents are offered supportive counselling and access to the child.*

Arrangement for wardship or adoption may ultimately be required, but should not be considered until the above steps have been undertaken. Persuasion in hospital is unlikely to be effective in changing the initial response and may be counterproductive.

PA-C59   CORRECT RESPONSE B

Peripheral cyanosis in an otherwise normal newborn is most often due to hypothermia resulting from exposure in the delivery area. *The infant's rectal temperature should be checked* and, if low, the infant should be wrapped and gently warmed. Oxygen is unnecessary and return of normal colour on warming eliminates the need for investigations, such as chest X-ray.

The normal respiratory rate and absence of abnormal respiration offer no suggestions of respiratory distress, while the cyanosis accompanying convulsions is generally central and due to hypoventilation during the seizure.

PA-C60   CORRECT RESPONSE A

Obesity affects 5–10% of Australian children. It is defined as weight above the 90th percentile. Less than half of untreated overweight infants will become obese adults. Despite their widespread use, evaluation of diet and exercise programmes has shown generally disappointing results. Underlying metabolic or endocrine disorders are rare, occurring in well under 10% of cases.

PA-C61   CORRECT RESPONSE B

Foods other than milk are not needed by the normal infant before 4–6 months of life. *Bottle-fed babies are more likely to be overweight than breast-fed babies.*

Postpartum psychosis may not always be a contraindication to breast feeding, but lithium therapy is a specific contraindication. Breast milk, like other milks, does not have a high iron content. Nevertheless, because breast milk iron is better absorbed, it suffices for optimal development in the first months of life unless the infant's birth weight was low. Test weighing before and after breast feeding may give a rough guide to milk intake, but is subject to errors. Considerable variation occurs between different feedings; milk flow may also be reduced due to the embarrassment of the mother in the test situation. Mothers anxious about the adequacy of their breast milk supply are especially vulnerable to discouragement from a test weigh.

PA-C62   CORRECT RESPONSE D

Hypernatraemic dehydration in childhood is often complicated by convulsions. Clinical diagnosis may be difficult, as tissue turgor may be normal. Rapid rehydration will aggravate the tendency to convulse. In the presence of circulatory failure, initial prompt establishment of circulatory volume by the use of an isotonic plasma volume expander will be needed. This type of dehydration is most common in older infants, with fluid lack associated with febrile illness.

PA-C63   CORRECT RESPONSE D

Glycosuria can have many causes, ranging from innocent conditions such as reduced renal threshold for sugar, to diabetic keto-acidosis requiring immediate diagnosis and management. *In an ill child it cannot be ignored and is a significant observation demanding further elucidation.*

Glycosuria does not necessarily indicate hyperglycaemia.

When associated with normal blood sugar, glycosuria may be an isolated tubular defect or part of a more complex disorder such as Fanconi syndrome, an inherited disorder of renal tubular function associated with vitamin D-resistant rickets, glycosuria and aminoaciduria. If blood sugar is not known, the significance of glycosuria cannot be assessed.

PA-C64   CORRECT RESPONSE A

Although hypothyroidism is now uncommon in Australian children because of a successful screening and management programme, it is important to be aware of *the critical role of thyroid hormone in longitudinal growth. Hypothyroidism is the most likely cause of growth retardation in this case with short stature and retarded bone age.*

Diabetes mellitus has little effect on longitudinal growth unless severe and poorly controlled.

There are several genetically different forms of congenital adrenal hyperplasia, some of which are associated with advanced bone age. Retarded bone age is not a feature.

Genetic short stature or constitutional short stature are terms applied to otherwise healthy short individuals with a family history of shortness. Bone age, if reduced at all, is usually proportionate to height age.

Psychological deprivation is a cause of short stature, but rarely of the degree described and, as with constitutional short stature, bone age is likely to be normal or proportionate to height age.

PA-C65   CORRECT RESPONSE A

All of the groups of disorders listed are potential causes of failure to thrive (failure to gain weight normally) in the first year of life, when weight gain is rapid. *In Australia, many studies have confirmed that the most common cause of failure to thrive in infancy is not an organic cause in the infant, but impaired parenting and subsequent undernutrition.*

Both gastro-oesophageal reflux and recurrent infection are common, but neither approaches the non-organic group as causes of failure to thrive. Malabsorption and endocrine/metabolic disorders are even less common causes of failure to thrive.

PA-C66   CORRECT RESPONSE C

Acute bronchiolitis is usually due to the respiratory syncytial virus. It occurs most commonly under the age of 6 months. Babies with minor symptoms may be nursed at home, *but inability to feed adequately is a major indication for hospitalisation*, as oxygen therapy and supportive fluids may be required. While beta-adrenergic agents are effective in older children with asthma, wheezing in bronchiolitis is associated with bronchiolar narrowing due to inflammation, rather than bronchospasm and does not respond to beta-adrenergic agents. Affected infants have a higher risk of further wheezing than unaffected infants in the same age group. It is unclear whether the viral bronchiolitis causes damage to the airways or whether abnormal airways predispose to the occurrence of bronchiolitis. Nevertheless, approximately half the affected infants subsequently have asthma.

PA-C67   CORRECT RESPONSE C

Osteomyelitis is by far the most likely diagnosis in this young child with constitutional symptoms, high fever and localised tenderness over bone. This question might be considered too easy for candidates at this level and indeed few failed to identify the correct response; however, the importance of the topic and the consequences of failure to make the diagnosis justify its inclusion.

Cellulitis would be a possible differential diagnosis, but the localised tenderness makes it less likely. Thrombophlebitis is rare in children and would not lead to the physical signs described. A fracture must be considered in a young child refusing to walk with a swollen lower limb and may give rise to some warmth of the fracture site and even a low grade fever, but would not account for a fever of 40°C. Osteosarcoma is very rare at this young age. It may be tender if rapidly growing and haemorrhagic and can also be associated with low grade, but not high-grade, fever.

PA-C68   CORRECT RESPONSE E

Of the organisms listed, **Escherichia coli** is the only common cause of neonatal meningitis. It should be noted that in recent years Group B streptococcus is at least as common a cause.

The more common causes of meningitis in older children, *Haemophilus influenzae*, *Streptococcus pneumoniae* and *Neisseria meningitidis,* are rare in the newborn period, while *Staphylococcus aureus* meningitis, where it occurs, is usually a complication of surgical breach of the meninges.

PA-C69   CORRECT RESPONSE A

Most children with measles can be safely treated symptomatically at home. There is no effective specific treatment and gamma-globulin is not helpful at this stage. There is no indication to give gamma-globulin to the sister, who is fully immunised. In unimmunised children over 12 months of age, measles vaccine given within 72 h of contact can prevent measles infection, because the incubation period of the vaccine strain is shorter than that of the wild strain.

It would be most inappropriate to advise the mother that he is 'over the worst of it'. He may be unwell for several more days and the significant complication rate makes it mandatory that appropriate medical supervision be arranged until he has recovered fully.

PA-C70   CORRECT RESPONSE D

Mild meningo-encephalitis is extremely common in mumps, although most often not identified because examination of the cerebrospinal fluid is not justified in most cases. Encephalomyelitis is fortunately a rare complication.

The association of onset of diabetes mellitus with mumps infection has been suggested in some studies, but is certainly not a common complication. Mumps orchitis is rare before puberty and although inflammation of salivary glands is common in mumps, sialectasis is not a sequel.

PA-C71   CORRECT RESPONSE D

Of the conditions listed, *cervical lymphadenitis* is the most likely cause of such a swelling. In this case there is a history of infection of the tonsils, which drain to the jugulodigastric group of lymph nodes deep in the upper anterior triangle of the neck, but such a history is often lacking, the infecting episode being silent. Such nodes may be tender, but often are not.

Tuberculous lymphadenitis and lymphoma are possible alternative diagnoses, but are of course much less common. They should be borne in mind when a cervical swelling does not run the expected course.

A branchial cyst rarely presents in young children and would not be firm. It is located deep to the sternomastoid protruding around its anterior border, while a thyroglossal cyst is a midline or near midline structure.

PA-C72   CORRECT RESPONSE A

This history and findings are most suggestive of **Giardia lamblia** *infestation*, which is extremely common in young children, particularly those in day-care. Coeliac disease is possible, but would usually have an earlier onset when gluten is introduced into the diet from about 6 months. Cystic fibrosis with significant malabsorption would present in early infancy, while *Campylobacter jejuni* and rotavirus infections present as acute gastroenteritis.

PA-C73   CORRECT RESPONSE B

Cloxacillin was developed for the treatment of staphylococcal infections. Of the conditions listed, only **osteomyelitis** is most often due to infection with *Staphylococcus aureus* and cloxacillin or a similar beta-lactamase resistant penicillin should be included in first-line therapy.

PA-C74   CORRECT RESPONSE C

Infectious mononucleosis is not associated with relapse after initial recovery although symptoms of tiredness may be prolonged for weeks in the initial illness. Suggestions that the girl has not had adequate rest and should have further absence from school are likely to reinforce the idea of physical illness rather than to assist recovery; the same is true of further tests.

Given that there are no other symptoms or signs apart from those mentioned, an emotional cause is most likely and should emerge on further inquiry, although both patient and mother deny the possibility at first interview. *At age 14 such a cause is best sought by interview with the patient alone.* Discussing her ill health privately with her parents is likely to be counterproductive.

PA-C75   CORRECT RESPONSE E

The appearance of the rash is petechial, rather than erythematous. While there are a number of possible explanations, there is a significant likelihood that the child has fulminating meningococcal septicaemia. This condition has a very high mortality, especially if diagnosis is delayed, so that the responses suggesting sending the patient home after initial treatment are all inappropriate.

Immediate hospital admission is required. The potential advantage of early treatment justifies an immediate initial dose of penicillin prior to hospitalisation as the preferred response, despite a small chance that subsequent blood culture may be negative. The evolution of the illness is so characteristic that this potential loss of precision in diagnosis is not of practical importance when balanced against the benefit of early treatment.

Because the rash of meningococcal septicaemia is occasionally mimicked in septicaemia of other causes, cefotaxime is added on arrival at hospital pending identification of the infecting organism.

PA-C76   CORRECT RESPONSE E

For many years **Haemophilus influenzae** *type B has been the most common organism to cause non-neonatal bacterial meningitis in children in Australia*, followed by *Neisseria meningitidis* and *Streptococcus pneumoniae*. *Staphylococcus aureus* meningitis, when it occurs, is usually a complication of an invasive procedure. Beta-haemolytic streptococcus is a very rare cause, unlike Group B streptococcus, which is a common cause in the newborn.

Widespread uptake of *Haemophilus influenzae* B vaccine has already been followed by decreased frequency of this cause of meningitis and it is to be hoped that by the time of publication *Haemophilus influenzae* may no longer be a common cause of meningitis in Australia.

PA-C77   CORRECT RESPONSE B

Although it can be difficult on clinical grounds to distinguish viral from bacterial tonsillitis, in this age group a beta-haemolytic streptococcus is the only likely bacterial cause of follicular tonsillitis. *An adequate course of penicillin is most effective in eradication of this organism,* so that B is the best response.

The concurrent presence of beta-lactamase-secreting bacteria in the pharynx may prevent eradication of beta-haemolytic streptococci by penicillin, so that in recurrent cases amoxycillin with clavulanic acid may be considered; however, this more expensive alternative would not be the first choice. There is no advantage from the broader spectrum of cefaclor, amoxycillin or Cotrimoxazole®.

PA-C78   CORRECT RESPONSE E

The sequence of events and X-ray are typical of staphylococcal pneumonia progressing to empyema.

Streptococcus pneumoniae (pneumococcus) is the most common bacterial cause of pneumonia in this age group and may produce a pleural effusion, but pneumatoceles are rare. The same applies to *Haemophilus influenzae,* which is an uncommon cause of pneumonia. *Klebsiella* species may cause pneumonia in the newborn, but *Klebsiella pneumoniae* is a rare cause after the newborn period and Group A streptococcus even rarer.

Staphylococcal pneumonia, common a generation ago, is now rare in infants in Australia.

PA-C79   CORRECT RESPONSE C

This is a typical description of viral 'croup', most commonly caused by the parainfluenza virus. Acute asthma in childhood may be associated with cough, but not with stridor; 'barking' cough is a feature of laryngeal inflammation. The larynx is not usually involved in group A streptococcal infection. A tracheal foreign body, however, may present in the manner described. It is important to consider this possibility, as it is commonly overlooked, mainly because of its relative infrequency. Although an important differential diagnosis, it is not the most likely cause of the symptoms. Acute epiglottitis is also an important cause of upper airway obstruction in this age group, but the symptoms differ in that the onset is usually over 3–4 h, cough is not prominent and fever is more severe. The voice is muffled and stridor is low-pitched and not confined to inspiration.

PA-C80   CORRECT RESPONSE C

The incubation period of mumps ranges from 14 to 24 days. In most patients, the parotid glands alone are affected, but submandibular gland involvement occurs frequently. *Meningoencephalitis can precede, occur simultaneously with or follow parotitis.* Although it is an important cause of male infertility, impairment of fertility is estimated to occur in less than 15% of patients with mumps orchitis. Laboratory confirmation of infection is generally unnecessary, but there is no reliable skin test to indicate immunity.

PA-C81 CORRECT RESPONSE C

The term 'croup' when unqualified refers to laryngotracheobronchitis, a virus infection in which the major risk is progression of airway obstruction to a point at which hypoxia occurs, with possible cardiorespiratory arrest.

Sedation is contraindicated in a child with croup, as it may produce respiratory depression and aggravate hypoxia.

Bronchodilators, as used for treatment of asthma, are generally ineffective in croup. Higher doses of inhaled adrenaline may give short-term relief of obstruction and may be used in hospital while preparing for mechanical relief of obstruction. This is not part of routine management.

Children with mild croup can be managed at home provided that the parents are good observers and understand that progression of obstruction, as indicated by sternal retraction at rest, is an indication for admission to hospital. In hospital or at home, close observation for evidence of hypoxia is indicated.

Tracheostomy is a satisfactory method for the relief of life-threatening obstruction, but is now rarely used. Nasotracheal intubation is preferred, but is required in fewer than 1% of cases.

Some texts still recommend the use of oxygen in the management of croup, but it is not accepted as part of routine treatment in Australia. If oxygen is routinely administered, it may conceal the development of progressive obstruction to a point where complete obstruction leads to cardiorespiratory arrest. Oxygen may, however, be given while preparations are made for the mechanical relief of obstruction.

PA-C82 CORRECT RESPONSE D

Herpes simplex infection in infancy is commonly associated with mouth ulceration and significant fever. Rubella occurs most commonly in school age children and the rash generally appears on the first day of the illness. Scarlet fever is now uncommon in Australia at any age. Should it occur, a high fever and significant toxicity would be expected.

The findings are typical of roseola infantum, an infection due to human herpes virus 6, which occurs predominantly in infants and is characterised by the appearance of the rash as the fever subsides.

Erythema infectiosum, also known as 'slapped cheeks' syndrome, has a distinctive rash and tends to occur in toddlers and young school age children. It is due to infection with human parvovirus.

PA-C83 CORRECT RESPONSE B

Viral gastroenteritis is the most common cause of gastroenteritis in infancy in Australia. It usually resolves within a few days, but *secondary lactase deficiency may cause persistent symptoms, including the development of watery acid stools which irritate the skin in the napkin area.* The stools contain reducing substances on testing. Secondary bacterial enteritis does not commonly complicate viral gastroenteritis. *Giardia lamblia* infestation is most commonly diagnosed in later childhood when it presents with persisting diarrhoea. Acute presentations occur uncommonly in infancy. Cow milk allergy, occurring within approximately 1 month of weaning, can mimic acute gastroenteritis, but this syndrome is much less common than infective diarrhoea. Coeliac disease does not usually present accutely, although it may rarely do so. In such cases, the acute presentation is superimposed on progressive failure to thrive and does not occur in a previously well infant.

PA-C84   CORRECT RESPONSE E

The history and findings are most suggestive of neuroblastoma. Neuroblastoma most commonly (65%) arises within the abdomen, usually in the adrenal gland, where it characteristically presents as an irregular mass. It is often non-tender, but may be tender if haemorrhagic. Extension across the midline helps to distinguish it from masses arising in kidney or even ovary, such as cystic dysplastic kidney or the rare large ovarian cysts. Retroperitoneal haematoma would be tender and non-mobile. Thalassaemia major may account for a protuberant abdomen due to liver enlargement and particularly splenic enlargement, but the history would be quite different.

PA-C85   CORRECT RESPONSE D

Acute lymphoblastic leukaemia is the most common childhood malignancy, representing approximately one-third of all neoplastic diseases in children.

With the exception of a small number of cases with identifiable 'unfavourable' histology, Wilms tumour is very responsive to modern combinations of chemotherapy, surgery and radiotherapy, with a cure rate approaching 80%.

Neuroblastoma is a highly malignant tumour of childhood. Screening techniques for early detection are under trial in some countries, but currently most cases are still diagnosed after the development of metastases, often very widespread.

Intracranial tumours in children most often arise in the cerebellum or brain stem and are thus infratentorial in origin. In this position they commonly obstruct the flow of cerebrospinal fluid, accounting for the frequency of symptoms of raised intracranial pressure at presentation.

Carcinoma is not the most common type of solid tumour in children; many childhood tumours are of soft tissue rather than epithelial origin.

PA-C86   CORRECT RESPONSE E

Sudden infant death syndrome remains the most common cause of death after the neonatal period under the age of 12 months, but by 3 years is rare.

Both infection and leukaemia are significant causes of death in early childhood, but less common than accidents. Viral pneumonia rarely causes death after infancy and the increasing cure rate of leukaemia has diminished its frequency as a cause of death.

Motor vehicle accidents have approached or exceeded drownings in frequency, but seat belt legislation has reduced motor accidents as a cause of death in recent years. *Drowning remains the most frequent cause of death among those listed.* Poisoning has been much reduced in recent years, probably because of public education and improved safety packaging. Similarly, legislation regarding swimming pool areas is aimed at reducing the frequency of drowning in young children.

SUMMARY OF CORRECT RESPONSES

CATEGORY & QUESTION NO.	CORRECT RESPONSE	CATEGORY & QUESTION NO.	CORRECT RESPONSE	CATEGORY & QUESTION NO.	CORRECT RESPONSE
PA-Q 1	A	PA-Q 32	E	PA-Q 63	D
PA-Q 2	E	PA-Q 33	D	PA-Q 64	A
PA-Q 3	B	PA-Q 34	E	PA-Q 65	A
PA-Q 4	D	PA-Q 35	B	PA-Q 66	C
PA-Q 5	E	PA-Q 36	C	PA-Q 67	C
PA-Q 6	C	PA-Q 37	A	PA-Q 68	E
PA-Q 7	A	PA-Q 38	C	PA-Q 69	A
PA-Q 8	D	PA-Q 39	A	PA-Q 70	D
PA-Q 9	A	PA-Q 40	A	PA-Q 71	D
PA-Q 10	D	PA-Q 41	E	PA-Q 72	A
PA-Q 11	E	PA-Q 42	A	PA-Q 73	B
PA-Q 12	D	PA-Q 43	B	PA-Q 74	C
PA-Q 13	A	PA-Q 44	B	PA-Q 75	E
PA-Q 14	A	PA-Q 45	C	PA-Q 76	E
PA-Q 15	D	PA-Q 46	E	PA-Q 77	B
PA-Q 16	B	PA-Q 47	B	PA-Q 78	E
PA-Q 17	D	PA-Q 48	A	PA-Q 79	C
PA-Q 18	E	PA-Q 49	A	PA-Q 80	C
PA-Q 19	B	PA-Q 50	A	PA-Q 81	C
PA-Q 20	E	PA-Q 51	E	PA-Q 82	D
PA-Q 21	C	PA-Q 52	C	PA-Q 83	B
PA-Q 22	C	PA-Q 53	C	PA-Q 84	E
PA-Q 23	D	PA-Q 54	D	PA-Q 85	D
PA-Q 24	E	PA-Q 55	D	PA-Q 86	E
PA-Q 25	D	PA-Q 56	B		
PA-Q 26	B	PA-Q 57	C		
PA-Q 27	D	PA-Q 58	D		
PA-Q 28	C	PA-Q 59	B		
PA-Q 29	A	PA-Q 60	A		
PA-Q 30	E	PA-Q 61	B		
PA-Q 31	A	PA-Q 62	D		

Obstetrics and Gynaecology Commentaries

and Summary of Correct Responses

TYPE

A

Commentaries OG-C1 to OG-C93

Correct Responses OG-Q1 to OG-Q93

OG-C-1   CORRECT RESPONSE C

The most accurate estimate of fetal gestational age is achieved by the use of ultrasound examination prior to 18 weeks of gestation. The earlier in the pregnancy that the crown–rump length (CRL) can be accurately measured, the more accurate the estimate will be. Ultrasound after 20 weeks of pregnancy becomes unreliable due to the slower rate of overall growth at that time and, like clinical examination, is particularly inaccurate after 30 weeks of gestation.

In the absence of an ultrasound scan assessment before 18 weeks, pelvic examination in the first trimester is the correct response. First trimester clinical assessments of uterine size provide a more accurate assessment of gestation than any of the other options given, despite the fact that pelvic examination in the first trimester can be difficult in obese women, those who do not relax well or those in whom the uterus is retroverted.

OG-C2   CORRECT RESPONSE C

Fetal movements are usually felt by 18 weeks (multigravida) and 20 weeks (primigravida), although some primigravid women do not feel movements until well after 20 weeks of gestation. Uterine size in late pregnancy is dependent upon many factors, including liquor volume, fetal size and maternal dimension. It is a very inaccurate assessment of gestation. Uterine size before 20 weeks is more accurate than that of late pregnancy and the earlier the assessment is performed the more accurate this is in defining gestation.

Engagement of the fetal head classically occurs in primigravida between 36 and 40 weeks of gestation, prior to the onset of labour; but if the position of the presenting part is occipitoposterior, engagement may not occur until labour supervenes. In multigravida, engagement usually does not occur until the time of labour.

In the absence of an ultrasound scan assessment and measurement of crown–rump length before 18 weeks, *first trimester clinical assessments of uterine size provide a more accurate assessment of gestation than any of the other options given*, despite the fact that pelvic examination in the first trimester can be difficult in obese women, those who do not relax well or those in whom the uterus is retroverted.

OG-C3   CORRECT RESPONSE E

Recurrent urinary infections, related to sexual activity, are best treated with antibiotic therapy either immediately before or after each act of intercourse. This will usually prevent further infection occurring. The most common antibiotics used are trimethoprim or nitrofurantoin. Prophylactic coitus-timed therapy is as effective as continuous therapy.

The infective organisms are vaginal organisms which reach the urinary tract due to urethral trauma (during intercourse); commonly bowel organisms are involved. Alteration of coital position rarely reduces the risk of recurrent infection.

Although cystoscopy and/or an intravenous urogram may be performed in some patients as part of the evaluation to exclude an underlying abnormality of the urinary tract, they are rarely necessary in a patient with coitus-related infection and are clearly much less important than prophylactic coitus-timed antibiotic therapy.

OG-C4   CORRECT RESPONSE E

All of the responses regarding pyelonephritis in pregnancy are correct except for immunity. The increased incidence of pyelonephritis in pregnancy is related to the dilatation and slower emptying of the urinary tract tissues, believed to be due to the high progesterone levels of pregnancy. *Pyelonephritis is not related to any change in the immune status.*

OG-C5   CORRECT RESPONSE C

Chlamydia infection in the non-pregnant state is usually treated with the tetracycline drug doxycycline, or **with erythromycin.** During pregnancy, tetracycline therapy is contra-indicated because of the incorporation into fetal bones and teeth. **Thus erythromycin is the drug of choice in pregnancy.**

OG-C6   CORRECT RESPONSE C

Group B streptococcal (GBS) infection in the fetus and infant occurs during birth as an ascending infection from the female genital tract colonised with the GBS organism (15% of the population are colonised but asymptomatic). Although only 1% of babies of colonised mothers develop significant infection, **when systemic infection does occur it is most difficult to treat and commonly results in a neonatal death.** Prophylactic penicillin therapy given in labour to the mother if she is GBS colonised and after delivery to the baby, virtually removes the risk of neonatal GBS infection. The organism is very sensitive to this antibiotic.

Infection can occur in the infant of any colonised woman, irrespective of maturity and normality; however, the risk is increased in patients in premature labour and in those with premature rupture of the membranes.

OG-C7   CORRECT RESPONSE C

The correct response is cytomegalovirus (CMV) infection. This is a common infection prior to the age of 30 years and is often virtually asymptomatic. When it occurs in early/mid pregnancy, it can produce devastating effects on the fetus. Toxoplasmosis is uncommon in Australia, although it is more common in France. Even there, however, CMV exceeds toxoplasmosis in incidence.

Herpes simplex infection of the fetus is very rare, except in women who have a primary herpetic infection during pregnancy and still have active virus shedding at the time of delivery. Contamination from the birth canal, resulting in fetal infection, can then occur.

Syphilitic infection is now extremely rare and routine serology screening and penicillin treatment will prevent any evidence of infection. Rubella infection, although previously common, is now also very rare because of the immunisation programmes involving all young girls and resulting in immunity to such infection prior to pregnancy.

The approximate incidence of non-bacterial fetal infection (intrauterine) is generally accepted to be:

- cytomegalovirus   1/200;
- toxoplasmosis   1/15 000;
- rubella   1/5 000;
- herpes simplex   1/8 000;
- syphilis   very rare.

OG-C8   CORRECT RESPONSE D

Staphylococcus aureus *is the organism of those listed which produces an exotoxin and produces 'toxic shock syndrome' associated with tampon usage.* Escherichia coli produces an endotoxin, not an exotoxin. *Clostridium welchii* produces endotoxins and exotoxins and can cause shock but not the 'toxic shock syndrome'. *Streptococcus agalactine* produces toxins but does not cause 'toxic shock syndrome'. *Mycoplasma hominis* does not produce a toxin at all.

OG-C9   CORRECT RESPONSE D

In general, whenever the abdomen is opened for an apparent clinical diagnosis of acute appendicitis and no other intra-abdominal cause is apparent on inspection, the appendix should be removed even if it is not visibly inflamed macroscopically. There is then no confusion in the future as to what was done and, in a proportion of cases, acute appendicitis can only be diagnosed on histological assessment. Thus the correct answer is *appendicectomy and incision closure.* Removal of a normal appendix is usually possible without major additional morbidity or technical problem.

Although sometimes access to the appendix is not possible until the baby is delivered by caesarean section and the resulting smaller uterus is displaced laterally or anteriorly, the likelihood of having to perform a caesarean section even at or after 36 weeks of gestation is small, as the position of the abdominal incision is changed to take the upward displacement of the appendix into account. In the absence of infection it would be unusual that the normal caecum and appendix could not be delivered into the abdominal wound and appendicectomy performed.

OG-C10   CORRECT RESPONSE D

Although there is immunological suppression in pregnancy, this does not result in suppression of the localising signs of acute appendicitis. The latter are more difficult to define because of displacement of the appendix by the ever-enlarging uterus. Other diseases that may result in confusion with appendicitis are hyperemesis gravidarum, urinary tract infection, ovarian cyst complications (particularly of the right ovary), red degeneration of a uterine fibroid and a small concealed placental abruption behind a right sided posterolateral placenta.

OG-C11   CORRECT RESPONSE E

Although acute appendicitis is often difficult to diagnose in pregnancy and failure to diagnose the condition can have disastrous consequences, the overall incidence is not increased in pregnancy and fatality is very rare. Difficulties in making the diagnosis are contributed to by the fact that the appendix is often behind the pregnant uterus, making the tenderness more difficult to localise. Also, the appendix is displaced upwards by the ever-enlarging uterus, thus confusing the clinician, who is used to expecting the pain to be in the right iliac fossa, as in non-pregnant women. *The site of maximal tenderness is higher, the later in pregnancy the condition occurs.* Other diseases that may result in confusion with appendicitis are hyperemesis gravidarum, urinary tract infection, ovarian cyst complications (particularly of the right ovary), red degeneration of a uterine fibroid and a small concealed placental abruption.

OG-C12   CORRECT RESPONSE C

This question intends to evaluate knowledge about viral hepatitis. All the responses are correct except response C, as *viral hepatitis during pregnancy due to hepatitis virus A, the usual infecting organism, is NOT teratogenic.*

OG-C13   CORRECT RESPONSE D

This woman has hepato–renal failure in late pregnancy, after vomiting of late pregnancy. The condition is life-threatening and urgent delivery is required to resolve the problem. *Pathological examination of the tissues shows acute fatty liver of pregnancy to be the most likely cause of this scenario.* Viral hepatitis would result in disordered liver function tests but not in renal failure. Alcoholic cirrhosis does not present this way.

Pre-eclampsia generally does not have the degree of liver function impairment observed and cholestasis of pregnancy has more elevation of the alkaline phosphatase levels with less hepato–cellular damage and usually no renal impairment. *The MOST likely diagnosis is acute fatty liver of pregnancy.*

OG-C14   CORRECT RESPONSE E

Pre-eclampsia (PE) is most common in primigravid women, with one-third of such women getting PE in the next pregnancy following severe PE in the first. For multigravid women who have never had PE in a previous pregnancy, the following causes must be sought:

- placental abnormality: hydatidiform mole, placental abruption;
- maternal medical disease: diabetes, essential hypertension, other forms of hypertension, chronic renal disease, systemic lupus erythematosus;
- fetal causes: multiple pregnancy, fetal hydrops.

The frequency of PE is not increased by placenta praevia.

OG-C15   CORRECT RESPONSE B

Multiple pregnancy is associated with an increased incidence of all the responses listed except feto–maternal haemorrhage. It should be noted that feto–fetal transfusion is reasonably common in uniovular twin pregnancies. Perinatal morbidity and mortality is 5–10-fold higher, postpartum haemorrhage (predominantly due to uterine atony) is markedly increased, intrauterine growth retardation of one or both twins is increased and umbilical cord prolapse (particularly that of twin 2) is increased.

OG-C16   CORRECT RESPONSE A

The correct response is 7 weeks gestation.

This question aims to determine whether candidates know when Rhesus negative women are likely to become immunised if they receive a feto–maternal transfusion of Rhesus positive fetal cells. *This can occur as early as 7 weeks gestation. Termination of pregnancy performed as early as 7 weeks of gestation has resulted in Rhesus immunisation*, so anti-D should be administered to all pregnant women who are Rhesus negative, at any gestation, when the appropriate indications exist.

OG-C17   CORRECT RESPONSE A

The severity of Rhesus and other blood group sensitisation in pregnancy can be assessed by:

- maternal serum antibody (e.g. anti-D) titres: these are relatively inaccurate unless the titres are very low, or very high and are only of considerable use in the first affected pregnancy. Amniotic fluid antibody titres are of no real additional value.
- previous obstetric performance: the condition tends to get worse with succeeding pregnancies.
- *liquor bilirubin levels at gestations of 26–34 weeks generally provide a good assessment. Before 26 weeks or when the sensitisation is Kell, liquor bilirubin levels are less accurate. Until the introduction of fetal blood sampling, they were the only valuable assessment available.*
- measurement of fetal haemoglobin in blood obtained at fetal blood sampling (20–36 weeks of gestation), in order that fetal blood transfusion can be given if the haemoglobin

is low. The procedure also allows the blood group of the fetus to be determined accurately and a direct Coombs' test to be performed to confirm the immunisation/sensitisation process. The test detects red cell antibodies either on the red cells (direct) or in the serum (indirect) by using rabbit anti-serum against human red cells.

- ultrasound: looking for ascites and/or hydrops, but these are late signs of severe immunisation.

Of the responses given, the best evaluation is achieved by response A.

OG-C18   CORRECT RESPONSE C

Although glycosuria in pregnancy may indicate abnormal glucose tolerance, it is much more likely to be just due to a decreased renal threshold for glucose in a normal pregnancy in a woman who is not diabetic, nor ever likely to develop diabetes. It is found in 25–50% of all pregnant women. Despite the fact that diabetes is only found in 2–3% of those with glycosuria in pregnancy, *a full glucose tolerance test should be performed when glycosuria is found on two or more occasions.*

OG-C19   CORRECT RESPONSE D

Although pancreatitis in the pregnant or non-pregnant woman can be associated with any of the responses given, *in pregnancy, the most common association is cholelithiasis.*

OG-C20   CORRECT RESPONSE C

Intrahepatic cholestasis (hepatosis) is common in the third trimester of pregnancy, usually being evidenced by pruritus of the abdominal wall and without any abdominal pain or tenderness. Liver function tests are often mildly abnormal with the predominant abnormality being an elevation of the alkaline phosphatase levels with minimal change in transaminase or bilirubin levels. Very high bilirubin levels are much more likely to be due to infectious hepatitis, not hepatosis.

The condition is associated with an increased risk of placental dysfunction resulting in perinatal hypoxia and death, although most women with this disorder are able to be safely managed during the pregnancy and safely delivered around term or slightly earlier. Following delivery, the condition rapidly resolves, although *it commonly recurs in subsequent pregnancy and may occur if the woman is given the combined oestrogen/progestogen oral contraceptive pill.* Excessive antacid use does not produce cholestasis.

OG-C21   CORRECT RESPONSE E

Hypertension in pregnancy can be treated with any of the drugs listed except thiazide diuretics. The actual drug used will vary according to the preference of individual physicians, the severity of the hypertension and whether the patient is still in the antenatal period, in labour or has recently delivered.

Diuretics should not be used because they result in a decrease in intravascular fluid volume, which is already often reduced in patients with pregnancy induced hypertension and/or pre-eclampsia. A further reduction in blood volume may well result in a decrease in placental perfusion and, thus, compromise the condition of the fetus.

OG-C22   CORRECT RESPONSE C

Although delivery may be by caesarean section, oxytocin may be used to stimulate labour, ultrasound may be used to assess the type of breech, fetal size and fetal head extension and radiological pelvimetry may be necessary to assess maternal size if vaginal delivery is contemplated, *the initial action must be to do a vaginal examination to exclude cord prolapse, which would require urgent action if diagnosed.* In the absence of cord prolapse, the other options would need consideration.

OG-C23   CORRECT RESPONSE A

This young woman may be unresponsive because of a head injury, severe shock due to blood loss or because of severe hypoxia. *The first assessment must be in regard to respiratory status:* ensuring the airway is adequate and patent and that she is breathing. She will die very quickly unless these are corrected.

The other assessments are followed in appropriate order: assessment of consciousness state, presence of bleeding and shock, assessment of fetal viability.

OG-C24   CORRECT RESPONSE D

The validity of cardiotocograph (CTG) assessment in premature labour has been questioned; however, when it is clearly abnormal, it is generally reflecting the fetal condition as accurately as when used later in pregnancy. In general, baseline tachycardia on its own is of little significance; loss of beat-to-beat variability can be due to hypoxia, sedation, or just fetal sleep. However, persistent late decelerations or severe variable decelerations can indicate severe fetal compromise.

The most ominous of the options given is thus, baseline 150 beats/min, poor variability and late decelerations.

Figures 46–50 show examples of five CTG tracings varying from a normal to a terminal trace. Fetal heart rate (normally 120–160 beats/min) and variability are recorded above, intra-uterine pressure and contractions are shown below.

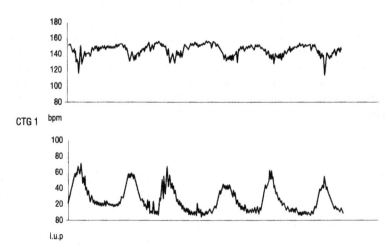

Figure 46 — CTG No. 1

No. 1 is a normal CTG with a normal baseline, good beat-to-beat variability and small early decelerations of no significance, which are probably due to head compression.

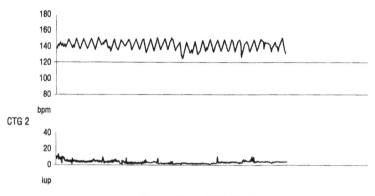

Figure 47 — CTG No. 2

No. 2 is a sinusoidal wave pattern which, although the rate is within the normal range, shows none of the other normal features and is usually indicative of profound anaemia in the fetus. This anaemia can be due to Rhesus or other blood group incompatibility, or a large fetomaternal haemorrhage.

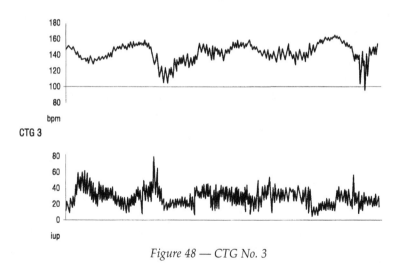

Figure 48 — CTG No. 3

No. 3 shows evidence of late decelerations after every contraction. The lowest point of the deceleration is well after the peak of the contraction and there is a variable time to full recovery.

This particular deceleration pattern, even where the rate still remains within the normal baseline values, is significant of intrauterine hypoxia in up to 25% of patients.

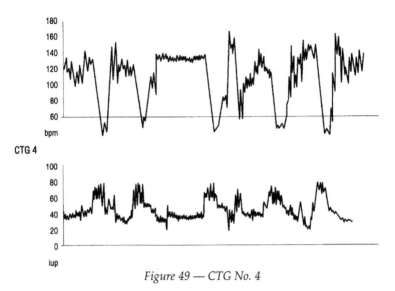

Figure 49 — CTG No. 4

No. 4 shows evidence of moderate and severe variable decelerations which, even on their own and associated with a normal baseline, are indicative of cord compression and may be an indication of fetal hypoxia.

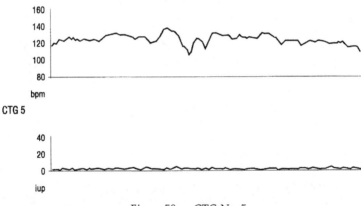

Figure 50 — CTG No. 5

No. 5 is a terminal trace. There is virtually no short-term variability with the heart rate just wandering across the paper. Sometimes it is very difficult to determine whether accelerations and decelerations are actually present when this form of trace is evident.

OG-C25   CORRECT RESPONSE E

The clinical scenario of painless vaginal bleeding of a significant volume, but normal fetal heart rate is most consistent with placenta praevia. In addition to admission, bed rest and the insertion of an intravenous line, the following observations and investigations are necessary:

• full blood examination to check baseline haemoglobin level and platelet count;

- cross-match blood in case further blood loss occurs;
- ultrasound examination to determine the placental site.

If placenta praevia is shown on ultrasound, observe and decide gestation time for delivery, watch subsequent progress for recurrent bleeding, but not after 38 weeks. Also, prepare for caesarean hysterectomy because of increased risk of placenta percreta after previous caesarean section.

If no placenta praevia on ultrasound, do:

- gentle speculum examination to exclude an incidental cause, such as cervical carcinoma;
- coagulation profile;
- close fetal monitoring on CTG and ultrasound assessment of subsequent fetal growth.

Of the responses given, rectal and vaginal examination are clearly contraindicated until ultrasound has shown a placenta praevia is not present, beta sympathomimetic agents are generally contraindicated unless the woman is actually in labour and immediate caesarean section is not required unless further heavy bleeding occurs. *The correct response is observation and further investigation as detailed above.*

OG-C26   CORRECT RESPONSE A

The pain could be due to red degeneration of a fibroid, concealed placental abruption or a complication in an ovarian cyst. The shock is most likely to be due to blood loss. A tense uterus is known to be associated with overdistension (polyhydramnios) or concealed placental abruption.

All clinical diagnoses listed are possible, but the most likely is concealed placental abruption. Spontaneous rupture of the uterus and amniotic fluid embolism are very rare during the antenatal period, a twisted cyst may result in continuous pain but not the signs of shock or a tense uterus, and red degeneration of a fibroid does not produce shock.

OG-C27   CORRECT RESPONSE E

The signs of progress of labour are:

- increased strength, duration and frequency of uterine contractions (if not on a syntocinon drip);
- descent of the fetal head into the pelvis (the head becomes less palpable above pubic symphysis);
- rotation of the fetal head as defined on abdominal palpation (occipito–transverse to occipito–anterior); this is difficult to define;
- increasing cervical dilatation, associated with shortening (effacement) of the cervix.
- rotation of the occiput (occipito–transverse to occipito–anterior) as assessed on pelvic examination;
- descent of the bony fetal head within and through the pelvis;
- above spines → spines → below spines → coccyx → vulva.

Effacement of the cervix may occur before the onset of labour, so *that the best sign of progress is a progressive increase in cervical dilatation.* Descent of the head can occur at any stage of labour, as can rotation of the head defined abdominally or on pelvic examination.

OG-C28   CORRECT RESPONSE A

Pelvic swellings, such as ovarian tumours, uterine fibroids or ectopic kidneys, if large enough and if they are unable to be displaced out of the pelvis, may result in obstruction of labour. A very distended urinary bladder can also prevent descent of the head. However, *a cystocele or rectocele is soft and readily pushed out of the way and thus is the correct response.*

OG-C29   CORRECT RESPONSE A

Shoulder dystocia is most commonly associated with *a large baby*, such as in a diabetic mother, or *when the pregnancy goes well past term.* Even where the baby weighs more than 4500 g, the incidence of shoulder dystocia is less than 30%. In clinical practice it is difficult to predict when this complication will occur unless the clinical examination shows a very large baby or this has been found on ultrasound assessment. There is a high incidence of shoulder dystocia associated with mid-forceps delivery, especially if a malposition (such as an occipito–posterior position) is not present.

Prolonged gestation is the only correct answer of those listed. Hydrocephalus may result in obstructed labour, but this is cephalo–pelvic disproportion; the obstruction which may occur with non-immune hydrops is not at the shoulder level but at the lower chest–abdominal level. Toxoplasmosis and intrauterine growth retardation result in smaller babies with less risk of obstruction and of shoulder dystocia.

OG-C30   CORRECT RESPONSE E

Elective low forceps delivery is usually uncomplicated with no adverse effects being seen in the baby. An increased incidence of vaginal tears occurs and the need for an episiotomy is greater. As a change in the incidence of maternal injury was not included in the responses provided, *none of the above responses is the correct answer.*

OG-C31   CORRECT RESPONSE E

The pudendal nerve arises from sacral segments 2, 3 and 4 of the spinal cord before passing laterally, over the ischial spines and into the ischio–rectal fossa and perineum. It contributes motor fibres to anal and perineal muscles and supplies sensory fibres to the labia and lower vagina. When used in obstetric practice, the pudendal block is usually achieved using 5–10 mL local anaesthetic injected just posterior to the ischial spine, with the needle being guided to that site transvaginally or through the perineum midway between the posterior fourchette and the ischial tuberosity.

OG-C32   CORRECT RESPONSE C

Epidural anaesthesia is generally contraindicated in the following circumstances:

- previous surgery to the vertebrae in the area concerned: the epidural can, however, be placed above or below such surgically attacked vertebrae;.
- skin infection in the region;
- significant maternal haemorrhage, because it may make the extent of haemorrhage more difficult to assess;
- where a coagulation/bleeding disorder has been diagnosed *(such as significant thrombocytopenia)* and the risk of epidural haemorrhage, possibly causing spinal cord compression, would be increased. *A platelet level less than 40×10^9/L (40 000 /mm³) puts the patient at significant risk;*
- some cardiac conditions, such as primary pulmonary hypertension, when the ability to

increase cardiac output to cope with the vasodilatation produced by the epidural, is markedly compromised; this is not usually the case with rheumatic heart disease such as mitral stenosis;

- where severe fetal distress has been diagnosed and it would be much faster to give a general anaesthetic to expedite immediate delivery.

Thrombocytopenia is the correct response. Hypertension is not in itself a contraindication, nor is previous caesarean delivery or anaemia.

OG-C33   CORRECT RESPONSE D

Postpartum haemorrhage is usually due to a failure of uterine contraction (uterine atony) or a laceration within the genital tract (perineal, vaginal, cervical or uterine). Overall, uterine atony is more common than a laceration as a cause.

Of the causes listed in the responses, *postpartum haemorrhage is least likely in an 8 h labour in a 21-year-old G1 P0 with mild pre-eclampsia.* The first option is likely to result in either uterine atony or genital trauma; the second and fifth options are associated with uterine atony; and the precipitate labour in option three is likely to result in a genital laceration.

OG-C34   CORRECT RESPONSE D

When bleeding occurs in pregnancy, the patient attempts to cope with this by vasoconstriction of peripheral beds, including the kidney. If this does not result in the restoration of circulating blood volume to normal, the pulse rate is increased. Ultimately hypotension results if the loss continues.

It is therefore possible to have a normal pulse rate, blood pressure and pulse pressure despite significant blood loss; however, the urine output declines if the blood volume is reduced. Overbreathing (air hunger) is a very late sign of hypovolaemia. *Urine output is the best sign for monitoring adequacy of blood volume replacement.*

OG-C35   CORRECT RESPONSE D

Postpartum haemorrhage is usually due to a failure of uterine contraction (uterine atony) or a laceration within the genital tract (perineal, vaginal, cervical or uterine).

Of the situations listed, two are likely to be associated with uterine atony (overdistension of the uterus and prolonged labour) and two are likely to be associated with lacerations (precipitate labour and delivery of an elderly grand-multigravida). *The only response NOT predisposing to postpartum haemorrhage is delivery of a growth-retarded infant.*

OG-C36   CORRECT RESPONSE E

The tests required for someone having a life-threatening postpartum haemorrhage usually include full blood examination, coagulation profile (platelet count, fibrinogen level, activated partial thromboplastin time (APTT) and prothrombin time (PT)) and the assessment of D-dimers or fibrin degradation products (FDP).

The assessment of haemoglobin level is useful in providing a basal haemoglobin level, but it is of little use in assessing the degree of loss or the need for blood transfusion unless the haemoglobin is low. The coagulation profile assessment, which takes 30–60 min to perform, clearly indicates the severity of any coagulopathy and what form of treatment is likely to be most appropriate. *Observation of clotting and estimation of the whole blood clotting time can be done by the bedside and provides very rapid information on whether the blood is clotting or not.* Where the blood does not clot or the time to clot is prolonged (> 8 min) the coagulation profile and fibrinolysis assessment are obviously next required. Thus, although each of the responses gives very useful information, the *response giving the most useful information in the shortest time is bedside observation of clotting and clotting time.*

OG-C37 — CORRECT RESPONSE C

Uterine inversion is a potentially lethal complication of pregnancy resulting in postpartum haemorrhage and shock, but where **the shock (believed to be due at least in part to autonomic stimulation consequent upon drawing the ovaries and their nerve supply into the inversion funnel) is out of proportion to the extent of blood loss.** Severe pain is unusual, as is the finding of a 'dimple' above the pubic symphysis or discovery of the uterine fundus at the introitus, in the absence of severe shock and bleeding.

OG-C38 — CORRECT RESPONSE A

Uterine inversion is an obstetric emergency as failure to correct it quickly may result in a maternal death from shock and haemorrhage. Where it is discovered immediately after it has occurred, it should be rapidly corrected manually before a tonic uterine contraction occurs. Under these circumstances the shock and bleeding cease. The correct answer is *to attempt immediate replacement of the uterus.* If the placenta is still attached to the fundus, it should not be removed until the inversion has been corrected or bleeding from the placental site is likely.

Where the uterus is firmly contracted it is not possible to manually replace the inversion except under anaesthesia unless the hydrostatic method is used. Both the manual and hydrostatic techniques take some time to be effective, during which time blood transfusion and circulatory support is usually required and a uterine relaxant may be necessary.

OG-C39 — CORRECT RESPONSE E

Maternal mortality in Australia occurs in approximately one in 10 000 pregnancies. The most common causes are severe pre-eclampsia or eclampsia, pulmonary thrombo-embolism, postpartum haemorrhage and anaesthetic accidents. **The condition with the highest maternal mortality complication rate is undoubtedly primary pulmonary hypertension.** Approximately 50% of such afflicted women do not survive pregnancy and the puerperium despite intensive care of the cardiopulmonary condition during and following the pregnancy.

The other maternal disorders mentioned require more specialised care in pregnancy but rarely result in a maternal death.

OG-C40 — CORRECT RESPONSE B

The only correct answer is vascular and lymphatic engorgement of the breasts, which is a normal characteristic of the puerperium. Colostrum secretion lasts for only 2–3 days until milk production commences. Ovulation rarely occurs within 2 weeks of delivery even in women who are not breast feeding; if placed on bromocriptine early ovulation may occur but still is rare within 2 weeks of delivery. The puerperium is associated with a transient leucocytosis, not leucopenia. The basal layer of the endometrium is not shed into the lochia; it is required to allow subsequent development of the endometrium during the follicular phase of the next cycle.

OG-C41   CORRECT RESPONSE D

Coagulase-positive Staphylococcus aureus *is the most common organism causing postpartum mastitis.* It is usually not sensitive to penicillin or amoxycillin, but is sensitive to flucloxacillin or erythromycin.

OG-C42   CORRECT RESPONSE D

Psychotic depression associated with pregnancy is most commonly seen during the puerperium when the high hormone levels of pregnancy have fallen precipitously.

OG-C43   CORRECT RESPONSE B

Rapid evaluation of the new-born infant at 1 min of age can be provided by the Apgar score. This grades 5 components from 0 to 2 (heart rate, respiratory effort, colour, muscle tone and reflex irritability), with a maximum (normal) score of 10.

Although a very low Apgar score at 1 and 5 min may be associated with significant hypoxia and may be a sign of perinatal asphyxia (with the possible development of seizures and neurological impairment), there are many other causes and adequate resuscitation will usually prevent long-term problems from occurring. *Clearly the initial treatment must be resuscitation ensuring an adequate airway, oxygenation and circulation.*

OG-C44   CORRECT RESPONSE A

This baby requires

- aspiration to ensure the airway is patent;
- additional oxygen by face mask or intubation;
- narcotic antagonist in view of recent administration of pethidine; to mother. *Naloxone is the best agent to use.* Nalorphine tends to reverse the narcotic, but has a sedative effect as well. Theophylline and caffeine are used for apnoea of prematurity, not narcotic suppression. Amphetamine is not used for this purpose.

OG-C45   CORRECT RESPONSE A

Growth-retarded infants show a reduction in size of most parts of their body; *however, the part least affected is the brain.* This information is of value in determining the presence of intrauterine growth retardation and identifying its cause. The biparietal head diameter (BPD) is the last fetal dimension as determined ultrasonically to be affected in asymmetric growth-retarded fetuses, such as those due to placental dysfunction. However, BPD it may be reduced along with other dimensions in the less common symmetric growth-retarded fetus such as that with intrauterine infection or abnormalities.

OG-C46   CORRECT RESPONSE B

The normal cord vessel pattern is two arteries and one vein. A two-vessel cord is the most likely cord abnormality associated with fetal malformation. Unless one of these was an artery and the other a vein, the fetus would not survive the first trimester of pregnancy. *Thus response B is correct: one artery and one vein.*

OG-C47   CORRECT RESPONSE C

The risk of a neural tube defect in the general population is probably around 1/1000, although the use of prophylactic folic acid therapy has reduced this incidence considerably. *Having had one neural tube defect, however, the incidence of a second (prior to the almost routine use of folic acid supplementation prior to and during pregnancy) was 2–5%.*

OG-C48   CORRECT RESPONSE C

The following drugs, when given in pregnancy have adverse effects on the fetus:

- diethylstilboestrol produces reproductive tract abnormalities in both male and female fetuses and an increased risk of clear cell carcinoma of the vagina in the female children produced;

- phenytoin can result in hydantoin syndrome (facial, nail and other abnormalities);

- tetracycline produces abnormalities due to incorporation into bones and teeth;

- danazol results in androgenisation of the female fetus.

Nalidixic acid is not considered to be teratogenic and can be used to treat urinary infections in pregnancy without adverse fetal effects.

OG-C49   CORRECT RESPONSE B

The following circulatory changes occur in the newborn baby after delivery:

- closure of umbilical vein and ductus venosus;

- opening up of the lungs to give massively increased pulmonary artery blood flow;

- *increased venous return from lungs results in functional closure of the atrial septal defect flap from the left atrial side, as the foramen ovale is a flap valve;*

- closure of the ductus arteriosus due to locally produced prostaglandins.

OG-C50   CORRECT RESPONSE A

The first response is correct as the spontaneous abortion rate increases progressively with age over 35 years.

Most abortions occur between 6–10 weeks of gestation, 60% are due to chromosome abnormalities (mostly trisomies) and diethylstilboestrol does increase the abortion rate due to an increased incidence of uterine abnormalities. Because of the progressive abortion of many pregnancies bearing chromosomally abnormal fetuses, the chromosome abnormalities detected in liveborn infants are different from that of spontaneous abortions (i.e. the worst ones are lost as abortions with the 'less severe' being born alive).

OG-C51   CORRECT RESPONSE C

It is important to be able to define the types of abortion as the management and treatment may be different. It should be noted that:

- not all abortions have had vaginal bleeding (e.g. missed abortion);

- uterine cramping is usually, but not invariably, associated with an inevitable abortion;

- the cervix is closed in threatened abortion, missed abortion and previous complete abortion, but open in inevitable abortion, incomplete abortion and recent complete abortion;

- products of conception may be found in the cervix in inevitable and incomplete abortion;

- the uterine size is as expected for gestation in threatened abortion, but smaller than expected in missed abortion, incomplete abortion and complete abortion;

- temperature above 37.8°C indicates probable septic abortion.

The most correct response in regard to the characteristics of inevitable abortion is vaginal bleeding with cramping and an open cervix.

OG-C52 **CORRECT RESPONSE B**

Cervical incompetence can present as follows:

- painless cervical dilatation;
- increased cervical mucous discharge associated with cervical dilatation;
- premature rupture of the membranes;
- second trimester miscarriage after a virtually painless labour;
- premature labour and/or delivery.

The correct answer is membrane rupture. Contractions are rare, the babies are often born alive and are usually of normal size, there is little if any vaginal bleeding (compared with other causes of miscarriage) and the discharge is not purulent unless there has been a prolonged time interval of significant cervical dilatation resulting in the development of chorioamnionitis.

OG-C53 **CORRECT RESPONSE B**

Amniocentesis is most commonly performed in the second trimester of pregnancy for genetic counselling purposes. The other alternative would be to do a chorion–villus biopsy (CVB) at approximately 10 weeks of pregnancy.

The chance of a miscarriage occurring after these procedures is generally agreed to be one in 200 for amniocentesis and 1 in 100 for CVB. The importance of this question is that clinicians should be able to balance the risk of the procedure against the risk of the disease they are attempting to diagnose.

OG-C54 **CORRECT RESPONSE B**

A 14-year-old girl with an imperforate hymen will have primary amenorrhoea, will probably have cyclical and recurrent lower abdominal pain, is likely to have a protruding mass evident in the hymenal region, will not have a normal appearing vagina and may develop a suprapubic abdominal mass and even acute urinary retention if the obstruction is not relieved and the haematocolpos becomes big enough. *All of the responses are, therefore, likely except for cyclic chills and fever, which are not a feature.*

OG-C55 **CORRECT RESPONSE A**

Danazol, a progestogen derived from testosterone, has predominantly androgenic side effects of weight gain, fluid retention, acne and voice change but it can certainly androgenise a female uterus if given during pregnancy. It has been shown to be effective in the treatment of endometriosis and menorrhagia and has been used with considerable success in patients with breast pain and discomfort due to *fibrocystic disease of the breast. It relieves this condition rather than exacerbating it.*

OG-C56 **CORRECT RESPONSE E**

In anorexia nervosa, the FSH levels are low or low–normal, but such levels are seen in patients with other causes for their secondary amenorrhoea apart from that associated with anorexia nervosa. *As such, FSH levels are not pathognomonic for anorexia nervosa.* Each of the other statements regarding anorexia nervosa is correct.

OG-C57   CORRECT RESPONSE E

Isotretinoin is a most effective agent for the long-term control of severe adolescent acne. It is generally only given for 6 months but often results in prolonged suppression of the process. If given during pregnancy, it is teratogenic. *It is therefore essential to exclude pregnancy before commencing therapy.* Disorders of other body systems are rare and other biochemical screening tests prior to commencement of therapy are unnecessary.

OG-C58   CORRECT RESPONSE D

Excitement during sexual activity is not affected by the menopause, fear of pregnancy, previous hysterectomy or the fact that the children have all left home (the empty nest syndrome). Each of these may reduce the desire for sex but do not affect the excitement phase during sexual activity.

Marital discord is likely to reduce both desire and performance and is the correct response.

OG-C59   CORRECT RESPONSE D

Intermenstrual bleeding or spotting is a common symptom in women during the first few months of treatment with an oral contraceptive pill. It usually resolves spontaneously if the pill is continued to be taken in the normal way. Where it does not resolve spontaneously after 3 months of therapy, the prescription of a pill with a higher oestrogen dosage, in this instance a constant dose 50 µg ethinyl oestradiol pill, such as Microgynon 50®, will usually eradicate this symptom.

The correct answer is, therefore, to continue medication and review in 2 months.

OG-C60   CORRECT RESPONSE D

The benefits of taking the combined oestrogen/progestogen oral contraceptive pill are:

- excellent contraception;
- reduced dysmenorrhoea;
- reduced iron-deficiency anaemia;
- reduced menstrual loss;
- reduced benign breast disease;
- reduced functional ovarian cysts;
- reduced ovarian and endometrial cancer;
- reduced pelvic inflammatory disease.

The cervical carcinoma incidence is not decreased. It appears to be slightly increased, but this is probably due to the increased sexual activity and not the ingestion of the contraceptive pill.

OG-C61   CORRECT RESPONSE C

The Pearl Index is used to assess the contraceptive failure rate. *It represents the number of pregnancies in 100 women using the particular contraceptive method for 1 year (i.e. pregnancies per 100 women years).*

OG-C62   CORRECT RESPONSE A

Tubal sterilisation is a common and very safe procedure in developed countries, with an expected peri-operative mortality of < 1:10 000. Tubal sterilisation is now usually performed laparoscopically, unless performed at the time of caesarean section or in the postpartum period when an open tubal ligation or excision is more commonly performed. When performed laparoscopically, the causes of death may be an intra-operative surgical mishap, such as major blood vessel or bowel trauma or damage diathermy burn. The other operative complication is that due to an anaesthetic complication. Sepsis and myocardial infarction are extremely rare life-threatening complications of sterilisation, as is tubal haemorrhage.

Although the risk of pulmonary embolism is increased after an open sterilisation procedure, especially when performed during the puerperium, there are now so few of these done that *the most common cause of death of those listed is anaesthesia*.

OG-C63   CORRECT RESPONSE D

The only cause of primary amenorrhoea among those listed is Turner Syndrome (45,XO). All of the other diagnoses listed usually cause secondary amenorrhoea, having had their menarche at the appropriate time.

Turner syndrome of ovarian dysgenesis is characterised by an outwardly female phenotype, incomplete and infertile gonads, short stature, webbed neck, wide carrying angle, congenital heart defects and the XO karotype.

OG-C64   CORRECT RESPONSE C

This woman has premature ovarian failure as indicated by the marked elevation of her FSH and LH levels. The amenorrhoea and 'hot flush' symptomatology are also consistent with this diagnosis. The fact that the prolactin level is normal is indicative of the fact that the double-floor of the sella turcica, as determined by polytomography, is probably just a normal anatomic variant.

Gonadotrophin-producing pituitary tumours are extremely rare, neurofibromatosis would not result in elevated FSH and LH levels, a non-hormone-producing pituitary tumour usually causes significant enlargement of the pituitary fossa and a craniopharyngioma would have suprasellar calcification on tomography, usually occurs at a much earlier age and would be associated with low FSH and LH levels.

OG-C65   CORRECT RESPONSE C

Dysmenorrhoea is common, often commencing approximately 2 years after the menarche when ovulatory cycles commence and continuing at least until the early 20s. It is less common after completion of a pregnancy or after cervical dilation, is commonly relieved considerably with anti-prostaglandin preparations, the oral contraceptive pill and sometimes placebo therapy, but may be due to organic causes such as a submucous fibroid, endometriosis, adenomyosis or pelvic inflammatory disease and necessitate specific treatment of these conditions. *Secondary dysmenorrhoea is not seen secondary to the onset of regular ovulation (this is primary dysmenorrhoea with the pain usually commencing prior to menses and persisting for the first 1–2 days of the period), but is secondary to one of the organic causes listed and often persists throughout the menses.*

OG-C66   CORRECT RESPONSE A

Galactorrhoea in a multigravid woman with normal prolactin levels and normal menstrual cycles is common and rarely requires therapy or further investigation; bromocriptine therapy is occasionally indicated, but only if the galactorrhoea is particularly profuse and troublesome.

Reassurance is the most appropriate management.

OG-C67 CORRECT RESPONSE A

This question does not attempt to pinpoint the timing of ovulation but whether ovulation has occurred. Responses C, D and E are used to detect the time of ovulation, although they do not confirm that ovulation did actually occur. Both a biphasic temperature chart and an elevated plasma progesterone do confirm ovulation; *however, the plasma progesterone measurement is the more accurate assessment.*

OG-C68 CORRECT RESPONSE B

Regular periods with some dysmenorrhoea is the best predictor of ovulation of those listed.

Ovulatory menstrual cycles are usually regular, have premenstrual abdominal and breast distension and sometimes acne, have increased mid-cycle mucus production and finally *dysmenorrhoea.* Sometimes mid-cycle bleeding, at the time of the fall in oestrogen levels, is also observed. None of these symptoms is absolutely indicative that the patient is ovulating nor are all symptoms present in all ovulating women.

OG-C69 CORRECT RESPONSE B

Although endometrial biopsy and basal body temperature assessment provide evidence of ovulation having occurred, they do not pinpoint the exact time when it occurred. Oestrogen estimations are of some value in pinpointing ovulation, as the pre-ovulatory oestrogen peak occurs approximately 36–48 h prior to ovulation, and the cervical mucus changes do reflect the oestrogen excretion and are maximal immediately prior to ovulation. Changes in oestrogen and mucus can occur without ovulation actually occurring and are an inaccurate method of pinpointing the time of ovulation, even when it does occur.

The mid-cycle LH surge occurs 12–36 h prior to ovulation, with a peak value being observed at approximately 24 h prior to ovulation. Of the options given, this is clearly the most exact method available.

OG-C70 CORRECT RESPONSE C

The mucus changes described, 14 days after the start of the last normal menstrual period, are most likely an indication of adequate oestrogen production immediately prior to ovulation. It is possible, however, that ovulation will not occur as the mucus is produced due to the effect of the oestrogen being produced, not the process of ovulation. In fact, at the time of ovulation, when the progesterone levels are already rising, the mucus becomes thick, cellular, non-elastic and reduced in amount. It is therefore not possible, on mucus assessment alone, to be certain ovulation will occur, that it would be normal, that a postcoital test would be normal (it could be abnormal for any number of reasons) or to evaluate the presence or absence of progesterone receptor. *The only correct answer is that she is producing an effective amount of oestrogen.*

OG-C71 CORRECT RESPONSE D

Hyperprolactinaemia is due to a deficiency in the release of hypothalamic dopamine (in approximately 70% of women), a pituitary or suprapituitary adenoma or tumour (in 25% of women), primary hypothyroidism (in 1% of women) and a variety of other uncommon causes in the remaining 4%.

Phenothiazines, polycystic ovaries and stress all exert their hyperprolactinaemic effect via hypothalamic dopamine production.

The only cause listed in the responses that does not produce hyperprolactinaemia is chronic pelvic inflammatory disease.

OG-C72   CORRECT RESPONSE E

Endometriosis is a condition seen commonly during the reproductive years, often associated with infertility, can sometimes be diagnosed because it can be seen at the vaginal vault or uterosacral nodules, can be felt on pelvic examination and almost never undergoes malignant change. *The most common sites of endometriosis are the ovaries, uterosacral ligaments and the pelvic peritoneum, particularly in the region of the Pouch of Douglas. The Fallopian tube is not the most common site.*

OG-C73   CORRECT RESPONSE C

Clomiphene citrate, used for ovulation induction, stimulates the pituitary gland to produce more FSH and LH and often results in ovulation or superovulation. Thus, it may produce:

- excessive oestrogen levels causing fluid retention and breast enlargement;
- hot flushes (vasomotor symptoms);
- development of more than one follicle and release of more than one ovum, causing multiple pregnancy (5–10% risk);
- inadequate ovulation; particularly corpus luteum dysfunction;
- enlarged ovaries with multiple cysts, pain and increased risk of torsion;
- hyperstimulation syndrome with ascites, hypovolaemia, haemo-concentration.
- The correct answer is *birth defects*, as *there is no evidence that clomiphene citrate increases the incidence of congenital malformations* over and above the incidence seen in anovulatory, infertile women not treated with clomiphene.

OG-C74   CORRECT RESPONSE E

Dyspareunia can be due to a number of causes including fear of pain (vaginismus), endometriosis, vulval or vaginal infection (particularly thrush and herpetic infection), vaginal introital narrowing such as seen with lichen sclerosis et atrophicus, or vaginal dryness due to oestrogen deficiency. *In a patient at the age of 48 years, the most likely cause is perimenopausal oestrogen deficiency.* Ovarian tumours, fibroids and uterine prolapse rarely result in dyspareunia.

OG-C75   CORRECT RESPONSE D

It is now known that the *menopause is genetically determined,* being unrelated to the age at menarche, occurring at the same age in women who have not ovulated regularly because of repeated pregnancies or constantly having their ovulation suppressed by the oral contraceptive pill and is not changing in developed countries despite improvement in nutrition and life style. Smoking does cause an earlier menopause, however, as does an abnormal chromosome state (XXX females), ovarian surgery or radiotherapy, some cytotoxic agents and some autoimmune processes.

OG-C76   CORRECT RESPONSE B

The only absolute contraindication for hormone-replacement therapy (HRT) of those listed is severe liver disease.

Cholelithiasis and pancreatitis are relative contraindications and HRT is certainly indicated in patients who have disordered lipoproteins or hypertension in an attempt to reduce their increased incidence of cardiovascular disease.

OG-C77 CORRECT RESPONSE E

Hot flushes are more common in women having a premature menopause, especially when surgically induced and in women with less endogenous oestrogen production (thin women). Responses A–D are, therefore, all associated with more hot flushes. *Low gonadotrophin-releasing hormone (GnRH) production is consistent with more endogenous oestrogen production and with less hot flushes.*

OG-C78 CORRECT RESPONSE C

The amount of calcium required for normal calcium balance after the menopause is approximately 1 g/day.

OG-C79 CORRECT RESPONSE A

Calcium supplementation, in postmenopausal women, is poorly absorbed and thus relatively ineffective in preventing bone loss even when administered with vitamin D, unless hormone replacement therapy with oestrogen *with or without* progestogen in adequate dosage is also given. Under such circumstances, the dose of calcium required is 1000–2000 mg/day.

OG-C80 CORRECT RESPONSE B

Genital chlamydial infection is sexually transmitted, *is commonly asymptomatic* until severe salpingitis or urethritis occurs and is a common cause of infertility due to tubal obstruction.

OG-C81 CORRECT RESPONSE D

The likely causes of the discharge observed are trichomonal vaginitis or bacterial vaginosis (gardnerella infection). *To perform smears of the vaginal discharge (KOH and wet smear) is correct, will enable the correct diagnosis to be made and will allow effective therapy to be commenced.* In general, therapy should not be commenced before the smears or swab are taken to make the correct diagnosis. Clotrimazole is an effective antithrush medication, but is not effective against trichomonas or gardnerella; the symptoms and signs are not those of gonococcal or chlamydial infection and syphilis infection is rarely associated with either trichomonal or gardnerella infection.

OG-C82 CORRECT RESPONSE E

Although all the organisms listed in the responses can result in severe shock if the infection is generalised and severe, by far *the most common micro-organism causing septic shock in obstetrics and gynaecology is* Escherichia coli.

OG-C83 CORRECT RESPONSE C

Adenomyosis is a common condition in women, but certainly not all women and is most often found *between the ages of 35 and 50 (fourth and fifth decades of life)*. It is usually associated with dysmenorrhoea and often dyspareunia, results in a slightly enlarged and tender firm uterus, but can only be definitively diagnosed by histologic examination of a biopsied or removed uterine specimen. Curettage does not usually allow this diagnosis to be made, although a core biopsy of the myometrium laparoscopically or via the uterine cavity would produce a specimen suitable for histological examination. Although endometriosis is more common in nulliparous women, this is not the case for adenomyosis, which is due to invasion of the muscle layer by the basal endometrium of the uterine cavity.

■   Because the adenomyotic glands respond poorly to hormonal suppression, hysterectomy has been the treatment of choice if the symptoms warrant treatment.

OG-C84 — CORRECT RESPONSE A

The clinical diagnosis is that of uterine fibroids, with mild uterine enlargement and menorrhagia. The menorrhagia may be due to an endometrial polyp, some other endometrial pathology, or a submucous fibroid, or may be due to the intramural fibroids felt clinically. Prior to making a decision regarding the use of surgical removal of a fibroid or the uterus, progestogen therapy for apparent dysfunctional bleeding or antiprostaglandin drugs to reduce menstrual loss, a *uterine curettage (± hysteroscopy) is required*. This may be both diagnostic and therapeutic and allows a subsequent rational decision to be made regarding the woman's care.

OG-C85 — CORRECT RESPONSE B

Menorrhagia in a 45-year-old woman is likely to be due to a disorder of ovulation, most likely that of anovulatory cycles, especially as the cycles have become irregular. Endometrial carcinoma is an uncommon cause of menorrhagia but usually causes postmenopausal bleeding. Fibroids, endometrial polyps and adenomyosis can certainly cause menorrhagia, although the cycles are usually regular and a dramatic change from previously normal cycles 6 months previously would be unusual.

OG-C86 — CORRECT RESPONSE E

A 5 cm unilocular ovarian cyst in a 25-year-old asymptomatic woman *is most likely to be a follicular cyst requiring observation but no active treatment.* If, in 6 weeks time, the cyst size is unchanged, the CA125 levels should be measured (likely to be elevated in serous cysts and endometriosis), a trial of hypothalamic/pituitary suppressive therapy with a combined oral contraceptive pill considered or laparoscopic assessment and/or removal of the cyst arranged.

OG-C87 — CORRECT RESPONSE E

Any ovarian enlargement initially detected in a woman after the menopause must be considered malignant until proven otherwise and *requires early surgical exploration and probable oophorectomy.*

OG-C88 — CORRECT RESPONSE E

A large right adnexal mass developing in a 60-year-old postmenopausal woman, *must be considered due to an ovarian malignancy until proven otherwise. This is not only the diagnosis to be excluded, but also the most likely diagnosis.* Endometrial carcinoma usually presents with postmenopausal bleeding but usually does not have any adnexal mass, although the uterus itself may be enlarged. Follicular cysts are very rare after the menopause, a benign ovarian tumour is less common at this age and a degenerating fibroid would be unusual, especially as the pelvic examination was normal 3 years previously.

OG-C89 — CORRECT RESPONSE C

The most common invasive malignancy found in the vagina is *extension of squamous carcinoma spread from the cervix.*

The other malignancies are found in the following decreasing order of frequency.

- metastatic adenocarcinoma from the endometrium;
- primary invasive squamous cell carcinoma of the vagina;

- clear cell adenocarcinoma (following diethylstilboestrol therapy);
- carcinoma of the urethra, Bartholin gland, or Gartner duct.

Carcinoma *in situ* is not an invasive malignancy, although it can progress to invasive malignancy.

OG-C90   CORRECT RESPONSE D

When narcotics are used for pain relief in women with advanced gynaecological malignancies, addiction may occur, but this is not a troublesome problem. Nausea is not usually a problem associated with long-term narcotic use, although it is often seen associated with short-term use in the postoperative period. Drowsiness and respiratory depression can be seen when very high doses of narcotics are used, but such doses are not usually given except in the terminal phase of the disease. It should also be noted that the doses given to many patients have to be increased markedly with time, with relatively little sedative or respiratory depressive effects being observed compared with those that would be expected in a non-addicted individual. *Constipation is by far the most common troublesome side effect.*

OG-C91   CORRECT RESPONSE C

The vulval swelling described is in the classical position of the left Bartholin duct and gland. *The spherical and non-tender nature of the swelling make it almost certainly a non-infected Bartholin cyst* rather than a Bartholin abscess, either of which would be best treated by marsupialisation.

An adenoma or tumour of the Bartholin gland is extremely rare, vulval carcinoma is not usually spherical and unchanging in size over some months. Sebaceous cysts are seen in the labia majora itself rather than in the position described and a Gartner duct cyst is within the vagina, being in the suburethral position low in the vagina and becoming more lateral the higher in the vagina it occurs.

OG-C92   CORRECT RESPONSE B

Urinary tract infection is the most common postoperative complication following major gynaecological surgery.

The frequency (in descending order) of the other postoperative complications listed is:
- vaginal vault haematoma;
- pneumonia;
- deep venous thrombosis;
- hydronephrosis due to ureteric damage or obstruction.

OG-C93   CORRECT RESPONSE D

Urinary incontinence in a 50-year-old woman is most likely to be either stress or urge incontinence. Incontinence due to the presence of a fistula would only be seen with an extensive malignancy of the cervix or as a complication following gynaecological surgery.

It is important to exclude a urinary tract infection and define the exact cause of the incontinence by urodynamic studies before embarking on surgical treatment of any associated prolapse or medical therapy of possible urge incontinence.

SUMMARY OF CORRECT RESPONSES

CATEGORY & QUESTION NO.	CORRECT RESPONSE	CATEGORY & QUESTION NO.	CORRECT RESPONSE	CATEGORY & QUESTION NO.	CORRECT RESPONSE
OG-Q 1	C	OG-Q 32	C	OG-Q 63	D
OG-Q 2	C	OG-Q 33	D	OG-Q 64	C
OG-Q 3	E	OG-Q 34	D	OG-Q 65	C
OG-Q 4	E	OG-Q 35	D	OG-Q 66	A
OG-Q 5	C	OG-Q 36	E	OG-Q 67	A
OG-Q 6	C	OG-Q 37	C	OG-Q 68	B
OG-Q 7	C	OG-Q 38	A	OG-Q 69	B
OG-Q 8	D	OG-Q 39	E	OG-Q 70	C
OG-Q 9	D	OG-Q 40	B	OG-Q 71	D
OG-Q 10	D	OG-Q 41	D	OG-Q 72	E
OG-Q 11	E	OG-Q 42	D	OG-Q 73	C
OG-Q 12	C	OG-Q 43	B	OG-Q 74	E
OG-Q 13	D	OG-Q 44	A	OG-Q 75	D
OG-Q 14	E	OG-Q 45	A	OG-Q 76	B
OG-Q 15	B	OG-Q 46	B	OG-Q 77	E
OG-Q 16	A	OG-Q 47	C	OG-Q 78	C
OG-Q 17	A	OG-Q 48	C	OG-Q 79	A
OG-Q 18	C	OG-Q 49	B	OG-Q 80	B
OG-Q 19	D	OG-Q 50	A	OG-Q 81	D
OG-Q 20	C	OG-Q 51	C	OG-Q 82	E
OG-Q 21	E	OG-Q 52	B	OG-Q 83	C
OG-Q 22	C	OG-Q 53	B	OG-Q 84	A
OG-Q 23	A	OG-Q 54	B	OG-Q 85	B
OG-Q 24	D	OG-Q 55	A	OG-Q 86	E
OG-Q 25	E	OG-Q 56	E	OG-Q 87	E
OG-Q 26	A	OG-Q 57	E	OG-Q 88	E
OG-Q 27	E	OG-Q 58	D	OG-Q 89	C
OG-Q 28	A	OG-Q 59	D	OG-Q 90	D
OG-Q 29	A	OG-Q 60	D	OG-Q 91	C
OG-Q 30	E	OG-Q 61	C	OG-Q 92	B
OG-Q 31	E	OG-Q 62	A	OG-Q 93	D

Psychiatry
Commentaries
and Summary of Correct Responses
TYPE
A

Commentaries PS-C1 to PS-C51

Correct Responses PS-Q1 to PS-Q51

PS-C1 CORRECT RESPONSE D

The correct answer to this question is gamma-aminobutyric acid (GABA*).*

The pharmacological actions of the benzodiazepines require the presence of GABA, an inhibitory amino acid neurotransmitter. Benzodiazepines have specific receptor sites which are closely associated with GABA receptors on presynaptic neuronal sites. These receptor sites are scattered throughout the central nervous system, being densest in the cortex but also present in the limbic system and the spinal cord. Benzodiazepines enhance the inhibitory action of GABA on its receptors which accounts for their effectiveness as anticonvulsant, muscle relaxant, anxiolytic and sedative agents.

Any effects of benzodiazepines on other neurotransmitters are only indirect.

PS-C2 CORRECT RESPONSE C

The correct answer to this question is that because the antipsychotic drug *chlorpromazine can cause parkinsonism,* this provides indirect evidence in support of the dopamine hypothesis of schizophrenia.

The dopamine hypothesis of schizophrenia attributes the positive features of the condition to overactivity of dopaminergic pathways, specifically the mesolimbic and mesocortical pathways to the temporolimbic and frontal cortex. There is good correlation between the affinity with which typical antipsychotic medications, for example haloperidol and chlorpromazine, bind to certain dopamine receptors (the D_2 receptors) and the drugs' effectiveness at relieving the positive symptoms of schizophrenia.

The extrapyramidal symptoms that frequently accompany antipsychotic drug therapy are caused by receptor blockade in the nigrostriatal dopaminergic system, which projects to the basal ganglia. A decrease in dopamine availability at receptors in the basal ganglia is associated with tremor, akinesia and muscle rigidity, as occur in patients with Parkinson disease.

Amphetamines may aggravate or produce a schizophreniform psychosis by increasing dopamine in the synaptic clefts of the mesolimbic and mesocortical systems.

Catatonia is a disturbance of motor activity which is neither specific to schizophrenia nor caused by intravenous diazepam.

The effectiveness or not of imipramine in depression is irrelevant to dopamine metabolism in schizophrenia. Electroconvulsive therapy may increase the effectiveness of phenothiazines, which should be continued as maintenance therapy in patients with schizophrenia or psychotic depression while receiving electroconvulsive therapy.

PS-C3 CORRECT RESPONSE A

One of the defining characteristics of childhood autism is its *onset within the first 30 months of life after a period of normal development.*

The earliest description of childhood autism was made in 1943 by Leo Kanner, Professor of Child Psychiatry at Johns Hopkins University Hospital. The core features of the condition are:

- A profound failure to develop social relationships. These children are aloof and indifferent to other people with a dislike of physical contact and affection. They avoid eye contact and are slow to smile or use facial expressiveness. They lack empathy and do not initiate interaction or play cooperatively.

- Language acquisition is delayed or absent (in 50%). When present, language is abnormal and idiosyncratic with echolalia (repetition of words or phrases), poor comprehension and abnormalities in tone, rhythm and pitch.

- Ritualistic and compulsive behaviours are common, typically unusual preoccupations and interests, intense attachments to objects, such as stones or pieces of cloth, restricted and stereotyped patterns of play and marked resistance to any change in their environment or routine. Tantrums and explosive outbursts may result when change is attempted.
- Stereotypical movements, such as rocking, finger twirling, spinning and tip-toe walking.

The prevalence rate in community surveys varies between 20 and 200 per 100 000, depending on the looseness of the criteria used to define the disorder. Boys are affected three times as often as girls.

Autistic behaviour may also occur in a diverse group of other conditions, including rubella, phenylketonuria, tuberosclerosis and the neurolipoidoses. Approximately 25% of autistic children develop epilepsy during adolescence.

The aetiology is unknown, but a primary cognitive deficit with an organic or genetic basis is most likely.

PS-C4   CORRECT RESPONSE C

The correct answer to this question is *mental retardation.*

The total prevalence of mental retardation (developmental disability) in the community is approximately 3% and approximately one-fifth of these will have moderate to profound retardation. *Most will manifest transient delay in normal speech development, but more or less normal language ability will be acquired by the majority.*

Deafness, cerebral palsy, infantile autism and social deprivation are other important causes of delayed speech. Most children can use words with meaning by 21 months of age, but by the time they start school 1% of children have serious speech retardation. The process by which language is acquired is complex and still poorly understood.

Deafness may develop before speech is learnt (prelingual deafness) or afterwards. Profound early deafness will interfere with speech and language development and the need to eventually communicate by sign language. It is important to recognise deafness as the cause of delayed speech development; early recognition and treatment can prevent otherwise inevitable further delay.

The essential feature of stammering is not delayed speech, but a disturbance in the normal fluency and time patterning of speech that is inappropriate for the individual's age. The disturbance in fluency interferes with academic or occupational achievement and with social communication. The severity of the disturbance varies with different situations and is worsened by stress and performance anxiety. There is strong evidence for genetic factors in the aetiology; the male : female ratio is 3 : 1. Recovery typically occurs spontaneously before the age of 16 years.

Elective (now selective) mutism is a rare condition, the essential feature of which is the persistent failure to speak in specific social situations, typically in school or with particular playmates. Speech and communication will be normal at other times. The condition usually develops between 3 and 5 years of age, after normal speech has been acquired, but it may not come to clinical attention until after the child enters school. The disturbance generally lasts only a few months, but it may persist for years. There is no evidence that any treatment is generally effective.

Speech and language disorders are central features of infantile autism, but autism is a relatively rare disorder with a prevalence of about 40 per 100 000.

PS-C 5 CORRECT RESPONSE E

The correct answer to this question is *all of the above features.*
Down syndrome is the most common cause of developmental disability (mental handicap) caused by a chromosomal abnormality (trisomy 21). The condition occurs in approximately one in 600–700 live births, but its incidence is decreasing because of increased detection by amniocentesis and subsequent termination of pregnancy. The level of mental handicap is extremely variable, from mild to severe.

The clinical picture is made up of a number of features, any of which may occur in normal people. The most characteristic features are:

- Moon-shaped facies with a small mouth and teeth, transverse furrowed tongue, high arched palate, oblique palpebral fissures and epicanthic folds in the eyes, a flattened occiput and face, short, squat nose and sparse, coarse hair.
- Hands that are short and broad with hyperextensible fingers; abnormalities of the thumb and little finger and a single transverse palmar crease.
- Hypotonia and hyperreflexia are common.

Associated clinical abnormalities include congenital heart malformations (usually septal defects) and duodenal atresia. The temperament of people with Down syndrome is usually gentle and good natured, but lively and affectionate. They are generally cheerful and sociable and many have a particular affinity for music, rhythm and dance.

PS-C6 CORRECT RESPONSE D

The correct answer to this question is that *Alzheimer-like changes in the brain develop in middle life.*

In 1959, Gerard Lejeune, a French paediatrician, discovered that the major chromosomal abnormality in 95% of cases of Down syndrome was a trisomy (three chromosomes instead of two) of chromosome 21. These cases are due to the failure of disjunction (separation) during meiosis, most commonly associated with increased maternal age when pregnant. The risk of recurrence in subsequent pregnancies is approximately 1%.

The remaining 5% of cases of Down syndrome are due to either a translocation involving chromosome 21 or to mosaicism. The disorder leading to translocation is often inherited and the subsequent risk of recurrence is 10%.

There is no association between temporal lobe epilepsy and Down syndrome. Previously infant mortality was high, but with improved medical care and surgical treatment of the associated heart and intestinal defects, survival into adult life is more common, with a significant percentage now living beyond 50 years of age. Signs of premature ageing and Alzheimer-like changes in the brain develop in the fourth and fifth decades.

PS-C7 CORRECT RESPONSE C

The correct answer to this question is *autosomal dominant.*

Huntington chorea was first described in 1872. Since then epidemiological studies have shown that the condition occurs worldwide in many countries and affects men and women equally. The prevalence is approximately five per 100 000. It is transmitted by a single autosomal-dominant gene located on the short arm of chromosome 4. This means that 50% of children of an affected parent will develop the disease and will in turn transmit the gene to their offspring in a similar ratio. The children of unaffected offspring are not at risk. Sporadic cases with no known family history occur and are presumed to be due to new mutations.

It is a progressive degenerative disease of cognition, emotion and movement, which produces neuronal loss in the frontal lobes, the caudate nucleus, putamen and the corpus striatum. A genetic test is now available to determine whether at-risk individuals will develop the disease, but should only be administered at specialised centres with resources to provide counselling and follow-up.

PS-C8   CORRECT RESPONSE B

The correct answer is the **Capgras syndrome.**

In the Capgras syndrome, the individual believes that a close acquaintance or relative has been replaced by a double or an impostor pretending to be that person. The abnormality is a delusion, not an hallucination and is a symptom rather than a syndrome. It is uncommon, but is most frequently associated with schizophrenia, affective disorder or organic lesions of the fronto–parietal lobe. The misidentified person is usually the individual's spouse or other relative.

Related to this, but rarer, is the Fregoli syndrome, named after an actor skilled in altering his facial appearance. For this condition, the individual patient misidentifies or recognises familiar people in various other people (strangers). This symptom is usually associated with schizophrenia.

De Clérambault syndrome (erotomania) is also rare. It is usually a disorder of women. The individual believes that an exalted person, typically an older man of high social standing or fame, is in love with her and communicates his love for her in obscure, indirect ways. The victim of the infatuation will then be pursued and stalked by the patient necessitating involvement of the police and eventually the courts. Although the delusion of love may remain unshakeable, sometimes it turns into a persecutory delusion and the patient becomes abusive and litigious. Most patients with erotomania suffer from schizophrenia.

Querulant paranoia is a form of delusional disorder which is characterised by complaints, claims and endless litigation directed at civil and political authorities usually by an individual or a family. The individual is passionate, angry, strong willed and unwilling to accept defeat in the courts. The web of litigation widens to include former lawyers, magistrates and judges who are perceived to have conspired or colluded to prevent acknowledgement or correction of the original or succeeding injustice.

Migration psychosis is the term applied to the development of paranoid symptoms in recent immigrants from a foreign country. Risk factors include enforced migration, torture and persecution in the country from which they are emigrating and language, cultural and religious dissonance. Migration to a foreign country is a stressful experience, but latent psychosis itself may stimulate some people to migrate, predisposing them to subsequent breakdown. This was not a factor in this scenario.

PS-C9   CORRECT RESPONSE C

The most appropriate response to this question is **a false belief.**

A delusion is a false, unshakeable idea or belief which is out of keeping with the person's educational, cultural and social background. It is held with extraordinary conviction and subjective certainty and is not influenced by rational argument or evidence to the contrary. Delusional beliefs are not arrived at through normal logical processes and, subjectively, are indistinguishable from true beliefs. The mechanisms or processes by which normal beliefs or delusions are formed and are tested are unknown.

Formal thought disorder is a series of disturbances in the ways that thoughts are linked together. Flight of ideas occurs when thoughts and conversation move quickly from one topic to another without first completing the topic or train of thought. It is characteristic of mania. Perseveration is the persistent and inappropriate repetition of the same thoughts or responses to a series of different questions and may occur in dementia. Loosening of associations denotes a loss of the normal structure of thinking. Conversation appears muddled and illogical and cannot be clarified by further inquiry. It most often occurs in schizophrenia.

Blunted affect implies that there has been a reduction in the normal range of emotional responsiveness and a lack of emotional sensitivity.

Auditory hallucinations are noises, voices or music heard and experienced in the absence of external stimuli and may have a similar quality to a true perception. In organic states, the auditory hallucinations may be unstructured sounds or elementary hallucinations, such as bangs, rattles, whistles or machinery-like, and are usually unpleasant and frightening. Hearing voices is characteristic of schizophrenia, but it may also occur in alcoholic hallucinosis and affective psychoses.

Passivity experiences are subjective disturbances in the control of thinking, which becomes so disorganised that thought processes are ascribed to outside influences. It is typically found in schizophrenia and the person experiences thoughts, feelings, impulses and actions as being foreign or alien and not within his control. Passivity experiences are examples of delusional thinking, but a delusion is **not** a passivity experience.

PS-C10   CORRECT RESPONSE C

The correct answer is *auditory hallucinations.*

For patients with schizophrenia, three types of auditory hallucinations are regarded as being diagnostic. These are audible thoughts (hearing one's own thoughts spoken out loud) voices heard arguing (usually two or more voices quarrelling with each other or discussing the patient in the third person) and voices giving a running commentary on the patient's activities. The commentary may occur just before, during or after the activity. Auditory hallucinations are generally private events, but simultaneous whispered vocalisations may sometimes be observed which correspond with the content of the voices. The 'voices' may be so insistent, compelling and interesting that ordinary conversations are considered boring in comparison. Sometimes the voices may give commands to the patient with such force that the patient feels compelled to carry them out. This may become a psychiatric emergency if the command involves harm to self or others.

Sociopathic personality is an outmoded term for antisocial personality, which is characterised by impulsivity, failure to make and sustain loving relationships, lack of remorse or guilt and failure to learn from adverse experiences. Patients with schizophrenia may coincidentally have antisocial or sociopathic personalities, but there is no direct link or association.

Depersonalisation is a peculiar change in self awareness such that the person feels unreal. It is difficult to put into words for the sufferer: it is 'as if' the person feels unreal, detached from his own experience and unable to feel emotion. Careful enquiry usually distinguishes descriptions of depersonalisation from delusional ideas. It may occur in schizophrenia, anxiety disorders and depression, but is not a characteristic or diagnostic symptom of any of these conditions.

Gender dysphoria occurs when there is a lack of congruence between biological sex and gender identity. Gender identity is usually clearly established as either male or female in early childhood, but occasionally there is a feeling of discomfort and inappropriateness about his or her biological sex, with a persistent wish to be of the opposite sex and a repudiation of his or her anatomy. Cross-dressing in childhood is quite common and is not pathological; and the vast majority of children who do cross-dress, eventually develop normal gender identity and sexual behaviour. Gender dysphoria is reserved for those individuals who experience anxiety, depression and suicidal ideation as a result of persistent gender identity disorders. Some people with schizophrenia have psychotic disturbances of gender identity as part of a global disturbance of self-image, but it is not a typical characteristic of the disorder.

PS-C11   CORRECT RESPONSE C

The correct answer to this question is *delusions of reference*.

Delusions of reference develop from ideas of reference; that is, that the person is special, or that 'people' are noticing, watching or gossiping about him (or her). Sufferers may believe that they are being talked about on the radio or that they are referred to in newspapers or television programmes; that they are being followed and their movements are being constantly monitored and that what they say is recorded. What they believe is far beyond the grounds of possibility, but they do not recognise their beliefs are false. It is a form of paranoid thinking that may progress to paranoid or grandiose delusions involving complex and bizarre plots, or special powers, talents and abilities. Delusions of reference commonly occur in schizophrenia and also in organic and affective disorders.

The essential feature of passive–aggressive personality is a pervasive pattern of negativistic attitudes and passive resistance to demands for adequate performance in social and occupational situations that begins by early adulthood and that occurs in a variety of contexts. These individuals habitually resent, oppose and resist demands to function at a level expected by others, most often in work situations, but also evident in social functioning. The resistance is expressed by procrastination, forgetfulness, stubbornness and intentional inefficiency, especially in response to tasks assigned by authority figures. These individuals feel cheated, unappreciated and misunderstood and chronically complain to others. They are sullen and argumentative and express envy and resentment towards others apparently more fortunate. They may alternate between hostile defiance and contrition with promises to perform better in the future. Passive–aggressive personality has no direct association with schizophrenia.

Illusions are misperceptions of external stimuli and are most likely to occur when consciousness or the general level of sensory stimulation are reduced. They are also likely when attention is not focused or when there is a strong affective state (usually fear or terror) accompanied by hyperarousal and hypervigilance. An illusion is a false perception of a real stimulus, whereas a hallucination is a false perception in the absence of any external sensory stimulus. Illusions are most commonly seen in states of fatigue or organic brain syndromes (delirium) and are not characteristic of schizophrenia.

Cataplexy is the sudden loss of muscle tone and temporary episodes of paralysis that occur as part of the narcolepsy syndrome. It may be precipitated by strong emotions. Other associated features are sleep paralysis and hypnagogic hallucinations. It should be distinguished from catalepsy, or waxy flexibility, which is a disorder of muscle tone which allows people to adopt awkward and uncomfortable positions without distress or discomfort for long periods of time, for example, lying for long periods with their head raised above a pillow. Catalepsy is rarely seen nowadays in patients with catatonic schizophrenia; cataplexy has no association with schizophrenia.

PS-C12   CORRECT RESPONSE C

According to the International Pilot Study of Schizophrenia conducted by the World Health Organisation in the 1970s and involving identical assessment, diagnosis and epidemiological enquiry in several First and Second World countries, the most frequent symptom of acute schizophrenia was *lack of insight*, which is the correct answer to this question.

Impaired insight is characteristic of schizophrenia. Most patients do not accept that they are ill and ascribe their experiences to the actions of other people or agencies. This usually results in lack of cooperation with doctors and nurses and an unwillingness or refusal to have treatment. Insight is a matter of degree and involves an awareness of one's own mental condition. Are the patients aware of or responsive to the concerns and observations of friends or relatives? If they do acknowledge certain beliefs, impulses, moods or behaviours, do they themselves regard them as morbid or abnormal? If they consider these phenomena as abnormal, do they consider they may be due to mental illness, as opposed to physical illness or the effects of diet, pollution or chemicals? If they accept that they have an illness, will they accept treatment or agree to assessment or hospitalisation? Many patients with schizophrenia will answer negatively to some or all of these questions, especially during their first few episodes of illness.

Insight is a complex construct and is not a single, easily quantifiable, or anatomically localisable function of the mind. Adequate insight presupposes intact intellectual and cognitive function, but it is not synonymous with intelligence. Insight has emotional components, is somewhat culturally bound and is influenced by defence mechanisms and personality. Insight may fluctuate with stress and level of arousal or with illness severity. Informed consent in the medical setting often requires mature judgement and decision-making capacity, as well as knowledge and insight. Insight is impaired by cognitive deficits, mood disorders and psychosis. Extreme lack of insight is usually associated with conversion disorders, factitious disorders, addictions, mania and schizophrenia. Insight should be viewed along a continuum, with many levels between insightfulness and a complete lack of insight. Frontal lobe and non-dominant parietal lobe lesions are frequently associated with significantly impaired insight.

Auditory hallucinations, delusions of persecution, flattened affect and ideas of reference are all characteristic of schizophrenia, but were less common features in the WHO international study.

PS-C13   CORRECT RESPONSE A

Typically, an amphetamine-induced psychosis is *paranoid* and may be indistinguishable from acute paranoid schizophrenia when it occurs following chronic use of amphetamines. Paranoid delusions are prominent, often with extreme fear and suspiciousness. Persecutory auditory hallucinations, hearing one's thoughts spoken aloud or feeling one's thoughts are being interfered with and other passivity experiences are common. Visual illusions and hallucinations may intrude at any time and tactile hallucinations of bugs or vermin crawling under the skin (formication) can lead to scratching and extensive skin excoriations. Anxiety, hostility and aggressiveness may accompany the paranoid ideation and ideas of reference requiring the use of restraint.

Depression may accompany acute use of amphetamines, but is more usually seen when the drug is withdrawn after a period of heavy use. Suicidal ideation may complicate amphetamine withdrawal and may persist for months. Suicide is a major risk.

Grandiosity is most commonly seen in amphetamine intoxication and may be part of 'the rush' induced by intravenous amphetamines. There are characteristic feelings of well-being and overconfidence and a heightened sense of sexual feeling and subjective 'profound thoughts'.

Amphetamine psychosis usually occurs with clear consciousness, but confusional episodes may occur. Upon recovery from the psychosis, there may be amnesia for parts of or for the whole episode.

Treatment of amphetamine psychosis involves secure hospitalisation, cessation of amphetamines and use of haloperidol or phenothiazines. Symptoms may be persistent for weeks or months and, upon recovery, acute psychosis may return on re-exposure to small doses of amphetamines.

PS-C14   CORRECT RESPONSE D

The most characteristic feature of alcoholic hallucinosis is *auditory hallucinations.* Typically, these occur in clear consciousness but they may be a continuation of hallucinations first experienced during withdrawal from alcohol. The hallucinations may also begin while drinking. Visual hallucinations are uncommon.

At first the hallucinations begin as simple sounds, such as whispering, muted laughter, the clink of glasses or single words, but they progress to formed sentences and frequently derogatory and offensive voices which accuse the sufferer of shameful actions. Command hallucinations may occasionally result in violence or suicide. Secondary paranoid delusions may develop. There is only a minor overlap with schizophrenia — in those with either a family history of schizophrenia or premorbid Cluster A personality traits.

Management involves withdrawal from alcohol and lifetime abstention. Antipsychotics may be used if hallucinations persist, but can usually be stopped within 3 months. Renewed drinking usually brings about a relapse.

The basis of alcoholic hallucinosis is uncertain, but is presumably related to alcohol-induced brain damage, perhaps of the temporal lobes or elsewhere in the limbic system.

PS-C15   CORRECT RESPONSE A

The most likely site of this man's brain lesion is the *frontal lobe.*

Characteristically, frontal lobe damage has distinctive effects on temperament and behaviour. Behaviour changes result in loss of normal socialisation, with disinhibition, over-familiarity, tactlessness and garrulousness, or apathy and loss of interest in the environment. Lesions of the basal orbital region are more likely to cause jocularity and euphoria which can easily deteriorate into irritability, whereas lesions of the dorsolateral areas most often cause apathy and loss of mental flexibility. Concentration and attention are impaired and there may be concrete thinking and a tendency to perseverate. There is loss of foresight and planning and judgement and insight are reduced. The actual symptoms depend on the size, location and bilaterality of the frontal lobe damage.

Clinically there is preservation of memory, but the digit span (the ability to recall series of numbers of increasing lengths, both forwards and backwards) is impaired. Digit span is a commonly used attentional test in the assessment of cognitive function. There may also be an inability to complete or copy various visual patterns, follow a maze, or complete a picture by joining up dots in sequence. Rapid sequential hand movements may also be impaired. With more extensive frontal lesions, a grasp or sucking reflex may be present. Incontinence, anosmia, akinesia and mutism develop later.

Lesions affecting the other cerebral areas listed will not produce the pattern of symptoms outlined in this scenario.

PS-C16   CORRECT RESPONSE E

The correct answer to this question is *all of the above conditions*, as depression can accompany each of the four conditions listed.

Depression frequently accompanies or complicates cerebrovascular thrombosis, haemorrhage or infarction. Lesions involving the left anterior hemisphere are reported to be most likely to be associated with depression. The depression is a mixture of adjustment disorder, grief reaction and organic impairment and may respond to conventional antidepressant therapy.

Aphasia is the loss of language function caused by lesions in specific cerebral areas. Broca (non-fluent/motor/expressive/anterior) aphasia accompanies pathology in the anterior speech area (the middle and inferior frontal gyri), most commonly due to left middle cerebral artery infarcts. Most patients have associated dysarthria and other motor deficits. Affectively, many of these patients are agitated and depressed.

In contrast, receptive or sensory or posterior aphasia (Wernicke aphasia) is produced by lesions in the superior temporal gyrus and the posterior temporo–parietal areas. The resultant speech is rambling, incomprehensible and full of neologisms. Affective abnormalities include euphoria and paranoid combativeness.

The prevalence rate of depression in Parkinson disease is 40% and is frequently associated with anxiety, irritability and pessimism, but little guilt or self-blame. Depression is more common in women with Parkinson disease, when the left hemisphere is involved, with earlier age of onset and when bradykinesia and gait instability are prominent. Mood changes in Parkinson disease respond to antidepressant therapy or electro–convulsive therapy.

Depression may be a feature of Alzheimer disease (presenile dementia) in the early stages when mood disturbance is common. As the disease progresses, between one-quarter and one-third of people will develop depression. It is important to distinguish depression from dementia, as depressive illness may produce a pseudodementia with patchy cognitive impairment and complaints of memory loss (which does not usually occur in dementia).

PS-C17   CORRECT RESPONSE C

The most likely explanation for the change in this man's mental state is *fat embolism syndrome.*

Minute globules of fat can often be demonstrated in the circulation following fractures of long bones (which have fatty marrows) and less commonly in association with soft tissue trauma, extensive burns, rapid decompression syndrome, cardiopulmonary bypass, diabetes, organ transplantation and neoplasms.

There are two main pathogenic hypotheses to explain fat embolism syndrome. Either or both of these may contribute. The mechanical theory suggests that free fat globules are able to enter the venous circulation and embolise to the lungs because of physical disruption to the bone and blood vessels at the fracture site. The chemical theory posits that a trauma-induced catecholamine surge results in either lipid mobilisation and the release of free fatty acids, which results in a toxic vasculitis, followed by platelet-fibrin thrombosis (and hence thrombocytopenia and disseminated intravascular coagulation) or the coalescence of chylomicrons into fat globules, which cause obstruction of small arterioles by macroaggregates of fat. Cerebral fat emboli and ischaemia, rather than hypoxaemia, produce the neurological damage.

Characteristic clinical features include a latent period of 12–72 h or more after injury before the sudden onset of fever, tachycardia, respiratory distress, clouding of consciousness, confusion, restlessness, delirium, stupor and most seriously, coma. Focal or generalised seizures may occur, as may aphasia and hemiparesis in association with more severe disturbances of consciousness. The central nervous system manifestations may occur without respiratory signs. Fine petechiae may be observed in the conjunctiva, retina or axillary folds.

The chest X-ray may be unremarkable, but fine stippling or bilateral hazy infiltrates similar to the adult respiratory distress syndrome, are often present. Hypoxaemia with a P_aO_2 of less than 60 mmHg is very common and may be the only laboratory abnormality, although thrombocytopenia and an evolving anaemia may occur. The most common cerebral CT findings are diffuse oedema, evidence of small infarcts appearing after one week and cerebral atrophy later.

This man was successfully treated with 40% oxygen by mask, supportive care, haloperidol and corticosteroids. However, there are no controlled trials which assess the benefit of corticosteroids in this condition. He made a complete recovery, but mortality can be as high as 40% and as many as 25% of patients have permanent neurological deficits. Restoration of normal arterial oxygen levels may not relieve the central nervous system symptoms and signs, which usually resolve 24–48 h after the pulmonary manifestations.

None of the other responses fits the clinical picture described in this scenario.

PS-C18   CORRECT RESPONSE D

The correct answer is to *arrange involuntary psychiatric admission, if he still refused voluntary admission.*

This is a serious episode of self-harm, with a potentially lethal outcome in a man with at least two recent major life events. He is depressed and the severity and duration of his depression, his intent underlying the overdose, his current mental state and psychosocial circumstances are all unclear. The situation is unstable. His cognitive functioning may be impaired and his previous refusal of psychiatric assessment makes urgent specialist assessment imperative.

He has a serious mental disorder and is a danger to himself at least. Further hospitalisation is essential in these circumstances.

It would be foolhardy to either increase or change his medication, to contact his wife or simply arrange for alcohol counselling. Any or all of these approaches may be the eventual outcome, but clearly psychiatric assessment, involuntary if necessary, is the most appropriate *initial* management.

PS-C19   CORRECT RESPONSE A

The correct answer to this question is that *she should be taken seriously and referred for treatment.*

It is a myth that people who talk about harming themselves or threaten suicide never carry out their stated intentions. Most people who harm themselves will have given prior warnings to friends, relatives or their doctors. An expressed intention to harm oneself is a cry for help, an indication that the person is not coping with the present circumstances and a plea that she be listened to, understood and helped to deal with her distress. The expressed intention is an invitation to explore the nature of the problems facing her, to assess her coping skills and other resources available to her.

It is poor counselling to reassure people who are considering self-harm that they will not do it. Unless exceptionally drastic measures are taken, it is impossible to prevent people from harming themselves at some future time when they are determined to do so. When people are so desperate that they are considering self-harm, reassurance that they will not do it may act as an incentive and a belief they are being patronised and that their concerns are not being taken seriously.

Genuine warmth and concern and gentle questioning about the depth of their despair will defuse their distress and will enable them to discuss their plans and preparations (if any) and the nature of their circumstances that has produced this decision. Most people will not harm themselves if they are given the chance to discuss their situation and consider alternatives.

Marital status is only one factor to be considered in assessing suicidal risk. A previous attempt at self-harm is a more worrying risk factor as is the presence of depression, alcohol or substance abuse, schizophrenia, severe or chronic anxiety, some forms of personality disorder, painful or debilitating physical illnesses, long-term unemployment, lack of social supports and a sense of hopelessness about the future. This is not an exhaustive list.

Diazepam is best used for acute anxiety states as a short-term treatment only. Tolerance usually develops rapidly and dosage may creep upwards if it is used beyond a fortnight. Benzodiazepines are effective anxiolytics, but used long term they may block or deter the development of innate coping strategies or discourage the learning of new ones. They must only be a considered treatment and not a reflex response to distress. Benzodiazepines are often prescribed to treat the doctor's anxiety and sense of clinical impotence when faced with a distressed patient.

PS-C20   CORRECT RESPONSE A

The correct answer to this question is *an overvalued idea.*

An overvalued idea is an acceptable, comprehensible idea which is pursued by a patient beyond the bounds of reason. It has been defined as 'a solitary, abnormal belief that is neither delusional nor obsessional in nature, but which is so preoccupying that it dominates the life of the individual'. The idea causes disturbed functioning or suffering to the person or to others. The person's whole life may revolve around this one idea. It is usually associated with strong affect and an abnormal personality and shares similarities with passionate religious and political convictions. The background evidence on which an overvalued idea is held is neither necessarily unreasonable nor false.

In anorexia nervosa, the patient's conviction that she is overweight despite clear contrary evidence, is not considered delusional. The belief is preoccupying, acted on unquestioningly and leads the patient to engage in sustained abnormal behaviour. Although it may also be accompanied by a fear of gaining weight, this is not a phobia, as there is no excessive anxiety or arousal in the presence of food.

A delusion is qualitatively different from a normal belief or an overvalued idea. Delusions are a radical and irrational transformation of the meaning of events and are incomprehensible to the observer.

An obsession is experienced subjectively as senseless and irrational and is normally resisted by the sufferer. Ruminations are more complex obsessional thoughts which are repetitive, intrusive, unwanted and upsetting.

Other examples of overvalued ideas include some forms of morbid jealousy, hypochondriasis, querulous paranoid states and dysmophorphobia (disturbance of body image).

PS-C21   CORRECT RESPONSE E

The correct answer to this question is *all of the above conditions.*

Depersonalisation is a highly unpleasant experience, resulting from a peculiar change in self-awareness such that the individual feels detached, alienated or unreal. It is a common experience and frequently accompanies other mental disorders. Sufferers find it hard to describe the experience which may be accompanied by time distortion, changes in body image and a feeling of being outside one's body and observing one's actions, often from the ceiling above (autoscopy). Reality testing (the ability to determine the boundary between inner experience and the experience of the outer world) remains intact. Depersonalisation is often accompanied by derealisation, a sense that the external world and environment is strange or unreal.

Depersonalisation and derealisation may be experienced as transient phenomena lasting no more than minutes, in healthy adults and in children, especially when tired or when sleep-deprived. They are particularly common in panic disorder, **post-traumatic stress disorder**, **agoraphobia** and other anxiety disorders, depression and **schizophrenia** and are thus non-diagnostic. Acute intoxication and withdrawal from alcohol, hallucinogens and other substances also may result in depersonalisation.

Voluntarily induced experiences of depersonalisation and derealisation form part of meditative, **ecstatic** and **trance practices** that are prevalent in many cultures and religions.

A transient experience of depersonalisation and derealisation develops in approximately one-third of individuals exposed to life-threatening danger in traumatic accidents, violent crime or war/combat situations. Here, the onset is sudden and the course chronic and fluctuating.

Depersonalisation may also accompany epilepsy, particularly affecting the temporal lobes. There is no specific treatment and the aetiology is unclear. Some depersonalisation experiences are related to disturbances in arousal and consciousness.

PS-C22   CORRECT RESPONSE D

The correct answer to this question is *onset in winter, recovery in spring.*

Seasonal affective disorder is characterised by the onset and remission of major depressive episodes at characteristic times of the year. In most cases the episodes begin in autumn or winter and remit in spring. Less commonly, there may be recurrent episodes of depression in summer. The diagnosis does not apply to mood disorders in which the pattern is better explained by seasonally linked psychosocial stressors such as seasonal unemployment, school holidays or anniversary reactions. Seasonal depression typically represents as prominent irritability, hypersomnia, hyperphagia with carbohydrate craving, weight gain and energy loss. The majority of sufferers are women and younger age is a risk factor. There may be a link with latitudes closer to the poles where winter sunlight is weakest. Several clinical trials suggest that exposure to bright light (approximately 2500 lx) for several hours in the early morning and evening (to lengthen the winter photoperiod), relieves the symptoms. It is unclear whether this is merely a placebo effect.

It is postulated that the disorder is mediated by melatonin, which is secreted by the pineal gland and is responsible for controlling several diurnal rhythms. The diagnosis was popularised in the 1980s and was magnified by media reports of its prevalence, but interest in the condition has since waned.

PS-C23   CORRECT RESPONSE A

This is a straightforward definitional question. The correct answer is *identity disturbance, unstable relationships, inappropriate anger and impulsivity.*

Diagnostic criteria for borderline personality disorder do not include social withdrawal, magical thinking, high intelligence, reaction formation, neurasthenia, repression, hypochondriasis or cognitive impairment. One or more of these characteristics may occur coincidentally in people with borderline personality disorder, but are not central to the diagnosis.

People with borderline personality traits are major consumers of medical care and time and familiarity with the major features of the condition and its modes of presentation is essential.

PS-C24   CORRECT RESPONSE A

The correct answer to this question about a patient with a plethora of symptoms is *somatisation disorder.*

Somatisation refers to the psychological mechanisms underlying the formation of somatic symptoms. Somatisation disorder has a pattern of recurrent, multiple, clinically significant somatic complaints (resulting in medical investigation or treatment). The somatic complaints begin before the age of 30, occur over several years and cannot be explained by any known physical condition or the effects of any known substance.

Current DSM-IV diagnostic criteria for somatisation disorder require the presence of multiple symptoms affecting many different organ systems:

- four pain symptoms;
- two gastrointestinal symptoms;
- one sexual symptom;
- one neurological symptom.

If there is an associated general medical condition, the physical complaints or resulting social or occupational impairments are in excess of what would be expected from the history, physical findings or laboratory investigations.

Somatisation disorder is more common in women than in men and there are genetic, environmental and personality factors which increase the risk of developing the disorder. There may be overlap with antisocial personality disorder and alcohol or substance abuse. The symptoms (and the disorder) are neither intentionally produced nor feigned, thus excluding factitious illness. The course of somatisation disorder is chronic and fluctuating and rarely remitting.

The essential feature of hypochondriasis is the preoccupation with fears of having or the idea that one has a serious illness based on a misinterpretation of one or more bodily signs or symptoms. This unwarranted fear persists despite thorough examination, investigation, explanation and medical reassurance.

Conversion disorders are characterised by the presence of symptoms or deficits affecting motor or sensory functioning that suggest a neurological or other general medical condition. The initiation or exacerbation of the symptom or deficit is preceded by conflicts or other stressors. Conversion symptoms do not conform to known anatomical or physiological pathways, but follow an artless individual's conceptualisation of a disorder. Symptoms are produced unconsciously and may coexist with current or prior neurological pathology. They are more common in women and are much more common on the left side of the body. Conversion symptoms may be part of or may precede the later development of somatisation disorder.

Münchausen syndrome is a form of factitious disorder characterised by feigned dramatic presentations with symptoms suggesting surgical pathology accompanied by pathological lying and a tendency to transfer the presentation from hospital to hospital or 'doctor shop'. It is associated with severe character pathology and the active pursuit of the sick role.

PS-C25   CORRECT RESPONSE D

The symptoms in this patient are characteristic of **post-traumatic stress disorder.**

While it is possible that the patient may have depression and some cognitive impairment consistent with his age, these conditions are less likely to present in this way.

'Jet lag' should have resolved within days and 'culture shock' is a sociological term with no direct psychiatric significance.

PS-C26   CORRECT RESPONSE D

The history suggests that **psychological reaction to deafness** is the explanation. Deafness is a well documented predisposing factor to paranoid illness in elderly people. Characteristically, this complicates severe bilateral deafness resulting from middle ear disease and chronic mastoiditis, rather than perceptual deafness present from birth. Deafness produces social isolation through impaired communication. Tinnitus may produce or aggravate auditory hallucinations. Paranoid illnesses in the elderly are frequently superimposed on long-standing abnormal personality traits of suspiciousness, hypervigilance, over-sensitivity, social avoidance and friendlessness. Most deaf people do not become paranoid.

In this case, the premorbid personality is described as 'well adjusted' and his symptoms only began after his tinnitus and hearing loss developed. The history and clinical features do not support a diagnosis of early schizophrenia, organic brain syndrome or cerebral arteriosclerosis.

Methyldopa may cause transient sedation, involuntary movements, nightmares, depression and reversible mild psychoses. After 5 years of treatment, it is unlikely to be a factor in this situation.

PS-C27   CORRECT RESPONSE E

The correct answer is **all of the above features.**

The core clinical features of anorexia nervosa are:
- characteristic over-valued ideas about shape and weight;
- active maintenance of bodyweight 15% below the expected weight for the person's age, sex and height (or a Body Mass Index below 17.5);
- **amenorrhoea** in women (who are not taking the oral contraceptive pill).

Some patients with anorexia nervosa share clinical features in common with patients with bulimia nervosa. In these patients there will be a history of **binge eating** and self-induced vomiting to control weight.

Laboratory investigations show endocrine, haematological and electrolyte abnormalities, including **hypokalaemia** and metabolic alkalosis secondary to vomiting.

Associated psychopathology in anorexia nervosa includes depression, suicidal ideation, anxiety symptoms usually focused on eating; marked social withdrawal and **obsessional behaviour** concerning food, weight, diet and exercise. Many patients are perfectionistic and preoccupied with external appearance.

PS-C28   CORRECT RESPONSE D

This is the typical sleep disturbance associated with *anxiety and generalised anxiety disorder is the correct response.*

Although anxiety *may* be a feature of all of the alternatives, sleep disorder is not a defining characteristic of either borderline personality disorder or schizophrenia.

Sleep disorders with major depression are common and may share some of the characteristics described. What is more typical is early morning awakening, 2 or 3 h before the patient's usual waking time with an inability to get back to sleep because of low mood and morbid, pessimistic thoughts. The disturbance may be bimodal, with difficulty falling asleep as well. Some patients with major depression may oversleep, rather than wake early.

Nocturnal epilepsy is characterised by generalised seizures occurring while asleep, usually marked by involuntary vocalisation and then a Grand-mal fit. There may be blood on the pillow or accompanying enuresis if the patient has not woken or been observed. Deep postictal sleep may ensue.

PS-C29   CORRECT RESPONSE C

The most likely underlying problem in this man is *social phobia.*

Social anxiety may be an underrecognised predisposing factor in alcoholism capitalising on alcohol's anxiolytic effects. In this scenario, alcohol usage has only begun recently. The man has insight into his anxiety and is aware that his fears are irrational. There is nothing to support a diagnosis of schizophrenia and the pattern of anxiety symptoms focused on his work situation precludes agoraphobia at this stage.

In agoraphobia, anxiety is determined by distance from safety as well as by the proximity of the phobic stimulus. Agoraphobia affects a cluster of situations, of which the most commonly mentioned is fear of entering crowded places, but it may also include fears of confined spaces (supermarkets, cinemas, hairdressers), of public transport and of being far from home. The symptoms include both fear and marked avoidance of situations from which it might be difficult to escape or hard to get help in an emergency. Agoraphobics usually feel safe at home and become more fearful the further they venture away from a safe place.

Untreated or unrecognised social phobia may culminate in a panic attack, but that is not the situation here.

PS-C30   CORRECT RESPONSE E

The correct answer to this question is *all of the above disorders.*

Cognitive–behaviour therapy (CBT) is a package of active, structured treatments based on an integration of behavioural and cognitive principles, which has evolved in the past 25 years. Most psychiatric disorders have elements or symptoms for which cognitive or behavioural approaches are suitable.

Chronic pain is characterised by anxiety, depression and avoidance behaviours, all of which may respond to CBT. The aims are to gradually improve the patient's quality of life by reducing anxiety about pain and gently increasing exercise tolerance and enhancing control. Cognitive strategies focus on negative thoughts and stress that 'hurt does not necessarily equal harm'.

Social phobia is a complex phobia which centres on the fear of scrutiny and, hence, negative evaluation and criticism. Typical situations avoided are public speaking and eating, or writing under observation (as in a bank). Distressing thoughts and avoidance of social situations are characteristic. Treatment is multimodal: teaching anxiety management, challenging cognitions and video review of speaking, with graduated practical exercises to overcome avoidance behaviours.

Cognitive therapy was first used as an adjunctive treatment in non-psychotic, non-bipolar **depressive disorder**, to speed recovery and help prevent relapse, by teaching patients depression-management skills. Typical approaches include the scheduling of pleasant events, re-evaluating dysfunctional behaviour and the challenging of depressive attributions. Treatment is problem-oriented rather than focusing on the historical origins of symptoms.

Some form of CBT is the treatment of choice in **bulimia nervosa.** Techniques used include education about the disorder, self-monitoring of relevant thoughts and behaviour, the use of self-control measures to establish regular eating patterns and prevent dieting, vomiting and purging. Social skills and problem-solving strategies may also be used.

PS-C31   CORRECT RESPONSE C

The correct answer to this question is *obsessive–compulsive disorder.*

Cognitive behaviour therapies are forms of psychological treatment which attempt to alter symptoms and dysfunctional behaviours associated with psychiatric disorders. Exposure and response prevention are but two of several behaviour therapies used in the treatment of obsessive–compulsive disorder.

The core features of obsessional disorders are:

- the avoidance of objects or situations which trigger obsessions;
- obsessions (unwanted, intrusive thoughts, images or impulses);
- compulsive behaviours and thought rituals.

When obsessions occur, despite the use of avoidance, rituals usually result.

Exposure treatments are aimed at confronting patients with what is feared (and is causing anxiety), while encouraging them to block any behaviours which may prevent or terminate the exposure (response prevention). A review of their fears is encouraged, so that patients realise that the catastrophic or terrible consequences which they fear, do not occur.

Exposure can be conducted 'in situ', in actual situations that provoke anxiety; or by getting the patient to imagine such situations in a vivid way — 'in imagination'. Patients are then discouraged or dissuaded from carrying out their neutralising rituals for increasingly longer periods. They are warned to expect an increase in their fears initially, but are taught ways to challenge and overcome their anxiety until it declines naturally.

Cognitive–behavioural therapies may be used in each of the other conditions listed, but the treatment packages would not commonly include both exposure and response prevention.

PS-C32   CORRECT RESPONSE D

The correct answer to this question is that a phobia *may respond to systematic desensitisation.*

A phobia is a persistent unreasonable fear of and wish to avoid a specific object, activity or situation. The person recognises that the fear is irrational and is out of proportion to the real danger. Phobias are powerful and compelling by nature and may come to dominate a person's life. They are repetitive and resistance is typically minimal and unsuccessful. Although the sufferers recognise that their origin is internal from within themselves, they may feel controlled by them.

The fear may be of external stimuli, such as animal phobias, social phobia or agoraphobia, or internal stimuli of illness or contamination. The anxiety generated may lead to avoidance, which maintains the fear. Occasionally what begins as a specific phobia, for example 'of an animal or reptile', may generalise to a persistent dread of situations which have only a tenuous link with the original stimulus.

A delusion is a false, unshakeable idea or belief which is out of keeping with the patient's educational, cultural and social background and which is held with extraordinary conviction and objective certainty.

Phobic symptoms may occur in schizophrenia as a result of delusions or hallucinations, but are not frequent nor are they a defining characteristic of the disorder.

The treatment of choice in phobic disorders is cognitive behavioural therapy. One form of this involves the graduated exposure of the person to the feared stimulus or situation while practising relaxation and controlled breathing until the level of anxiety experienced is manageable or has dissipated. This is systematic desensitisation.

Benzodiazepines have little or no place in the routine management of phobias and their usage may delay or impede efforts to master symptoms using behavioural techniques.

PS-C33   CORRECT RESPONSE E

The correct answer is *phobic anxiety*.

Vaginismus is recurrent or persistent spasm of the perineal musculature of the lower one-third of the vagina that causes pain and interferes with coitus or attempted vaginal penetration with a tampon, finger or speculum. In some women, even the anticipation of vaginal penetration may result in muscle spasm. Like all forms of sexual dysfunction, its prevalence is unknown, but is more common among women of high socioeconomic groups.

It may be a lifelong condition or it may be acquired after a period of normal sexual functioning; for example, associated with scarring following an episiotomy. It may be limited to certain types of stimulation, situations or partners or it may be generalised.

Sexual responsiveness may not otherwise be impaired, but if severe and persistent, vaginismus may be a cause of non-consummation of marriage. The disorder is more often found in younger than in older females, with negative attitudes towards sexual relationships. A sexual trauma such as rape or childhood sexual abuse can be the cause. A strict upbringing that equates 'sex with sin' may be a factor.

It is not commonly associated with schizophrenia, depression, borderline personality disorder or obsessive–compulsive disorder. The spasm may commonly be the result of a phobic anxiety response to anticipated or actual vaginal penetration made worse by the presence of an inexperienced partner. Once the disorder is established, its course is usually chronic.

PS-C34   CORRECT RESPONSE E

The correct answer to this question is postpartum psychosis typically *demonstrates all of the above characteristics.*

Postpartum psychosis occurs in apporximately one in 500 births and is more common in primiparous women, those with a prior history of major psychiatric illness and those with a *family history* of major psychiatric illness. There is no clear relationship between psychosis and obstetric factors. The onset is usually within the first 30 days of delivery, but rarely in the first 2 days. There is no evidence that hormonal or endocrine changes in women with postpartum psychosis are different from other women in the puerperium.

Three types of clinical pictures may occur; organic, affective and schizophrenic, but most are **affective**, with a high proportion of manic disorders. The **onset is usually abrupt with severe insomnia**, followed by confusion, fluctuating agitation and labile mood. Mothers with delusional ideas may believe their infant is deformed, evil or possessed and infanticide is a major risk. Postpartum schizophrenia may be accompanied by command hallucinations to kill the infant. Depressed or schizophrenic mothers may attempt to harm themselves.

Optimal care is provided in special mother and baby units, where there is close observation of the mother and supervision of her continued care of the infant.

Electroconvulsive therapy is the treatment of choice for severe depression, because it is rapidly effective, but is also used early on in mothers with schizophrenic features who are not responding quickly to antipsychotics. Antidepressants are used for less severe depressive disorders and lithium (or another antimanic agent) and antipsychotics are used for mania.

Most patients fully recover from postpartum psychosis, but the recurrence rate for depressive illness after subsequent childbirth may be as high as 20%. There is a **significant risk of relapse of mood disorder in later life independent of further pregnancies.**

PS-C35   CORRECT RESPONSE E

The correct answer is **lithium carbonate.**

There are dangers and risks associated with prescribing or using all of the psychotropic drugs during pregnancy. However, lithium carbonate is definitely teratogenic in the first trimester and should always be suspended, preferably **before** an intended pregnancy. The mother's mood and mental state during the pregnancy will need close monitoring and her early warning signs of relapse inquired after. Lithium may be resumed in the latter stages of pregnancy if the mother's mental state and clinical condition warrant this.

Other psychotropic drugs are **relatively** contraindicated during pregnancy. With methadone, mothers are encouraged to remain on it during the first trimester. If they wish to withdraw and are at low risk of relapse, the methadone can be gradually withdrawn during the second trimester. Mothers (on methadone) are encouraged to breast feed to prevent or minimise withdrawal or abstinence in the neonate.

PS-C36   CORRECT RESPONSE D

The correct answer to this clinical situation is to administer **benztropine.**

Here the clinical problem is an acute dystonic reaction to a neuroleptic, most probably haloperidol or fluphenazine. Acute dystonia typically occurs within the first few days of commencing neuroleptic treatment and has been reported in 20% of young males who are receiving high potency drugs.

The reactions are characterised by sustained, involuntary muscle spasm, most often involving the facial, head or neck muscles. Examples include spasm of the masticatory muscles (trismus), orbicularis oculi (blepharospasm), oculogyric crises (fixed upward gazing of the eyes: 'the look-ups'), torticollis, dysarthria, dysphonia and dysphagia. Such spasms are painful and very distressing and may be undetected or misdiagnosed. The exact pathophysiological mechanism underlying acute dystonia is not clear.

Treatment of acute dystonia is swiftly effective with parenteral anticholinergics such as benztropine 2 mg by intramuscular or intravenous injection. If there is no prompt relief, the dose should be repeated in 30 min. Anticholinergic drugs are then continued for a week or longer afterwards. The choice of neuroleptic or the dose may need to be reviewed, especially if the symptoms recur: then the dose should be reduced, or treatment should be changed to a lower potency neuroleptic.

Chlorpromazine and haloperidol are both neuroleptics that may induce dystonia and are contraindicated in this emergency situation. Phenytoin will have no benefit, whereas diazepam may lessen the distress, but will not stop the dystonic reaction.

PS-C37   CORRECT RESPONSE D

The correct answer to this question is *physostigmine.*

Anticholinergic delirium may be produced by a variety of psychotropic drugs either taken in combination or in overdosage. Drugs most commonly implicated include tricyclic antidepressants, low potency neuroleptics especially thioridazine and chlorpromazine; the anticholinergic antiparkinsonian drugs (benztropine, procyclidine, benzhexol), some antihistamines and antispasmodics, such as hyoscine. Emergency treatment of bradycardia with atropine, particularly in elderly patients, may also precipitate the anticholinergic syndrome.

The delirium is characterised by agitation, confusion, motor restlessness, dysarthria, myoclonus, hallucinations (including visual) and convulsions. Systemic manifestations of the anticholinergic syndrome include tachycardia, dry mouth and other mucous membranes, fever, dilated and sluggishly reactive pupils, blurred vision, warm, dry skin, reduced or absent bowel sounds with ileus and urinary retention.

Physostigmine salicylate, an anticholinesterase inhibitor that crosses the blood–brain barrier, can be diagnostically useful if an anticholinergic delirium is suspected. Its usefulness is limited by its short duration of action and its toxicity. Its only therapeutic use is in otherwise uncontrollable anticholinergic delirium which is producing life-threatening behaviours.

Physostigmine is administered intravenously in doses of 1–2 mg slowly over 2–3 min. If no response occurs, the dose can be repeated in 30 min. If a toxic response to physostigmine occurs, such as bronchoconstriction, convulsions, bradycardia or worsening confusion, then its effects can be reversed with intravenous atropine sulphate, 0.5 mg for every 1 mg of physostigmine administered.

If there is a good response to physostigmine, the lowest effective dose can be repeated once after 30 min. It is not recommended that further dosing with physostigmine be continued thereafter. Often, the patients in whom it may be used will be quite sick and in need of intensive care support.

Anticholinergic delirium has a good prognosis. Atropine and benztropine will make anticholinergic delirium worse, succinyl choline is a muscle relaxant used in anaesthesia and phentolamine is an alpha-adrenergic antagonist used for hypertensive crisis.

PS-C38   CORRECT RESPONSE E

The correct answer is *all of the above conditions.*

Lithium salts have been used for over a century to treat various conditions. Lithium bromide was prescribed as a sedative then and lithium chloride was briefly popular as a salt substitute to treat hypertension in the 1940s. Lithium carbonate was first used to treat mania and manic excitement in 1949 by John Cade, an Australian psychiatrist. Lithium carbonate is still the treatment of choice for **acute episodes of mania**, but its primary use is in the **prophylaxis of bipolar affective disorder** — to prevent recurrence of either mania or depression.

Lithium is also recommended as combination therapy with high dosage tricyclic antidepressants in the management of **treatment-refractory depression.**

The use of lithium in the treatment of aggression in people with developmental disability is somewhat controversial, with mixed reports of its effectiveness in children and adolescents. The American literature **recommends its use in aggressiveness associated with developmental disability**, conduct disorder and pervasive development disorder.

Lithium affects many physiological systems, but its mode of action is unclear. It has effects on sodium, calcium and magnesium transport across cell membranes and also alters noradrenaline and serotonin metabolism. It also inhibits adenylcyclase and may, thus, unmask latent Parkinson disease or exacerbate established symptoms. Adenylcyclase inhibition accounts for the renal and thyroid side-effects of lithium.

PS-C39   CORRECT RESPONSE D

The correct answer to this question is that **lithium carbonate is neither habit forming nor addictive.**

Lithium carbonate has only been used routinely in the management of bipolar affective disorder since the 1960s. It is rapidly and completely absorbed from the gastrointestinal tract and serum levels peak within 1–1½ h of oral administration. There is no evidence that it is more or less effective in women, except that lithium carbonate is less effective in patients with rapid-cycling mood disorders, the majority of whom are women.

Advanced age alone does not compromise responsiveness to lithium, but associated physical illnesses and other medications, special diets and age-related changes in glomerular filtration rates predispose to an increased sensitivity to side effects. Long-term therapy with lithium for children and adolescents with bipolar mood disorder is also problematic because of concern about the potential for adverse side effects.

Long-term treatment does not cure bipolar affective disorder, so the discontinuation of lithium significantly increases the risk of further relapse. Maintenance levels are usually lower than those necessary in acute treatment. The maximum benefits of lithium maintenance may not become evident until treatment has been continued for long enough to show that relapses become less severe and less frequent than at first.

If lithium is discontinued, there is some evidence that previous lithium responders may fail to respond to the reintroduction of lithium therapy. Hence, the decision to cease successful lithium maintenance therapy should be carefully considered and the patient informed of the risks.

PS-C40   CORRECT RESPONSE D

The correct answer to this question is **lithium.**

Although lithium has been measured in many body fluids, only serum or plasma levels are used in clinical practice. The periodic determination of the serum lithium level is an essential aspect of patient care, but it should always be used in concert with sound clinical judgement. Early signs of lithium intoxication can still be present in patients with lithium levels within the normal laboratory range, especially in elderly patients. The level should be measured in the morning, 12 h (plus or minus 30 min) after the last dose the night before, and after 4 or 5 days of consistent dosage when a steady state condition should exist.

Opinions on the value of measuring plasma levels of tricyclic antidepressants vary widely. The only tricyclic antidepressant for which there is an accepted, well-defined therapeutic range is nortriptyline. There is little agreement on other drugs. In general, plasma levels of tricyclic antidepressants should be used only when there is doubt about patient compliance or to confirm toxicity due to overdose or adverse interactions.

Similarly, plasma level monitoring of the antipsychotic agents has been of only limited usefulness in both clinical and research settings. Some phenothiazines have complex metabolic pathways and plasma levels may not give an accurate picture because of the presence of active metabolites. With the exception of clozapine, there is little to be gained from routine measurement of plasma levels, except in situations where patients have failed to respond to what is usually an adequate dose, when it is important to distinguish toxic drug side effects from illness symptoms and deficits, in the very young, the elderly and the medically compromised in whom the pharmacokinetics of the antipsychotics may be significantly altered or when non-compliance is suspected or when compliance has been compelled by a court order.

Most benzodiazepines undergo multiple biotransformations prior to elimination and many of their metabolites are also clinically active. No therapeutic windows have been empirically established and validated. Plasma levels of the parent drug or its active metabolites are not used routinely in the management of patients treated with benzodiazepines, but plasma levels may be used to confirm compliance.

Plasma levels of the monoamine oxidase inhibitors are not measured routinely in clinical practice.

PS-C41   CORRECT RESPONSE D

The correct answer to this question is *haemodialysis.*

In acute overdosage of lithium, initially elevated levels of serum lithium concentrations can be misleading, as distribution into the tissues occurs over several hours. An initial highly toxic level (e.g. > 3 mmol/L) can fall to 1 mmol/L with final distribution, so repeated measurement of serum lithium levels and serial mental status examinations are essential in the assessment of toxicity.

Symptoms of lithium overdose include apathy, lethargy, tremor, slurred speech, ataxia and muscle fasciculations, which may progress to choreoathetosis, convulsions, coma and death. There may be residual neurological sequelae.

In addition to intensive supportive care, the treatment of choice for serious intoxication is haemodialysis. Dialysis must be considered in any patient with convulsions or coma, or when serum lithium levels at equilibrium are 4 mmol/L and above. Dialysis is the only route of elimination in patients with renal failure.

Sodium and water depletion and dehydration lead to marked increases in renal reabsorption of lithium and, hence, raised serum concentrations. Diuretics must not be used in the treatment of lithium overdosage.

Administration of intravenous saline may promote lithium excretion, but the value of forced saline diuresis is unclear and it is not recommended.

Oral L-tryptophan is of no value and activated charcoal does not absorb lithium and is also useless.

PS-C42   CORRECT RESPONSE C

Fluoxetine (Prozac®) is a *selective serotonin re-uptake inhibitor* (SSRI) and was the forerunner of several newer antidepressant SSRIs now available for general pharmaceutical prescription in Australia. Similar drugs include paroxetine (Aropax®) and sertraline (Zoloft®).

Clinical trials have shown that the efficacy of the SSRI antidepressants is equal to the tricyclic antidepressants. The half-life of fluoxetine and its metabolites is considerably longer than the other available SSRIs.

The SSRI antidepressants are usually given once daily (at least initially) and are well absorbed orally. Dosage may need to be reduced in the elderly and in patients with renal or hepatic impairment.

Side effects are generally much less of a problem than with tricyclic antidepressants, but include insomnia, anxiety, agitation, headache, nausea, diarrhoea and sexual dysfunction (mainly ejaculatory disturbance).

The SSRIs do not interact with alcohol, do not significantly impair psychomotor function and have low lethality in overdosage.

PS-C43   CORRECT RESPONSE A

Clozapine is an oral atypical antipsychotic drug which was approved for use in Australia in 1993 for the treatment of *treatment-refractory schizophrenia.*

Originally developed in the 1960s, it was withdrawn from general usage in 1975 after reports of fatal agranulocytosis associated with its use. Following the publication of an influential study in 1988, which showed that it was superior to chlorpromazine in patients with chronic schizophrenia who had not responded to haloperidol, clozapine was resurrected. It has since been hailed as the first major advance in the treatment of schizophrenia for 30 years.

It has a low potential for extrapyramidal side effects, but it commonly causes drowsiness and sedation, hypersalivation, tachycardia, dizziness and vertigo, headache, gastro-intestinal side effects and toxic delirium. The major concern still is leucopenia and agranulocytosis.

The main method of countering and averting agranulocytosis has been weekly white blood cell counts and the supply of a week's medication at a time. There is currently no means of predicting which patients will develop leucopenia, but it may be more common in the Ashkenazim Jewish population. The crude incidence of agranulocytosis is 0.6%. Although agranulocytosis may not develop for a year, 85% of cases occur within 9 months of beginning treatment. The onset is gradual and rapid recovery follows early detection and drug withdrawal.

The starting dose is 25–75 mg daily in divided dosage, gradually increasing to a target dose of 300–450 mg daily in 25–50 mg daily increments. Treatment should be continued for 6 months before deciding that response is inadequate. Clozapine should be withdrawn gradually over 2 weeks to minimise rebound exacerbation of psychosis.

Clozapine is contraindicated in patients with myeloproliferative disorders, severe central nervous system depression and a previous history of leucopenia or agranulocytosis. Caution should be shown in patients with prostatomegaly, narrow angle glaucoma, arrhythmias and underlying cardiovascular disorders, or a history of paralytic ileus or seizure disorders. It may interact with benzodiazepines, anticonvulsants and cimetidine, and concomitant use of other drugs with a significant risk of agranulocytosis is contraindicated.

PS-C44   CORRECT RESPONSE C

This scenario describes many of the characteristic features of opiate withdrawal.

The correct answer to this question is **heroin.**

Recreational or occasional use of marijuana (cannabis) does not produce an abstinence or withdrawal syndrome in most users. Chronic high dose usage may produce a withdrawal syndrome characterised by anorexia, irritability, insomnia and restlessness, 'hot flashes', sweating and hiccups, most often compared with a bout of influenza.

Lysergic acid diethylamide (LSD) does not produce a withdrawal syndrome, but recreational or repeated use may produce a 'bad trip' characterised by visual hallucinations, perceptual distortions and intense emotions of a frightening and unpleasant nature. Long after use of the drug a 'flashback' recurrence of part or all of the original LSD experience may occur with subjective distress similar to a panic attack.

Usage of cocaine or amphetamines may precipitate a 'stimulant psychosis', which is indistinguishable from acute paranoid schizophrenia and is characterised by paranoia and persecutory delusions in clear consciousness, together with ideas of reference and auditory or visual hallucinations. These symptoms remit with rest, sedation and the absence of further use of the offending drug. Post-withdrawal depression may require antidepressant treatment.

PS-C45   CORRECT RESPONSE A

The correct answer to this question is **rhinorrhoea.**

If a narcotic drug is suddenly withdrawn or antagonised by parenteral naloxone, there is a period of rebound hyperactivity of previously suppressed functions while the person adjusts to this drug-free state. In opiate withdrawal, there is rebound hyperactivity of the catecholaminergic and serotonergic systems, which are directly or indirectly responsible for most of the subjectively unpleasant experiences of going 'cold turkey'.

The features of withdrawal syndrome are broadly similar across all the natural and synthetic opiates, although the time course of the withdrawal syndrome varies according to the duration of action of the particular opiate. Classic symptoms include abdominal cramps, nausea, diarrhoea, goose flesh, sweating, sleeplessness, irritability, rhinorrhoea, excessive lachrymation and uncontrollable yawning. The severity of the withdrawal syndrome increases up to a peak at approximately 36–48 h, following which there is a gradual decline in severity of symptomatology down to a baseline level of ongoing distress during the protracted withdrawal syndrome. The flawed hero of Irvine Welsh's novel, *Trainspotting*, describes graphically the subjective misery of heroin withdrawal.

Detoxification may be attenuated by using steadily reducing doses of oral methadone linctus or oral clonidine. With clonidine, mild dizziness from postural hypotension and insomnia are common side effects, but clonidine is reduced rapidly after a few days.

PS-C46   CORRECT RESPONSE E

The correct answer to this question is **all of the above disorders.**

Electroconvulsive therapy (ECT) is a procedure in which generalised seizures lasting 25–150 s by the passage of an electric current through the brain under general anaesthesia and muscle relaxation are used for therapeutic purposes. A seizure must occur for ECT to be effective. There is no evidence that ECT is effective because it is perceived as a punishment or that it enhances repression by causing confusion. Modern ECT practice is neither painful nor threatening.

Electroconvulsive therapy is not effective in chronic schizophrenia, but can *be quite beneficial in patients with recent onset of schizophrenia* especially when characterised by depressive delusions, delusions of control and reference, perplexity and suicidal thoughts. Paradoxically, depression that is secondary to schizophrenia is not as responsive to ECT. Concurrent antipsychotic medication may potentiate the benefits of ECT in patients with acute schizophrenia.

A small number of ECT treatments often reverse *catatonic stupor.* Catatonia is a non-specific symptom that can occur in mood disorders, schizophrenia, cognitive disorders, medical and neurological disorders and various combinations of each of these disorders. Electroconvulsive therapy is effective regardless of the diagnosis or aetiology of the syndrome. Electroconvulsive therapy is also the most rapidly effective treatment for lethal catatonia, a syndrome aggravated by antipsychotics and associated with neurological signs, cardiovascular collapse, coma and increased serum levels of creatinine kinase, catecholamines and cortisol.

Electroconvulsive therapy is at least as effective as lithium in the treatment of mania and particularly so in patients with *lithium-resistant manic episodes.* Clinical experience suggests that bilateral ECT is more effective in this condition.

The primary indication for ECT is major depression. It is usually considered when medication cannot be tolerated or may be dangerous, but it is the treatment of choice for severely depressed patients who require a rapid response because of high suicide or homicide risk, extreme agitation, inanition or stupor. Electroconvulsive therapy is also appropriate for some *puerperal depressive disorders* when it is important that the mother should return quickly to the care of her baby.

Electroconvulsive therapy may also be used in cycloid psychoses and various atypical psychoses. Some clinicians have reported that ECT has been successful in severe forms of obsessive–compulsive disorders, anorexia nervosa, chronic pain disorders and some forms of delirium. These disorders are not usually regarded as an indication for ECT.

Electroconvulsive therapy may also be used in lethal catatonia and Parkinson disease, but is NOT an effective treatment for dysthymia, substance abuse, personality disorder, anxiety disorders or hypochondriasis.

PS-C47   CORRECT RESPONSE D

The correct answer is *discharge to community based alternatives to hospitalisation.*

Prior to the 1960s there were virtually no alternatives to the care and treatment of patients with serious mental illnesses outside large mental hospitals. The rehabilitation facilities that existed were hospital-based and it was politically expedient in terms of service cost to 'warehouse' patients in large institutions. Psychiatrists and nursing staff were long accustomed to working and living their professional lives in a rigid hierarchy where they enjoyed considerable power and prestige.

By the early 1960s, many Western countries were undergoing significant social and philosophical changes with a new-found emphasis on freedom, individual rights, the removal of legal and bureaucratic restrictions and a challenge to the hospital-based power of psychiatrists. Funding became available for pilot programs for community based treatment, rehabilitation and accommodation alternatives and the social and community psychiatry movement developed. The motivation for health departments and governments to move patients to the community was not entirely altruistic, as it enabled reductions in the staffing and size of hospitals and hence the costs of running the mental health system were reduced. Deinstitutionalisation became internationally popular as a cost-saving measure, but frequently at the expense of the quantity and quality of patient care.

The availability of effective psychopharmacological treatments such as chlorpromazine, imipramine and lithium contributed to the discharge of patients from mental hospitals, but they only accelerated the movement which had already begun. A common problem noted in long-stay mental hospital patients was apathy, which was falsely attributed to their prolonged hospitalisation. It was assumed that a return to independent community living would abolish this symptom, but it soon became clear that apathy was a major negative consequence of chronic schizophrenia and that major resources were needed to manage apathetic patients in community settings.

In Australia, there is a patchy network of community based resources and alternatives to hospital-based psychiatric services. Most of the large psychiatric hospitals throughout the country have either been significantly reduced in size or closed altogether, at the insistence of various governments and health departments, over the objections of patients, relatives and mental health professionals. Psychiatric units have been decentralised and are now often based in general hospitals. Hostels, halfway houses, independent community living group homes and various other forms of supported accommodation have been established, but demand far exceeds supply. Living skills centres, community rehabilitation workshops and drop-in centres have slowly developed, but generally they are understaffed and under-resourced and based in large cities. Services in country areas and smaller cities and towns are non-existent.

There have been no studies that have conclusively shown patients are better off or happier living in the community. There is no evidence that the wider, non-mentally ill community cares about the fate and welfare of people with mental illness.

The other alternative answers to this question were clearly incorrect and bear no relevance to deinstitutionalisation.

PS-C48   CORRECT RESPONSE D

Transference, in the context of a therapeutic relationship, refers to *the feelings a patient may have about a doctor or therapist based on the patient's childhood relationships.*

The relationship between a doctor or therapist and a patient is present from the start of any therapy and becomes more important as treatment lasts longer or is carried out more frequently, or is more intense. In most forms of psychotherapy this relationship forms the cornerstone of treatment, helping to sustain the patient through difficulties and to motivate him or her to overcome problems.

The 'therapeutic alliance' is the ordinarily good relationship that any two people need to have in cooperating over some joint task. In the medical context, it means establishing a good rapport with a patient. It is fostered by friendliness, courtesy, reliability and a willingness to actively listen to a patient's problems. It is the conscious, realistic component of any treatment relationship.

As treatment progresses, unrealistic or unconscious elements are superimposed on the relationship. Patients may begin to experience feelings towards the doctor or therapist as if he or she were a significant figure from the patient's past. The intimacy of the situation causes the patient to transfer to the doctor or therapist feelings or attitudes originally experienced in other important previous relationships, usually parents, but also siblings, grandparents, teachers or childhood heroes. This is transference.

When the doctor/therapist is perceived to be a good figure and feelings of hope, trust and love are generated, the transference is positive. When the feelings generated are anger, mistrust or hate, the transference is negative.

A doctor is expected to remain an impartial professional and yet display genuine concern about the most intimate personal problems of patients. Despite training and supervision, it is not always possible to balance detachment and concern, and the doctor may displace onto patients his or her own fantasies, feelings and attitudes related to other important figures in the doctor's life. This process is countertransference.

PS-C49   CORRECT RESPONSE B

The correct answer is that reassurance *should only be offered when the patient's concerns have been fully understood and investigated.*

Reassurance is one of the basic elements of supportive psychotherapy in patients with chronic illness for whom cure or basic change are not seen as realistic goals. The aims of supportive counselling are:

- the promotion of the patient's best possible psychological, social and occupational functioning;
- the bolstering of self-confidence and self-esteem;
- the promotion of the patient's contact with reality;
- the prevention of relapse;
- the transfer of support from the professional to family, friends and self-help or support groups.

The mere act of active and concerned listening, paying attention and responding to verbal and non-verbal cues, enabling the patient to fully explain his or her problems and difficulties and emphasising the here and now can result in significant relief of distress.

The key elements of supportive counselling, apart from active listening, include explanation and direct advice and guidance, given in uncomplicated, non-technical language (perhaps supplemented by writing important points down and the use of handouts), the ventilation of feelings, such as anger, frustration and despair, and reassurance.

Reassurance is valuable, but premature reassurance given before the patient has fully explained the situation can destroy the patient's confidence in you as a therapist. False reassurance is equally damaging. It may be effective initially, but will eventually prove fruitless because of the loss of basic trust upon which all treatment depends.

PS-C50   CORRECT RESPONSE D

The correct answer to the question is *that HIV antibody testing should not be performed routinely on patients, but only after obtaining their informed consent and after appropriate pretest counselling.*

The knowledge that one's HIV status is positive can be completely devastating to a person who is unprepared and unsuspecting. The critical interview must be handled with tact and sensitivity by a skilled and experienced counsellor and be followed up by ongoing psychotherapeutic support and appropriate information. These aspects assume even greater importance if the test has been performed without the patient's knowledge and consent.

All patients have a right to privacy and an assurance of confidentiality. It is a serious breach of confidentiality to inform other patients of this man's HIV status and may attract a complaint of misconduct if it was done maliciously and wilfully. There is no need for this man to be nursed in a separate, sterile area of the ward unless he has a coincident infectious disease which requires isolation in its own right.

Lithium carbonate does not lower immunity to infection and whether this man should have AZT at this stage may be debatable. There is current controversy about the use of AZT alone in patients with HIV infection.

The human immunodeficiency virus may cause a leucoencephalopathy as part of late stage AIDS, which may present as an affective disorder with either manic or depressive symptoms.

PS-C51 CORRECT RESPONSE A

The only correct answer to this question is that *sexual relationships between doctors and patients are prohibited by medical codes of practice*, including the Hippocratic oath. An official policy statement issued by the NSW Medical Board in 1992 in relation to Medical Practitioners and Sexual Misconduct is representative of Australian Practice Standards and affirms that:

> It is an absolute rule that a medical practitioner who engages in sexual activity with a current patient is guilty of professional misconduct.

While not detracting from the fundamental impropriety of such activity, the sanction applied, as a result of a finding of misconduct, may vary according to the circumstances of each case. Factors to be considered include the degree of dependence in the (particular) doctor–patient relationship, evidence of exploitation, the duration of the professional relationship and the nature of the medical services provided.

The rule refers to current patients. Although the termination of the doctor–patient relationship prior to sexual activity may be raised as a defence, its strength will be dictated by the factors referred to in the preceding paragraph, as well as by the time lapse after the end of the professional relationship. (There is currently no generally accepted 'waiting period' after which sexual relations can be commenced with former patients, thus escaping professional censure.)

This rationale has been supported in many other contexts by medical disciplinary authorities. Reasons for the rule include the following.

- the doctor–patient relationship depends on the patient having absolute confidence and trust in the doctor;
- the doctor is in a unique position regarding physical and emotional proximity: patients are expected to disrobe and to allow doctors to examine them intimately;
- the doctor–patient relationship is not one of equality: in seeking treatment, the patient is vulnerable. Exploitation of a patient is an abuse of power;
- breaches of the doctor–patient relationship have often caused severe psychological damage to the patient;
- the community expectation of the medical professional is one of utmost integrity. The community must be confident that personal boundaries will be maintained and that patients are not at risk;
- improper sexual conduct by doctors brings community censure and damages the credibility of the medical profession as a whole;
- the onus is on the doctor to behave in a professional manner. It is unacceptable to seek to blame the patient if a sexual relationship develops (most such relationships are initiated by doctors, not patients);
- personal involvement with the patient will often lead to a clouding of clinical judgement and the risk of peer condemnation and professional isolation.

The view that changing social standards require a less stringent approach is rejected. The nature of the professional doctor–patient relationship must be one of absolute confidence and trust. It transcends social values and no standard other than the highest can be acceptable.

ANNOTATED MULTIPLE CHOICE QUESTIONS

SUMMARY OF CORRECT RESPONSES

CATEGORY & QUESTION NO.	CORRECT RESPONSE	CATEGORY & QUESTION NO.	CORRECT RESPONSE	CATEGORY & QUESTION NO.	CORRECT RESPONSE
PS-Q 1	D	PS-Q 18	D	PS-Q 35	E
PS-Q 2	C	PS-Q 19	A	PS-Q 36	D
PS-Q 3	A	PS-Q 20	A	PS-Q 37	D
PS-Q 4	C	PS-Q 21	E	PS-Q 38	E
PS-Q 5	E	PS-Q 22	D	PS-Q 39	D
PS-Q 6	D	PS-Q 23	A	PS-Q 40	D
PS-Q 7	C	PS-Q 24	A	PS-Q 41	D
PS-Q 8	B	PS-Q 25	D	PS-Q 42	C
PS-Q 9	C	PS-Q 26	D	PS-Q 43	A
PS-Q 10	C	PS-Q 27	E	PS-Q 44	C
PS-Q 11	C	PS-Q 28	D	PS-Q 45	A
PS-Q 12	C	PS-Q 29	C	PS-Q 46	E
PS-Q 13	A	PS-Q 30	E	PS-Q 47	D
PS-Q 14	D	PS-Q 31	C	PS-Q 48	D
PS-Q 15	A	PS-Q 32	D	PS-Q 49	B
PS-Q 16	E	PS-Q 33	E	PS-Q 50	D
PS-Q 17	C	PS-Q 34	E	PS-Q 51	A

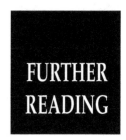

FURTHER
READING

Suggested Textbooks

There are many medical textbooks available and most of them are of high standard. They range from quite short texts, which cover essential knowledge, to long and comprehensive treatises which most people use as reference books. The AMC has drawn up the following list, as a guide to some useful texts. They are not intended as prescribed reading.

Medicine

Andreoli TE. *Cecil Essentials of Medicine*, 4th edn. Saunders, Philadelphia, 1997. ISBN 0721666973.

Edwards C, Bouchier IA (eds). *Davidson's Principles and Practice of Medicine*, 17th edn. Livingstone, Edinburgh,1995. ISBN 0443049610.

Harrison TR. *Harrison's Principles of Internal Medicine*, 13th edn. Revised by KJ Isselbacher. McGraw, New York, 1994. ISBN 0070323704.

Larkins R. *Clinical Skills: The Medical Interview, Physical Examination and Assessment of the Patient's Problems*. Melbourne University Press, Melbourne, 1993. ISBN 0522844677 (paperback).

Lau LSW. *Imaging Guidelines*, 2nd edn. Reprint Victorian Medical Postgraduate Foundation Inc. and Royal Australasian College of Radiologists, Melbourne, 1995. ISBN 0646138936.

Schwartz GR. *Principles and Practice of Emergency Medicine*, 3rd edn. Lea & Febiger, Philadelphia, 1992. ISBN 081211373X.

Talley NJ, O'Connor S. *Clinical Examination: A Systematic Guide to Physical Diagnosis*, 3rd edn. Maclennan & Petty, Sydney, 1996. ISBN 0864331029 (paperback).

Speight M, Holford NHG (eds). *Avery's Drug Treatment: Principles and Practice of Clinical Pharmacology and Therapeutics*, 4th edn. Adis International, Auckland, 1997. ISBN 0864710364.

Weatherall DJ, Ledingham JGG, Warrell DA (eds). *Oxford Textbook of Medicine*, 3rd edn. Oxford University Press, New York, 1995. ISBN 0192621408.

Wyngaarden JB, Smith LH, Bennett C (eds). *Cecil Textbook of Medicine*, 19th edn. Saunders, Philadelphia, 1992. ISBN 0721629318 (set).

Surgery

Clunie GJA, Tjandra JJ, Francis DMA. *Textbook of Surgery*. Blackwell Science Asia, Melbourne, 1997. ISBN 0 86793 353 4.

Forrest AP. *Principles and Practice of Surgery — A Surgical Supplement to Davidson's Principles and Practice of Medicine*, 3rd edn. Churchill Livingstone, Edinburgh, 1995. ISBN 0443048606.

Hunt PS, Marshall VC. *Clinical Problems in General Surgery*. Butterworths, Sydney, 1991. ISBN 0409492132.

Scott PR. *An Aid to Clinical Surgery*, 5th edn. Churchill Livingstone, Edinburgh, 1994. ISBN 0443045666.

Morris PJ, Malt RA. *Oxford Textbook of Surgery*. Oxford University Press, New York, 1994. ISBN 0192618008 (two volume set).

Paediatrics

Hull D, Johnston D. *Essential Paediatrics*, 3rd edn. Churchill Livingstone, Edinburgh, 1993. ISBN 0443047820.

Robinson MJ, Roberton DM. *Practical Paediatrics*, 3rd edn. Churchill Livingstone, Melbourne, 1994. ISBN 044304869X.

Obstetrics and Gynaecology

Beischer NA, Mackay EV. *Obstetrics and the Newborn: An Illustrated Text,* 2nd edn. WB Saunders, Sydney, 1986. ISBN 003900242X.

Llewellyn-Jones D. *Fundamentals of Obstetrics and Gynaecology. Volume 1 Obstetrics. Volume II Gynaecology,* 6th edn (combined volume). Mosby, London, 1994. ISBN 0723420009.

Mackay EV, Beischer NA, Pepperell R, Wood C. *Illustrated Textbook of Gynaecology*, 2nd edn. WB Saunders, Sydney, 1992. ISBN 0729512118.

Psychiatry

Gelder M, Gath D, Mayou R. *The Oxford Textbook of Psychiatry*, 3rd edn. Oxford University Press, 1996. ISBN 0192625012 (paperback); ISBN 0192662504 (hardback).

American Psychiatric Association. *DSM-IV: Diagnostic and Statistical Manual of Mental Disorders*, 4th edn. American Psychiatric Association, Washington DC, 1994. ISBN 0890420629 (paperback); ISBN 0890420610 (hardback).

Miscellaneous

Guidelines from Victorian Medical Postgraduate Foundation Therapeutics Committee.

'Analgesic Guidelines', 2nd edition, 1992
'Antibiotic Guidelines', 9th edition, 1996
'Cardiovascular Drug Guidelines', 2nd edition, 1995
'Gastrointestinal Drug Guidelines', 1st edition, 1994
'Psychotropic Drug Guidelines', 3rd edition, 1996
'Respiratory Drug Guidelines', 1st edition, 1994

Manual of Use and Interpretation of Pathology Tests, 2nd edn. The Royal College of Pathologists of Australasia, 1977. ISBN 0959335528.

MIMS Australia, Bi-monthly or Annual Subscription

Journals

In addition to the major texts, journals should be read selectively, using editorials, annotations and review articles. The following journals are suggested as source material: *Australian Family Physician, Australian Prescriber, British Medical Journal, British Journal of Hospital Medicine, Current Therapeutics, Lancet, Medical Journal of Australia, New England Journal of Medicine.*

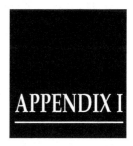
SUMMARY OF QUESTION CLASSIFICATIONS SHOWING FUNCTIONS AND SYSTEMS

KEYS AND DESCRIPTORS

Discipline

ME — Medicine
SU — Surgery
PA — Paediatrics
OG — Obstetrics and Gynaecology
PS — Psychiatry

Function/process

A   Aetiology, epidemiology, genetics
B   Anatomy, physiology, pathology, pathogenesis
C   Clinical manifestations
D   Diagnosis and investigations
E   Treatment and prevention of disease
F   Complications and outcome
G   Ethical, legal, social, economic, humanistic, historical aspects

Systems/regions/subspecialties

1   Integument/dermatology
2   Head and neck/eye/ENT
3   Nervous system/neurology
4   Musculoskeletal/orthopaedics/rheumatology
5   Circulatory system/heart/vessels
6   Respiratory system/lungs/chest wall
7   Gastrointestinal system/abdomen/abdominal wall
8   Breast/endocrine system
9   Reproductive system (male/female)
10 Haemopoietic system/haematology/blood/blood products
11 Renal system/urology
12 Mental state/intellectual function/behavioural problems
13 Major psychiatric disorders/drug and alcohol abuse
14 Developmental abnormalities
15 Nutrition/metabolism
16 Infectious diseases
17 Clinical pharmacology
18 Clinical oncology
19 Clinical immunology
20 Critical care/anaesthesia
21 Community medicine/public health

CATEGORY & QUESTION NO.	FUNCTION CODE	SYSTEM CODE: PRINCIPAL CLASSIFICATION	CATEGORY & QUESTION NO.	FUNCTION CODE	SYSTEM CODE: PRINCIPAL CLASSIFICATION
ME-Q 1	E	1	ME-Q 35	E	4
ME-Q 2	C	1	ME-Q 36	B	5
ME-Q 3	E	1	ME-Q 37	C	5
ME-Q 4	E	1	ME-Q 38	C	5
ME-Q 5	E	1, 19	ME-Q 39	D	5
ME-Q 6	A	2, 14	ME-Q 40	E	5
ME-Q 7	C	2, 8	ME-Q 41	E	5
ME-Q 8	C	2	ME-Q 42	B	5
ME-Q 9	F	2	ME-Q 43	B	5
ME-Q 10	C	2	ME-Q 44	B	5
ME-Q 11	C	3	ME-Q 45	C	6
ME-Q 12	C	3	ME-Q 46	C	6
ME-Q 13	C	3	ME-Q 47	B	6
ME-Q 14	E	3	ME-Q 48	B	6
ME-Q 15	C	3	ME-Q 49	B	6
ME-Q 16	D	3	ME-Q 50	C	6
ME-Q 17	A	3	ME-Q 51	B	6
ME-Q 18	A	3	ME-Q 52	B	6
ME-Q 19	C	3	ME-Q 53	C	6
ME-Q 20	A	3	ME-Q 54	D	6
ME-Q 21	C	3	ME-Q 55	D	6
ME-Q 22	E	3, 4	ME-Q 56	D	6
ME-Q 23	C	2, 4	ME-Q 57	C	6, 16
ME-Q 24	C	3, 4	ME-Q 58	C	6, 16
ME-Q 25	C	3, 4	ME-Q 59	D	6, 16
ME-Q 26	B	3	ME-Q 60	D	6, 16
ME-Q 27	B	3	ME-Q 61	E	6
ME-Q 28	E	3, 17	ME-Q 62	C	6
ME-Q 29	C	4	ME-Q 63	E	6
ME-Q 30	D	4	ME-Q 64	E	6, 16
ME-Q 31	C	4	ME-Q 65	B	7
ME-Q 32	C	4	ME-Q 66	C	7
ME-Q 33	D	4	ME-Q 67	E	7
ME-Q 34	D	4	ME-Q 68	D	7

CATEGORY & QUESTION NO.	FUNCTION CODE	SYSTEM CODE: PRINCIPAL CLASSIFICATION
ME-Q 69	B	7
ME-Q 70	F	7
ME-Q 71	C	7
ME-Q 72	A	7, 16
ME-Q 73	E	7
ME-Q 74	C	7
ME-Q 75	A	7
ME-Q 76	B	7
ME-Q 77	D	7
ME-Q 78	C	7
ME-Q 79	D	7
ME-Q 80	A	7
ME-Q 81	C	7
ME-Q 82	C	8
ME-Q 83	C	8
ME-Q 84	D	8
ME-Q 85	B	8
ME-Q 86	B	8
ME-Q 87	C	10
ME-Q 88	D	10
ME-Q 89	D	10
ME-Q 90	D	10
ME-Q 91	A	10
ME-Q 92	A	10
ME-Q 93	D	10
ME-Q 94	E	10
ME-Q 95	E	10
ME-Q 96	D	10
ME-Q 97	B	11
ME-Q 98	D	11
ME-Q 99	D	15
ME-Q 100	E	11
ME-Q 101	D	11
ME-Q 102	E	11

CATEGORY & QUESTION NO.	FUNCTION CODE	SYSTEM CODE: PRINCIPAL CLASSIFICATION
ME-Q 103	C	11
ME-Q 104	F	15
ME-Q 105	D	16
ME-Q 106	C	16
ME-Q 107	A	16
ME-Q 108	D	16
ME-Q 109	A	16
ME-Q 110	A	16
ME-Q 111	C	16
ME-Q 112	B	17
ME-Q 113	E	17
ME-Q 114	E	17
ME-Q 115	B	17
ME-Q 116	A	17
ME-Q 117	B	17
ME-Q 118	E	17
ME-Q 119	F	17
ME-Q 120	D	17
ME-Q 121	F	17
ME-Q 122	E	17
ME-Q 123	E	19
ME-Q 124	B	19
ME-Q 125	B	19
ME-Q 126	A	1, 3
ME-Q 127	E	1
ME-Q 128	F	1
ME-Q 129	B	3
ME-Q 130	B	3
ME-Q 131	E	3
ME-Q 132	C	3
ME-Q 133	C	3
ME-Q 134	C	3
ME-Q 135	F	3
ME-Q 136	C	3

CATEGORY & QUESTION NO.	FUNCTION CODE	SYSTEM CODE: PRINCIPAL CLASSIFICATION
ME-Q 137	B	3
ME-Q 138	E	3
ME-Q 139	B	3
ME-Q 140	B	3
ME-Q 141	B	3
ME-Q 142	E	3, 17
ME-Q 143	E	3, 17
ME-Q 144	C	4
ME-Q 145	C	4
ME-Q 146	D	4
ME-Q 147	C	5
ME-Q 148	C	5
ME-Q 149	B	5
ME-Q 150	E	5
ME-Q 151	E	5
ME-Q 152	E	5
ME-Q 153	E	5
ME-Q 154	E	5
ME-Q 155	E	5
ME-Q 156	E	5
ME-Q 157	C	5
ME-Q 158	E	5
ME-Q 159	E	5
ME-Q 160	E	5
ME-Q 161	E	5
ME-Q 162	D	6
ME-Q 163	B	6
ME-Q 164	B	6
ME-Q 165	C	6
ME-Q 166	D	6
ME-Q 167	C	6
ME-Q 168	C	6
ME-Q 169	C	6
ME-Q 170	E	6

CATEGORY & QUESTION NO.	FUNCTION CODE	SYSTEM CODE: PRINCIPAL CLASSIFICATION
ME-Q 171	B	7
ME-Q 172	B	7
ME-Q 173	A	7
ME-Q 174	E	7
ME-Q 175	D	7
ME-Q 176	E	18
ME-Q 177	B	7
ME-Q 178	B	8
ME-Q 179	D	8
ME-Q 180	B	8
ME-Q 181	D	8
ME-Q 182	D	8
ME-Q 183	F	9
ME-Q 184	F	9
ME-Q 185	D	10
ME-Q 186	C	11
ME-Q 187	A	14
ME-Q 188	D	15
ME-Q 189	E	16
ME-Q 190	D	16
ME-Q 191	A	16
ME-Q 192	C	17
ME-Q 193	E	17
ME-Q 194	E	17
ME-Q 195	F	17
ME-Q 196	F	17
ME-Q 197	F	17
ME-Q 198	E	17
ME-Q 199	F	17
ME-Q 200	E	18
ME-Q 201	F	19
ME-Q 202	C	19
ME-Q 203	D	19
ME-Q 204	D	19
ME-Q 205	C	19

CATEGORY & QUESTION NO.	FUNCTION CODE	SYSTEM CODE: PRINCIPAL CLASSIFICATION
SU-Q 1	A	1
SU-Q 2	E	1
SU-Q 3	E	1
SU-Q 4	C	1
SU-Q 5	D	1
SU-Q 6	C	1
SU-Q 7	C	1
SU-Q 8	C	1
SU-Q 9	F	1
SU-Q 10	A	1
SU-Q 11	C	1
SU-Q 12	C	2
SU-Q 13	D	2
SU-Q 14	B	2
SU-Q 15	D	2
SU-Q 16	C	2
SU-Q 17	D	2
SU-Q 18	C	2
SU-Q 19	C	2
SU-Q 20	C	3
SU-Q 21	C	3
SU-Q 22	C	3
SU-Q 23	C	3
SU-Q 24	C	3
SU-Q 25	B	3
SU-Q 26	C	4
SU-Q 27	C	4
SU-Q 28	C	4
SU-Q 29	C	4
SU-Q 30	F	4
SU-Q 31	C	4
SU-Q 32	D	4
SU-Q 33	C	4
SU-Q 34	C	4

CATEGORY & QUESTION NO.	FUNCTION CODE	SYSTEM CODE: PRINCIPAL CLASSIFICATION
SU-Q 35	D	4
SU-Q 36	C	5
SU-Q 37	D	5
SU-Q 38	C	5
SU-Q 39	F	5
SU-Q 40	F	5
SU-Q 41	F	5
SU-Q 42	C	5
SU-Q 43	C	5
SU-Q 44	C	5
SU-Q 45	D	5
SU-Q 46	D	5
SU-Q 47	E	6
SU-Q 48	F	6
SU-Q 49	F	6
SU-Q 50	D	7
SU-Q 51	E	7
SU-Q 52	D	7
SU-Q 53	D	7
SU-Q 54	F	7
SU-Q 55	C	7
SU-Q 56	E	7
SU-Q 57	C	7
SU-Q 58	E	7
SU-Q 59	C	7
SU-Q 60	D	7
SU-Q 61	C	7
SU-Q 62	C	7
SU-Q 63	D	7
SU-Q 64	D	7
SU-Q 65	D	7
SU-Q 66	D	7
SU-Q 67	D	7
SU-Q 68	F	7

CATEGORY & QUESTION NO.	FUNCTION CODE	SYSTEM CODE: PRINCIPAL CLASSIFICATION	CATEGORY & QUESTION NO.	FUNCTION CODE	SYSTEM CODE: PRINCIPAL CLASSIFICATION
SU-Q 69	F	7	SU-Q 103	C	18
SU-Q 70	C	7	SU-Q 104	C	18
SU-Q 71	C	7	SU-Q 105	E	18
SU-Q 72	B	7	SU-Q 106	B	18
SU-Q 73	F	7	SU-Q 107	E	20
SU-Q 74	D	7	SU-Q 108	C	1
SU-Q 75	C	7	SU-Q 109	B	1
SU-Q 76	C	7	SU-Q 110	C	1
SU-Q 77	C	8	SU-Q 111	C	1
SU-Q 78	E	8	SU-Q 112	C	2
SU-Q 79	C	8	SU-Q 113	C	2
SU-Q 80	C	8	SU-Q 114	C	2
SU-Q 81	C	9	SU-Q 115	B	2
SU-Q 82	E	9	SU-Q 116	C	2
SU-Q 83	C	9	SU-Q 117	A	2
SU-Q 84	D	10	SU-Q 118	C	3
SU-Q 85	C	10	SU-Q 119	C	3
SU-Q 86	D	10	SU-Q 120	C	3
SU-Q 87	C	10	SU-Q 121	C	3
SU-Q 88	D	11	SU-Q 122	C	3
SU-Q 89	D	11	SU-Q 123	C	4
SU-Q 90	D	11	SU-Q 124	C	4
SU-Q 91	E	11	SU-Q 125	C	4
SU-Q 92	C	11	SU-Q 126	C	5
SU-Q 93	B	15	SU-Q 127	D	5
SU-Q 94	E	15	SU-Q 128	B	5
SU-Q 95	E	15	SU-Q 129	C	5
SU-Q 96	B	15	SU-Q 130	C	5
SU-Q 97	E	16	SU-Q 131	C	6
SU-Q 98	E	16	SU-Q 132	C	7
SU-Q 99	C	16	SU-Q 133	A	7
SU-Q 100	F	16	SU-Q 134	C	7
SU-Q 101	B	18	SU-Q 135	C	7
SU-Q 102	C	18	SU-Q 136	C	7

CATEGORY & QUESTION NO.	FUNCTION CODE	SYSTEM CODE: PRINCIPAL CLASSIFICATION
SU-Q 137	F	7
SU-Q 138	D	7
SU-Q 139	B	7
SU-Q 140	C	7
SU-Q 141	C	7
SU-Q 142	D	7
SU-Q 143	A	7
SU-Q 144	D	7
SU-Q 145	C	7
SU-Q 146	B	7
SU-Q 147	A	7
SU-Q 148	A	7
SU-Q 149	C	7
SU-Q 150	C	7
SU-Q 151	C	7
SU-Q 152	C	7
SU-Q 153	C	7
SU-Q 154	C	7
SU-Q 155	C	7
SU-Q 156	C	7
SU-Q 157	C	8
SU-Q 158	B	8
SU-Q 159	C	8
SU-Q 160	E	8
SU-Q 161	C	8
SU-Q 162	C	9
SU-Q 163	B	9
SU-Q 164	B	10
SU-Q 165	C	10
SU-Q 166	D	10
SU-Q 167	C	10
SU-Q 168	C	10
SU-Q 169	A	10
SU-Q 170	B	11

CATEGORY & QUESTION NO.	FUNCTION CODE	SYSTEM CODE: PRINCIPAL CLASSIFICATION
SU-Q 171	B	11
SU-Q 172	D	11
SU-Q 173	B	11
SU-Q 174	C	11
SU-Q 175	C	11
SU-Q 176	E	15
SU-Q 177	F	15
SU-Q 178	B	15
SU-Q 179	B	16
SU-Q 180	E	16
SU-Q 181	C	16
SU-Q 182	B	16
SU-Q 183	E	16
SU-Q 184	F	17
SU-Q 185	C	18
SU-Q 186	F	19
SU-Q 187	E	20

CATEGORY & QUESTION NO.	FUNCTION CODE	SYSTEM CODE: PRINCIPAL CLASSIFICATION
PA-Q 1	E	1
PA-Q 2	C	2
PA-Q 3	E	2
PA-Q 4	C	3
PA-Q 5	E	3
PA-Q 6	F	3
PA-Q 7	C	3
PA-Q 8	E	3
PA-Q 9	C	3
PA-Q 10	A	4
PA-Q 11	C	4
PA-Q 12	C	4
PA-Q 13	C	4
PA-Q 14	E	5
PA-Q 15	C	5
PA-Q 16	E	5
PA-Q 17	E	5
PA-Q 18	C	1
PA-Q 19	F	6
PA-Q 20	B	6, 16
PA-Q 21	C	6
PA-Q 22	D	6
PA-Q 23	C	6
PA-Q 24	C	6
PA-Q 25	D	6
PA-Q 26	E	7
PA-Q 27	C	7
PA-Q 28	E	7
PA-Q 29	C	7
PA-Q 30	F	7
PA-Q 31	D	7
PA-Q 32	D	7
PA-Q 33	C	7
PA-Q 34	C	7

CATEGORY & QUESTION NO.	FUNCTION CODE	SYSTEM CODE: PRINCIPAL CLASSIFICATION
PA-Q 35	E	7
PA-Q 36	C	7
PA-Q 37	C	7
PA-Q 38	A	7
PA-Q 39	E	7
PA-Q 40	C	8
PA-Q 41	C	9
PA-Q 42	C	10
PA-Q 43	C	10
PA-Q 44	C	10
PA-Q 45	E	10
PA-Q 46	F	11
PA-Q 47	C	11
PA-Q 48	E	11
PA-Q 49	C	11
PA-Q 50	E	14
PA-Q 51	C	14
PA-Q 52	D	14
PA-Q 53	F	14
PA-Q 54	C	15
PA-Q 55	C	15, 20
PA-Q 56	C	14
PA-Q 57	D	14
PA-Q 58	D	14
PA-Q 59	A	20
PA-Q 60	C	15
PA-Q 61	C	15
PA-Q 62	C	15
PA-Q 63	E	15
PA-Q 64	E	14
PA-Q 65	F	15
PA-Q 66	B	16
PA-Q 67	B	16
PA-Q 68	B	16

CATEGORY & QUESTION NO.	FUNCTION CODE	SYSTEM CODE: PRINCIPAL CLASSIFICATION
PA-Q 69	E	16
PA-Q 70	C	16
PA-Q 71	C	16, 2
PA-Q 72	G	16, 7
PA-Q 73	A	16
PA-Q 74	C	16
PA-Q 75	C	16
PA-Q 76	C	16
PA-Q 77	A	16
PA-Q 78	E	16
PA-Q 79	E	16
PA-Q 80	C	16
PA-Q 81	D	16
PA-Q 82	A	16
PA-Q 83	D	16, 17
PA-Q 84	A	18
PA-Q 85	C	18
PA-Q 86	G	21

CATEGORY & QUESTION NO.	FUNCTION CODE	SYSTEM CODE: PRINCIPAL CLASSIFICATION
OG-Q 1	C	9
OG-Q 2	C	9
OG-Q 3	C	11
OG-Q 4	C	11
OG-Q 5	C	16
OG-Q 6	C	16
OG-Q 7	C	16
OG-Q 8	A	9
OG-Q 9	E	9, 7
OG-Q 10	D	9, 7
OG-Q 11	D	9, 7
OG-Q 12	C	9, 7
OG-Q 13	F	9, 7
OG-Q 14	E	9
OG-Q 15	C	9
OG-Q 16	F	9, 19
OG-Q 17	C	9
OG-Q 18	B	9
OG-Q 19	C	9
OG-Q 20	A	9
OG-Q 21	D	9
OG-Q 22	D	9
OG-Q 23	E	9
OG-Q 24	C	20
OG-Q 25	E	20
OG-Q 26	E	9
OG-Q 27	D	9
OG-Q 28	D	9
OG-Q 29	E	9, 20
OG-Q 30	D	9
OG-Q 31	D	20
OG-Q 32	C	20
OG-Q 33	C	9
OG-Q 34	D	9

CATEGORY & QUESTION NO.	FUNCTION CODE	SYSTEM CODE: PRINCIPAL CLASSIFICATION
OG-Q 35	D	9
OG-Q 36	E	9
OG-Q 37	D	9
OG-Q 38	D	9
OG-Q 39	A	9
OG-Q 40	C	9
OG-Q 41	E	9
OG-Q 42	E	9, 13
OG-Q 43	E	9, 14
OG-Q 44	D	9, 14
OG-Q 45	E	9, 14
OG-Q 46	C	9, 14
OG-Q 47	C	9, 14
OG-Q 48	D	17
OG-Q 49	D	14
OG-Q 50	F	14
OG-Q 51	E	14
OG-Q 52	E	14
OG-Q 53	F	14
OG-Q 54	C	9
OG-Q 55	D	17
OG-Q 56	F	12, 15
OG-Q 57	C	1
OG-Q 58	E	9
OG-Q 59	F	9
OG-Q 60	C	9
OG-Q 61	D	9
OG-Q 62	D	20
OG-Q 63	D	9
OG-Q 64	E	8
OG-Q 65	D	8
OG-Q 66	D	8
OG-Q 67	E	9
OG-Q 68	F	9

CATEGORY & QUESTION NO.	FUNCTION CODE	SYSTEM CODE: PRINCIPAL CLASSIFICATION
OG-Q 69	D	9
OG-Q 70	C	9
OG-Q 71	D	8
OG-Q 72	D	9
OG-Q 73	E	17
OG-Q 74	D	9
OG-Q 75	E	9
OG-Q 76	D	9
OG-Q 77	E	9
OG-Q 78	B	9
OG-Q 79	F	9
OG-Q 80	E	16
OG-Q 81	E	16
OG-Q 82	F	16
OG-Q 83	C	9
OG-Q 84	D	9
OG-Q 85	D	9
OG-Q 86	D	9
OG-Q 87	D	9
OG-Q 88	D	9
OG-Q 89	C	18
OG-Q 90	D	18
OG-Q 91	D	9
OG-Q 92	D	9
OG-Q 93	E	11

CATEGORY & QUESTION NO.	FUNCTION CODE	SYSTEM CODE: PRINCIPAL CLASSIFICATION	CATEGORY & QUESTION NO.	FUNCTION CODE	SYSTEM CODE: PRINCIPAL CLASSIFICATION
PS-Q 1	D	12	PS-Q 35	A	13
PS-Q 2	D	13	PS-Q 36	D	13
PS-Q 3	F	13	PS-Q 37	D	13
PS-Q 4	D	13	PS-Q 38	E	13
PS-Q 5	E	13	PS-Q 39	E	13
PS-Q 6	E	13	PS-Q 40	C	13
PS-Q 7	C	13	PS-Q 41	D	12
PS-Q 8	D	3, 12	PS-Q 42	C	12
PS-Q 9	D	3, 13	PS-Q 43	C	16
PS-Q 10	C	3, 12	PS-Q 44	C	12
PS-Q 11	E	13	PS-Q 45	D	12
PS-Q 12	D	13	PS-Q 46	C	13
PS-Q 13	E	12	PS-Q 47	C	13
PS-Q 14	E	12	PS-Q 48	C	13
PS-Q 15	D	13	PS-Q 49	D	12
PS-Q 16	D	12	PS-Q 50	E	12, 16
PS-Q 17	F	13	PS-Q 51	E	12
PS-Q 18	D	12			
PS-Q 19	F	12			
PS-Q 20	C	13			
PS-Q 21	B	13			
PS-Q 22	A	12			
PS-Q 23	C	12			
PS-Q 24	C	12			
PS-Q 25	C	12			
PS-Q 26	A	12			
PS-Q 27	A	13			
PS-Q 28	C	9			
PS-Q 29	C	13			
PS-Q 30	C	13			
PS-Q 31	C	13			
PS-Q 32	C	13			
PS-Q 33	C	13			
PS-Q 34	C	12			

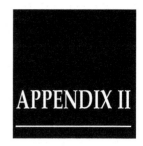

ALTERNATIVE MCQ FORMATS

Variations of MCQ formats include *extended matching questions*. Clinical vignettes require to be matched against a group of alternative diagnoses or tests, as shown below:

Uses of diagnostic imaging

After careful clinical assessment, it was felt that *further diagnostic imaging* was indicated for the following patients (Q1–22). Please select the **MOST APPROPRIATE INITIAL TEST** for each of these patients from the list (A–L) below. **Select ONE test only for each patient. Each test may provide the answer to more than one question.**

- **A** Conventional X-ray studies employing contrast media
- **B** Computed tomography (CT) scan with or without contrast media
- **C** Dual energy X-ray absorptiometry (DEXA) scan
- **D** Duplex–Doppler ultrasound
- **E** Imaging-guided biopsy
- **F** Mammography
- **G** Magnetic resonance imaging (MRI)
- **H** Nuclear medicine imaging (NMI)
- **I** Transrectal ultrasound (TRUS)
- **J** Transvaginal ultrasound (TVUS)
- **K** Ultrasound
- **L** Plain X-ray studies

Diagnostic imaging questions

Q1 A 40-year-old woman with suspected gall-bladder disease.

Q2 An 18-year-old cyclist who was hit by a car resulting in loss of consciousness. He is now drowsy and responds incoherently to questions. There are no focal neurological signs.

Q3 A 70-year-old man with a history of transient ischaemic attacks (TIA). On clinical examination, a loud carotid bruit was found on the left side.

Q4 A 45-year-old woman who last year had a wrist fracture following minor trauma. She also suffers from asthma, requiring long-term steroid therapy. In the past she had a hysterectomy and bilateral salpingo-oophorectomy.

Q5 A 32-year-old woman with multifocal neurological signs suggestive of demyelination. A CT scan was normal.

Q6 A 45-year-old woman who presents with the recent onset of a uninodular thyroid swelling. Examination reveals a 5 cm palpable nodule occupying most of the right lobe; no abnormality is felt in the rest of the gland. A needle aspirate (FNAC) has yielded a small amount of blood.

Q7 A middle-aged man with a painful swollen calf and thigh, suspected of suffering from deep venous thrombosis (DVT).

Q8 An 80-year-old patient with sudden onset of haemoptysis following total hip replacement 8 days earlier. The chest X-ray is normal.

Q9 A 20-year-old suffering from Crohn disease who presents with the finding of a palpable, tender swelling in the right iliac fossa.

Q10 A 40-year-old female patient presents with ill-defined right upper quadrant pain. Upper abdominal ultrasound revealed a 1 cm well-defined, solitary echogenic mass in the right lobe of the liver. The radiological provisional diagnosis is an incidental haemangioma.

Q11 A 35-year-old patient presenting with jaundice and abnormal liver function tests.

Q12 A 23-year-old man with recurrent haematuria and left-sided pain suggestive of renal colic. Plain films were taken and were unremarkable, as was an ultrasound assessment for a previous episode.

Q13 A 20-year-old woman with an irregular menstrual cycle whose last normal menstrual period (LNMP) was 6 weeks earlier. She thinks she may be pregnant. She presents with mild lower abdominal pain and spotting. Ultrasound of the abdomen and pelvis has failed to demonstrate an intrauterine gestational sac or an adnexal mass.

Q14 A 25-year-old-female with a readily palpable mass in the right breast.

Q15 A 40-year-old labourer with a chronically painful shoulder. Plain X-ray films were normal.

Q16 A 40-year-old man with an attack of acute low back pain precipitated by lifting, without any radiation. There are no clinical signs of nerve root impingement.

Q17 An 18-year-old Australian Football League footballer with persisting pain in the left forefoot. Plain X-ray films are reported as normal.

Q18 An 8-year-old girl with a proven urinary tract infection, her first such episode.

Q19 A 35-year-old male with a history of alcohol abuse presenting with central abdominal pain and distension. A provisional diagnosis of acute pancreatitis has been made.

Q20 A 65-year-old man found to have a mildly enlarged prostate on rectal examination. There was marked elevation of serum prostate-specific antigen (PSA).

Q21 A 50-year-old woman presents with an acute history of colicky abdominal pain, followed by vomiting, distension and constipation. She has a past history of abdominal hysterectomy for benign disease.

Q22 A 55-year-old woman has a mammogram (her first) within a mass screening programme. A focal cluster of branching microcalcifications is seen in the upper and outer quadrant of her right breast associated with increased parenchymal density 10 mm in diameter. The lesion is assessed as a possible early cancer, and can be seen on a recall ultrasound. No abnormality can be detected on clinical examination.

Answers to diagnostic imaging questions

A1   The correct answer is **K**.
Ultrasound is ideal for suspected gall-bladder stones, choledocholithiasis or cholecystitis. It can be used in patients who are vomiting, patients with peritonitis, and in pregnancy.

A2   The correct answer is **B**.
A *CT head scan* is indicated to exclude cerebral contusion or extracerebral collection. Plain film (skull X-ray) is a poor alternative and is **NOT** indicated if CT is available.

A3   The correct answer is **D**.
Duplex–Doppler ultrasound is used to assess the degree of carotid stenosis. Angiography is reserved for those patients with significant (usually >70%) stenosis who are considered suitable candidates for surgery.

A4   The correct answer is **C**.
Dual energy X-ray absorptiometry is used to diagnose and quantify the degree of osteoporosis in patients at risk, as after oophorectomy and steroid therapy.

A5   The correct answer is **G**.
Magnetic resonance imaging (MRI) is more sensitive than CT in detecting demyelinating plaques and stigmata of multiple sclerosis.

A6   The correct answer is **K**.
Ultrasound is used as the first imaging technique, to help diagnose the nature of the uninodular thyroid swelling, for example, recent haemorrhage into a colloid cyst or a solid solitary lesion. Ultrasound also helps determine whether the swelling is truly uninodular, or whether other impalpable nodules exist elsewhere, suggesting a dominant nodule in a multinodular goitre. If a solid lesion is demonstrated, further functional assessment with a radionuclide scan may be indicated. Independent of imaging results, aspiration cytology is the key diagnostic test in determining the requirement for surgery.

A7   The correct answer is **D**.
Duplex–Doppler ultrasound is non-invasive and accurate in diagnosing deep venous thrombosis (DVT), especially femoropopliteal DVT. When Doppler studies are unavailable or are indeterminate or equivocal, conventional venography is used.

A8   The correct answer is **H**.
The results of the prospective investigation of pulmonary embolism diagnosis (PIOPED) study confirm that *radionuclide scan (NMI)* is the key diagnostic procedure in diagnosing pulmonary embolism/infarction. A radionuclide scan will confirm or exclude the diagnosis in most cases. The perfusion study is performed after an intravenous injection of ^{99m}Tc-macroaggregated albumin. The ventilation scan involves the use of an aerosol of ^{99m}Tc-DTPA, sulphur colloid or ^{133}Xe. In a positive study, a perfusion defect is seen without a ventilation defect: a mismatched defect. 'Normal' and 'high probability' scans are reliable and can be used to make decisions regarding the use of anticoagulants. Patients with 'intermediate/ indeterminate' and 'low probability' scans require further confirmation with pulmonary angiography.

A9   The correct answer is **B**.
Computed tomography (CT) is better than ultrasound in assessing the iliac fossae due to the presence of bowel gas in this region which hinders ultrasound

study. A CT can diagnose bowel wall thickening in patients with inflammatory bowel disease and can help distinguish an inflammatory mass from an abscess. The diagnostic accuracy of an abdominal CT scan can be improved further by combining CT with oral and intravenous contrast material, giving information diagnostically superior to conventional X-ray studies using contrast.

A10 The correct answer is **B**.

A benign liver haemangioma is quite a common incidental finding on US. These lesions have a characteristic appearance on a *dynamic CT scan*, with enhancement by intravenous contrast medium.

A11 The correct answer is **K**.

Ultrasound is used to differentiate obstructive from hepatocellular jaundice. It is also useful in detecting the level of obstruction.

A12 The correct answer is **A**.

Intravenous urography (IVP) is still the best way to definitively exclude an obstructive uropathy. Ultrasound is useful if obstruction is associated with dilatation of the renal pelvis. Incomplete obstruction may not be evident on US. In addition IVP demonstrates the exact level of obstruction.

A13 The correct answer is **J**.

In this patient the aim is to establish whether the patient is pregnant (serum beta–HCG) and whether there is an intrauterine pregnancy. The likelihood for coexistence of an intrauterine and ectopic pregnancy is approximately 1 in 30 000; thus, if an intrauterine gestational sac is demonstrated, the chance of an ectopic pregnancy is very small. *Transvaginal ultrasound* is useful in cases of early pregnancy of uncertain dates. It can detect a gestational sac 3–4 days prior to the transabdominal US technique.

A14 The correct answer is **K**.

Females under 30 years of age usually have dense, featureless parenchyma on mammography, making interpretation difficult. *Ultrasound* is the preferred means to confirm the presence of a palpable mass in these patients and to differentiate normal parenchyma from a cyst or fibroadenoma.

A15 The correct answer is **K**.

Musculoskeletal ultrasound using high-frequency probes dedicated for the examination of superficial tissues is very useful in excluding partial or complete rotator cuff tendon tear.

A16 The correct answer is **L**.

Plain films of the lumbar spine give a good overall assessment of the lumbo-sacral region. A CT is indicated only in a small selection of patients when conservative treatment fails or nerve root or thecal compression are suspected.

A17 The correct answer is **H**.

A radionuclide bone scan is a very sensitive means of diagnosing a metatarsal stress fracture.

A18 The correct answer is **K**.

Children with bacteriologically proven urinary tract infection (UTI) have a high incidence of abnormalities requiring further treatment. Vesicoureteric reflux (VUR) is the most common abnormality (30%). Imaging is indicated after the first proven infection, with the aim to detect reflux, obstructive uropathy and renal scarring. *Renal ultrasound* is the modality of first choice in children for evaluating the kidneys, as it provides excellent anatomical information, is non-invasive and does not involve contrast material. Renal ultrasound is excellent at detecting hydronephrosis and most significant congenital anomalies. It can be readily repeated in patients with vesicoureteric reflux to ensure that renal growth is normal and to detect developing scars. Micturating cystourethrography (MCU) is indicated in all children under 4 years of age after the first UTI. It is the only way to detect VUR and anomalies of the male urethra. In older children, an MCU is normally not performed if the US is normal unless there is a history of repeated or complicated UTI.

A19   The correct answer is **B**.
A CT of the abdomen is used to image and diagnose acute pancreatitis. An abdominal ultrasound may be impaired by bowel gas in association with localised or general ileus. A CT scan is useful in showing enlargement of the pancreas, oedema and peripancreatic fluid collection. With contrast enhancement, CT can help in diagnosing areas of pancreatic necrosis.

A20   The correct answer is **I**.
Transrectal ultrasound (TRUS) is used to assess internal prostate architecture. If there is a significant difference between the serum prostate-specific antigen (PSA) and prostate size based on clinical or ultrasound examination, the possibility of an underlying malignancy is high. A TRUS will also assist imaging-guided biopsy by targeting focal hypoechoic areas.

A21   The correct answer is **L**.
Plain abdominal X-rays, together with a chest X-ray to display the diaphragm, are still the most helpful initial investigation in diagnosing intestinal obstruction. They often indicate the site (small or large bowel) and sometimes indicate the cause of the intestinal obstruction. Once the diagnosis of obstruction is made, if surgery is not immediately required, additional information can be provided by the use of contrast films using water-soluble gastrografin from above or below.

A22   The correct answer is **E**.
The aims of mammographic screening are to detect, by imaging, early breast cancers before they present clinically and to treat these screen-detected cancers optimally, usually by breast-conserving surgery, in the expectation (confirmed by several studies) of better results in these early tumours. Many benign conditions can mimic the mammographic signs of cancer and need to be differentiated. If diagnostic tests were 100% sensitive and 100% specific, no cancers would be missed and no benign lesions would be unnecessarily removed. *Imaging-guided biopsy* of these lesions increases diagnostic reliability. Using either ultrasound or stereotactic X-ray imaging, the lesion is identified and needle aspiration cytology (FNAC) or tissue core biopsy is done. A positive diagnosis of cancer facilitates a planned operation on a fully informed patient.

Questions such as those shown above have application in MCQ, and also in clinical vivas and objective structured clinical assessments. These types of questions are not currently used in the AMC MCQ assessments. These examples are included as an alternative aid for self assessment in the important field of diagnostic imaging.

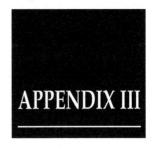

MEDICAL EPONYMS

The medical eponyms that follow were all drawn from this selection of MCQ. They are included for interest, not as examination material. Their diverse origins encompass all disciplines and a range of nationalities spanning the globe, highlighting the universality of medicine and its rich history. Their origins also reflect the ethnic diversity of the Australian population and of the many overseas-trained doctors who have successfully completed the AMC examination assessments over the past years to join and enhance the Australian health care work force.

Thomas Addison (1793–1860)   Addison disease

English physician at Guy's Hospital. He described adrenal insufficiency in 1855. Addison, Bright and Hodgkin comprised an illustrious trio at Guy's in the mid-19th century. It was the French physician, Armand Trousseau, who first referred to adrenal failure as 'Addison disease'.

Karl Albrecht (1856–1894)   Hamartoma

German anatomist. He originated the term 'hamartoma', and also described a small bone in the sphenoid–occipital region of the cranium.

Alois Alzheimer (1864–1915)   Alzheimer disease

German psychiatrist and neurologist. He published his classic description of presenile dementia in 1907. He was a contemporary of the neurologist Wilhelm Erb, neuropathologist Franz Nissl and psychiatrist Emil Kraepelin.

Virginia Apgar (1909–1974)   Apgar Score

American anaesthetist. She described score (out of 10) for clinical well-being of newborn babies at 1 min after birth.

Norman Rupert Barrett (1903–1979)   Barrett epithelium, Barrett ulcer

British thoracic surgeon who was born in Adelaide. In 1950 he described an area of replacement of oesophageal squamous epithelium by columnar epithelium resembling gastric mucosa, believed to be an acquired reparative or metaplastic response to oesophageal reflux of gastric contents. Ulceration can occur in the area and the lesion is considered premalignant.

Caspar Bartholin (1655–1738)   Bartholin gland, Bartholin cyst

Danish anatomist and physician. He described the bilateral glands situated near the vaginal introitus.

Sir Charles Bell (1774–1842)   Bell palsy, Bell sign, long thoracic nerve of Bell

English surgeon and anatomist at Middlesex Hospital in London. Also an accomplished artist, he attended the wounded at Waterloo, where he painted the battle scenes as well as performing surgery.

Edward Hallaran Bennett (1837–1907)   Bennett fracture

Professor of Surgery in Dublin. In 1882 he described a fracture dislocation of the metacarpal bone of the thumb.

Christian Albert Theodor Billroth (1829–1894)   Billroth I and II gastrectomy

Professor of Surgery at the University of Vienna. He performed the first successful distal partial gastrectomy in 1881. His work, and that of his pupils, heralded the development of modern gastrointestinal surgery. Distal gastrectomies are called Billroth I when gastro-duodenal reconstruction is used, Billroth II when gastrojejunal. He introduced concepts of surgical auditing and peer review and wrote on modern surgical education. He was an accomplished musician and close friend of Johannes Brahms.

John Templeton Bowen (1857–1941)   Bowen disease

American dermatologist at Harvard. He described *in situ* carcinoma of skin in 1912.

Alexander Breslow (1928–1980) and Wallace Clark Jr (b. 1924)   Staging of melanoma

American pathologists. In 1970 Breslow described the correlation with tumour thickness in determining prognosis. This is perhaps more easy to assess than the depth of invasion, as measured by Clark and reported in 1969.

Richard Bright (1789–1858)   Bright disease

English physician at Guy's Hospital. He described the clinical features of post-streptococcal nephritis with proteinuria in 1836.

Pierre Paul Broca (1824–1880)   Broca area, Broca aphasia (motor aphasia)

Professor of Surgery in Paris. He introduced hypnosis to surgery. In 1861 he developed the concept of left hemisphere dominance for motor control of speech and localised the area to the left inferior frontal gyri.

Sir Benjamin Collins Brodie (1783–1862)

English surgeon who pioneered the surgery of varicose veins.

Sir David Bruce (1855–1931)   Brucellosis, a disease contracted from the bacterium (*Brucella abortus*) causing infectious abortion in cattle

English physician and a founder of the study of tropical medicine. Identified the organism causing Malta fever in humans (*Brucella melitensis*) and the involvement of trypanosomes in sleeping sickness transmitted by the tsetse fly.

Denis Parsons Burkitt (1911–1993)   Burkitt lymphoma

English surgeon. In 1957 he identified the tumour that bears his name while practising in Uganda. He is also known for his work on high fibre diets in the prevention and treatment of gastrointestinal disease.

Sir Frank MacFarlane Burnet (1899–1985)   *Coxiella burnetii,*
and Herald Rae Cox (b. 1907)   **Q fever**

Burnet was an Australian scientist who received the Nobel Prize for Medicine in 1960 for originating the clonal theory of antibody production. Burnet also discovered the causative organism of Q (for Query) fever in 1937. Cox, an American virologist, isolated the organism at about the same time. The genus created to contain the rickettsial agent was named after Cox and the species after Burnet.

Julius Caesar (102–44 BC)   **Caesarean section**

In ancient times, incising the abdominal wall and uterus of the mother to give birth of an infant could be done on the death of a pregnant woman and was a legal obligation of clinicians in Roman law. Julius Caesar was said, probably incorrectly, to have been born thus.

Albert Leon Calmette (1863–1933)   **Bacillus Calmette–Guérin,**
and Camille Guérin (1872–1961)   **BCG**

French bacteriologists. They developed vaccination using an attenuated strain of tubercle bacilli at the Pasteur Institute in Paris in 1921 after discovering in 1908 that virulent bovine tubercle bacilli became less virulent on being cultured in a bile-containing medium. The hazards of a living vaccine were tragically demonstrated at Lübeck, when over 70 infants died of tuberculosis after vaccination with an improperly prepared vaccine.

Jean Marie Joseph Capgras (1873–1950)   **Capgras syndrome**

French psychiatrist. In 1923 he first described the delusion, more common in women, that close relatives or friends are replaced by impostors.

Anders Celsius (1701–1744)   **Celsius temperature scale**

Swedish astronomer and Professor of Astronomy at the University of Uppsala. He originated the centigrade thermometer scale in 1742, using as fixed points the freezing and boiling points of water.

Aulus Cornelius Celsus (53 BC–AD 7)   **Four cardinal signs**
of inflammation

Roman clinician during the time of the Emperor Tiberius. He wrote numerous treatises on medicine, described four classical signs of inflammation (calor, dolor, rubor, tumor) and was known as the Roman Hippocrates.

Jean-Martin Charcot (1825–1893)   **Charcot neuropathic joint,**
Charcot-Marie-Tooth disease:
peroneal muscular atrophy,
hereditary sensorimotor neuropathy

French neurologist and father of modern neurology. Described destructive arthropathy, usually secondary to neurosyphilis but also seen with diabetes, syringomyelia and leprosy. Described in 1886 (with his pupil Marie), peroneal muscular atrophy: hereditary wasting of the limbs confined to peripheral muscles below the knee and elbow, also associated with sensory or pyramidal involvement.

Pierre Marie (1853–1940)   **Charcot-Marie-Tooth disease**
French neurologist; pupil of Charcot.

Howard Henry Tooth (1856–1925)   **Charcot-Marie-Tooth disease**
English physician at St Bartholomew's Hospital London. He described the disease in 1886 independently of Charcot and Marie.

Gatian de Clérambault (1872–1934)   **de Clérambault syndrome**

French psychiatrist. He described the syndrome of erotomania, the delusional belief that a prominent public figure, usually older, is profoundly in love with the person, with either nil or brief acquaintance.

Edward Cock (1805–1892)   **Cock peculiar tumour**

Surgeon at Guy's Hospital in London. He was a renowned teacher and nephew of Sir Astley Cooper. His 'peculiar tumour' described an infected sebaceous cyst.

Sir Abraham Colles (1773–1843)   **Colles fracture, Colles perineal fascia**

Professor of Surgery in Dublin. He was first to describe, in 1814, the clinical features of the wrist fracture that bears his name.

Robin Royston Amos Coombs (b. 1921)   **Coombs test**

Professor of Immunology at Cambridge. He developed a test detecting red cell antibodies on the red cells (direct) or in the serum (indirect) by using a rabbit anti-serum against human red cells.

Sir Astley Paston Cooper (1768–1841)   **Cooper ligaments of the breast, iliopectineal ligament**

Surgeon and anatomist to St Thomas's and Guy's hospitals, London. He first described, in 1829, the fascial suspensory ligaments of the breast that bear his name.

Hans Gerhard Creutzfeldt (1885–1964)   **Creutzfeldt-Jakob**
Alfons Jakob (1884–1931)   **syndrome or disease**

German neurologists. In 1921 they independently described a syndrome of progressive encephalopathy with mental deterioration and psychosis, now thought due to a prion.

Burrill Bernard Crohn (1884–1983)   **Crohn disease**

American gastroenterologist who, in 1932, described with his colleagues Ginzburg and Oppenheimer, the disease they called regional ileitis, which has subsequently been known as Crohn disease.

Thomas Stephen Cullen (1868–1953)   **Cullen sign**

Baltimore gynaecologist who, in 1922, described the sign of umbilical discolouration as a feature of ruptured ectopic pregnancy.

Harvey Williams Cushing (1869–1939)   **Cushing syndrome, hypercortisolism**

Professor of Surgery at Harvard, Surgeon-in-Chief at Peter Bent Brigham Hospital in Boston and founder of the modern discipline of neurosurgery. He was the first to describe the clinical features of 'pituitary basophilism' in 1932.

Augusta Déjérine-Klumpke (1859–1927)   **Klumpke (T1) paralysis**

French neurologist and notable exemplar, against much opposition, for the role of women in medicine. Described the features of lower brachial plexus paralysis involving T1, often due to birth injury and particularly following breech delivery. With her husband Joseph Déjérine (1849–1917), also a neurologist, she performed research on the anatomy of nerve centres and founded a research institute in his memory.

Christian Johann Doppler (1803–1853)   Doppler effect

Austrian physicist who described the Doppler phenomenon in 1842, that the pitch of sound waves from a moving body is higher when the body is approaching the listener. This has had subsequent wide applications in radar, navigation, medicine and astronomy. Duplex–Doppler vascular imaging combines the Doppler principle and ultrasound to identify and quantify disturbances of flow.

James Douglas (1675–1742)   Recto-uterine pouch

Scottish physician and anatomist.

John Langdon Haydon Down (1828–1896)   Down syndrome

English physician who described 'Mongolism' in his Letsom lectures in 1866.

Guillaume Duchenne (1807–1875)   Duchenne muscular dystrophy

French neurologist who in 1868, described pseudohypertrophic infantile muscular dystrophy, an X-linked recessive disorder commencing before 5 years of age and involving pelvic and calf muscles with fatty infiltration initially giving pseudohypertrophy.

Cuthbert Esquire Dukes (1890–1977)   Stages A–C of colonic cancer

English pathologist at St Mark's Hospital, London.

Baron Guillaume Dupuytren (1777–1835)   Dupuytren disease or contracture

French surgeon who described this condition in 1831. He was an unpopular man once described as 'the first of surgeons, the last of men'. When Marjolin was appointed his assistant, Dupuytren purportedly addressed him coldly, 'Your appointment entitles you to operate when I am absent or ill. I am never absent and never ill'.

Ludwig Edinger (1855–1918) and Carl Friedrich Otto Westphal (1833–1890)   Edinger–Westphal nucleus

German neurologists. In 1885 in the fetus (LE) and in 1887 in the adult (CW), they described the nucleus beneath the aqueduct of Sylvius that gives rise to the pupillo–constrictor fibres of the oculomotor nerve.

Michael Anthony Epstein (b. 1921) and Yvonne Barr (b. 1932)   Epstein-Barr virus

Contemporary British virologists who isolated a new human herpes-like virus from cultured Burkitt lymphoma cells, since known as Epstein–Barr virus (EBV). It is the causative organism of infectious mononucleosis (glandular fever) and is believed to play a role in various human cancers, including Burkitt lymphoma and nasopharyngeal carcinoma.

Theodor Escherich (1857–1911)   *Escherichia*, the genus of Gram-negative enteric organisms

Munich paediatrician and bacteriologist. In 1885 he wrote the first account of *Bacillus coli* infections in children.

Gabriel Fallopio (1523–1562) **Fallopian tube or oviduct**
Italian anatomist and botanist, pupil of Vesalius and Professor of Anatomy in Padua.

Étienne Louis Arthur Fallot (1850–1911) **Fallot tetralogy**
French physician from Marseilles who described the syndrome (congenital cyanotic heart disease with pulmonary stenosis, ventricular septal defect, right ventricular hypertrophy, overriding aorta) in 1888.

Guido Fanconi (1882–1979) **Fanconi syndrome**
Zürich paediatrician. In 1931 he described an inherited metabolic disorder comprising renal tubular acidosis, aminoaciduria and vitamin D-resistant renal rickets.

Augustus Roi Felty (1895–1964) **Felty syndrome**
American physician who, in 1924, described the syndrome of pancytopenia and splenomegaly associated with rheumatoid arthritis.

Miller Fisher (b. 1910) **Miller Fisher syndrome: variant of Guillain-Barré syndrome**
Contemporary Canadian neurologist, who first reported the variant in 1956.

Jean Alfred Fournier (1832–1914) **Fournier gangrene**
French venereologist who described, in 1883, the condition of fulminating scrotal infection leading to cutaneous gangrene, frequently associated with diabetes.

Carl Friedlander (1847–1887) **Friedlander bacillus, pneumonia**
German bacteriologist, who discovered a bacillus causing pneumonia and who died at an early age from pulmonary tuberculosis.

Nikolaus Friedrich (1825–1882) **Friedrich ataxia**
Heidelberg neurologist. In 1863 he described a hereditary spinocerebellar degenerative disease with ataxia, diminished tendon reflexes, pes cavus, upgoing plantars and nystagmus.

Leopoldo Fregoli (1867–1936) **Fregoli syndrome or delusion**
Italian-born actor, famous for his ability to alter his facial appearance. Pioneer of the one-man show as a quick-change artist, mimic, singer and dancer. His name describes a delusional syndrome whereby strangers are misidentified as close acquaintances.

Herman Gardner (1912–1982) ***Gardnerella*: genus of pleomorphic Gram-negative bacteria**
American obstetrician and gynaecologist whose name was given to the bacteria that is found in the normal female genital tract and that can also cause bacterial vaginitis.

Hermann Treschow Gartner (1785–1827) **Gartner duct — lower remnant of mesonephric duct. Gartner cyst — cystic swelling of the vaginal remnant of Gartner's duct**
Copenhagen surgeon and anatomist who first discovered 'his' duct in a sow!

Gentian   **Gentian violet — aniline dye**

Named because its colour resembles the blossoms of the gentian plant, which in turn was named after King Gentius of Illyria (2nd century BC) who reportedly discovered that an extract of the root was an antidote for poisons.

Alfred Mathieu Giard (1846–1908)   **Giardiasis — the disease due to**
Giardia lamblia, a protozoal
organism causing diarrhoea

French biologist; the genus *Giardia* of intestinal zooflagellates was named in his honour.

Wilhelm Dusan Lambl (1824–1895)   **Giardia lamblia**

Czechoslovakian physician who, in 1860, was the first to describe the causative agent of Giardiasis in man.

Hans Christian Joachim Gram (1853–1938)   **Gram stain**

Danish physician who introduced his method of differential staining of bacteria with crystal violet in 1884. Bacteria taking up the stain are Gram positive, others are Gram negative.

Robert James Graves (1797–1853)   **Graves disease**

Irish physician. He described exophthalmic goitre in 1835.

Georges Charles Guillain (1876–1951)   **Guillain–Barré**
Jean Alexander Barré (1880–1967)   **syndrome**

French neurologists who, in 1916, published their description of an acute symmetrical lower motor neuron paralysis commencing distally and which travels proximally. It may involve the bulbar region and the diaphragm and is usually self-limiting with complete recovery. Also known as Landry–Guillain–Barré syndrome.

Jean Baptiste Octave Landry (1826–1865)   **Landry paralysis**

French physician who described an ascending paralysis in 1859, now linked with Guillain-Barré syndrome as Landry-Guillain-Barré syndrome.

Gerhard Henrik Armauer Hansen (1841–1912)   **Hansen disease**

Norwegian physician who devoted his professional life to the study of leprosy and identified the causative organism in 1873.

Alexis Frank Hartmann (1898–1964)   **Hartmann solution**

American paediatrician from St Louis who developed lactated Ringer's solution for intravenous use.

Henri Hartmann (1860–1952)   **Hartmann operation**
of sigmoid colectomy

French surgeon and Professor of Surgery at the Hôtel Dieu in Paris. He described, in the 1920s, operative excision of rectal and sigmoid colon cancer with closure of the lower rectal stump at or below the peritoneal reflection and with a terminal colostomy. The term is now used to describe a similar procedure used for complications of diverticular disease.

Robert Hartmann (1831–1893)   **Hartmann pouch**
of gall-bladder

German anatomist who described the dilatation of the gall-bladder neck below the cystic duct as it enters the bile duct.

Hakaru Hashimoto (1881–1934)   **Hashimoto auto-immune thyroiditis**

Japanese surgeon who published his description of chronic thyroiditis (struma lymphomatosa) in 1912.

William Heberden (1710–1801)   **Heberden nodes**

British physician. The description of the hard arthritic nodules named after him was published posthumously in 1802.

Lawrence Joseph Henderson (1879–1942) and Karl Albert Hasselbach (1874–1962)   **Henderson–Hasselbach equation**

Boston and Copenhagen biochemists, respectively. Henderson developed the chemical equations and nomograms used to describe blood buffer systems, which Hasselbach subsequently converted, in 1916, to logarithmic form.

Eduard Heinrich Henoch (1820–1910) and Johann Lucas Schönlein (1793–1864)   **Henoch–Schönlein purpura**

German physicians. Henoch–Schönlein purpura is a purpuric eruption without thrombocytopenia associated with abdominal colic and intussusception, and joint pains and swellings. In 1837 Schönlein described a form of purpura associated with pain in the joints and his pupil Henoch extended these observations and descriptions in 1868.

Harold Hirschsprung (1830–1916)   **Hirschsprung disease**

Danish paediatrician who published his description of congenital megacolon in 1888.

Thomas Hodgkin (1798–1866)   **Hodgkin disease**

English physician from Guy's Hospital who, in 1832, described the form of lymphoma associated with enlargement of the spleen and lymph nodes, which was subsequently named after him.

Johann Friedrich Horner (1831–1886)   **Horner syndrome**

Swiss ophthalmologist who, in 1869, described the syndrome of cervical sympathetic paralysis.

John Hunter (1728–1793)   **Hunterian subsartorial canal, perforating vein, chancre, ligation**

English surgeon, one of two medical brothers. Founded, virtually singlehanded, the disciplines of surgical anatomy, physiology, pathology and experimental surgery. Pioneered proximal ligation in treatment of arterial aneurysm.

George Sumner Huntington (1851–1916)   **Huntington chorea**

Third generation New York physician; described in 1872 a syndrome of hereditary chorea with uncontrollable tics, usually appearing in middle age and accompanied by mental deterioration.

Sir Jonathan Hutchinson (1828–1913)   **Hutchinson melanotic freckle**

English surgeon with major interests in syphilis and dermatology who described the clinical features of lentigo maligna in 1857.

Moritz Kaposi (1837–1902)   **Kaposi sarcoma**
Hungarian dermatologist who first described the clinical features of this sarcoma in 1872.

Bernhard Kayser (1869–1954)   **Kayser–Fleischer ring**
and Bruno Otto Fleischer (1848–1909)
German ophthalmologists who were first to describe the brown ring around the iris due to copper deposition in Wilson disease.

Mrs Kell   **Kell blood group**
Red cell antigen present in approximately 10% of the population which may cause haemolytic reactions after multiple transfusions. Named, as was the Duffy blood group, after the first patient in whom the antigen was recognised.

Theodor Albrecht Edwin Klebs (1834–1913)   *Klebsiella* **genus of enteric bacteria**
German bacteriologist who was the first to identify a number of pathogenic bacteria and introduced paraffin embedding for tissue sections.

Sergei Sergeyevich Korsakoff (1853–1900)   **Korsakoff psychosis, syndrome**
Russian neuropsychiatrist who initiated the principles of non-restraint in patient management. In 1887 he first described the syndrome of mental deterioration, memory loss and confabulation, seen as a sequel of chronic alcoholism.

Baron Joseph Lister (1827–1912)   **Listerism, the practice of antiseptic surgery; listeriosis, infection, typically meningitis in newborns due to bacteria of genus** *Listeria*
Professor of Surgery in Glasgow, Edinburgh and London who introduced antiseptic principles to surgery. His *Lancet* paper in 1867 'A new method of treating compound fractures' was one of the most significant in the history of medicine. He, John Hunter and Thomas Willis are buried in Westminster Abbey.

Marcello Malpighi (1628–1694)   **Malpighian corpuscles**
Professor of Medicine at Bologna and founder of microscopical anatomy. He described the corpuscles of lymphoid tissue around the arterial branches within the spleen.

Charles Mantoux (1877–1947)   **Mantoux test**
French physician who showed that the intradermal response to tuberculin, which he described in 1908, was more sensitive than that using a subcutaneous injection. The Mantoux test induces a delayed hypersensitivity reaction following intradermal injection of tuberculin in a person previously exposed to tuberculosis or immunised with BCG vaccine.

Antonin Bernard Jean Marfan (1858–1942)   **Marfan syndrome**
French paediatrician who, in 1896, described the syndrome marked by arachnodactyly, dislocation of the crystalline lens of the eye and abnormal flexibility of the joints. Marfan syndrome is a disorder of collagen and elastic tissue. Patients have characteristically long and narrow facies with high-arched palates and an arm span greater than height, double-jointedness, subluxation of the lens and aortic regurgitation predisposing to dissection of the aorta.

Jean-Nicolas Marjolin (1780–1850)   **Marjolin ulcer**

A much respected amiable, honourable and erudite French surgeon whose name is applied to squamous cell carcinoma developing in a chronic benign ulcer, such as an old unhealed burn or a wound scar. He was Dupuytren's assistant at the Hôtel Dieu in Paris, tolerating Dupuytren's disdain and arrogance for several years. Marjolin, in a tract on ulcers, did not describe clearly the association of cancer with a burn scar; whereas Dupuytren did so in his own writings. Robert Smith of Dublin later incorrectly, but lastingly, bestowed the eponym on Marjolin rather than on Dupuytren.

Charles McBurney (1845–1913)   **McBurney point**

American surgeon. A pioneer in the diagnosis and treatment of appendicitis who described, in 1889, the pressure point subsequently named in his honour.

Johann Friedrich Meckel (1781–1833)   **Meckel diverticulum —
                                                persistence of
                                                vitellointestinal duct**

Professor of Anatomy and Surgery at Halle; followed his father in that position.

Medusa   **Caput Medusae**

In Greek mythology, gorgon with hair of writhing snakes. Medusa was slain by Perseus.

Prosper Ménière (1799–1862)   **Ménière syndrome**

French otolaryngologist who described, in 1861, the syndrome of labyrinthine vertigo associated with nausea, vomiting, tinnitus, nystagmus and hearing loss.

Giovanni Battista Monteggia (1762–1815)   **Monteggia fracture**

Italian anatomist and surgeon who described a fracture in the proximal part of the ulna with dislocation of the head of the radius.

Giovanni Battista Morgagni (1682–1771)   **Testicular hydatid of
                                                Morgagni, diaphragmatic
                                                foramen of Morgagni**

Professor of Anatomy at Padua, founder of pathological anatomy.

Baron Karl Friedrich Hieronymus   **Münchausen syndrome**
von Münchausen (1720–1797)

Münchausen was a retired German cavalry officer who told a number of preposterous stories about his heroic exploits to guests of his estate in Hesse. These were subsequently published by an impecunious family friend, RE Raspe, in England in a book *Baron Münchausen's Narrative of his Marvellous Travels and Campaigns in Russia*. Münchausen syndrome was coined as a name by Richard Asher, a British physician, to describe a syndrome of factitious illness, with doctor-shopping, using vivid and imaginative symptoms to obtain medical care, hospitalisation or drugs.

Albert Ludwig Sigesmund Neisser   *Neisseria*, **genus of
(1885–1916)**   **Gram-negative organisms that
                                                contains the organism responsible
                                                for gonorrhoea**

German physician and bacteriologist who discovered the causative organism of gonorrhoea in 1897.

Ruggero Oddi (1864–1913)   sphincter of Oddi

Italian physiologist who, in 1887, described sphincteric fibres around the termination of the bile duct as it enters the duodenum.

Robert Bayley Osgood (1873–1956) and Carl Schlatter (1864–1934)   Osgood–Schlatter disease

American and German surgeons respectively. In 1903 they independently described apophysitis of the tibial tubercle, typically in early adolescent males, nowadays a frequent consequence of playing basketball.

Sir William Osler (1849–1919)   Osler disease, Osler–Weber disease: hereditary haemorrhagic telangiectasia

Renowned Canadian-born physician, medical aphorist and educator. Filled Chairs of Medicine successively at four universities: McGill, Pennsylvania, Johns Hopkins and Oxford. Hereditary haemorrhagic telangiectasia is a rare but important vascular anomaly, inherited as an autosomal dominant, with multiple small telangiectases of the skin, mucous membranes, gastrointestinal tract and internal organs. It is associated with recurrent episodes of bleeding, particularly upper gastrointestinal, with haematemesis and melaena.

Frederick Weber (1863–1962)

English physician who independently described the syndrome of inherited telangiectasia (see also Sturge–Weber syndrome).

Sir James Paget (1814–1899)   Paget disease of bone — osteitis deformans; Paget disease of nipple — eczematoid lesion due to cutaneous infiltration from an underlying ductal carcinoma; Paget disease of penis — carcinoma *in situ*

English surgeon at St Bartholomew's Hospital, London, who discovered trichinosis in muscle while dissecting as a medical student. Made numerous outstanding contributions to surgical pathology and surgery.

Henry K Pancoast (1875-1939)   Pancoast syndrome, tumour

American radiologist. He was appointed to the first American Chair of Roentgenology (later radiology) at the University of Pennsylvania in 1912. He described, in 1932, the syndrome of brachialgia, atrophy of muscles of the hand and Horner syndrome observed in apical lung tumours (pulmonary sulcus tumour), which involved the lower brachial plexus.

George Nicholas Papanicolou (1883–1962)   Papanicolou (PAP) smear or test for cervical cancer

American pathologist who developed the technique of the cervical smear in the 1930s, which was the forerunner of cytological testing for cancer.

James Parkinson (1755–1824)   Parkinson disease, parkinsonism

English physician who published his essay on the shaking palsy (paralysis agitans) in 1817.

Raymond Pearl (1879–1940)　　　　　　　　　**Pearl Index**
Biologist and mathematician, Professor of Biology at Johns Hopkins University. He described an index of contraceptive efficacy, measured as pregnancies per 100 women-years of treatment.

Hugh Spear Pemberton (1890–1956)　　　　　**Pemberton sign**
Liverpool physician and renowned teacher who described the 'Sign of Submerged Goitre 'in a brief letter to *The Lancet* in 1946: 'elevate both arms till they touch the side of the head; after a moment or so congestion of the face, cyanosis, and lastly distress become apparent'. The sign has also, but mistakenly, been attributed to John de Jarnett Pemberton (1887–1968), a Mayo Clinic surgeon who wrote extensively on thyroid surgery, including retrosternal goitres, in the 1920s.

George Clemens Perthes　　**Perthes disease — osteochondritis**
(1869–1927)　　　　　　　　　**juvenalis of femoral head;**
　　　　　　　　　Perthes test — for deep venous occlusion
German surgeon, who described osteochondritic hip deformity. He also described a test for assessing patency of the deep venous system of the leg: a venous tourniquet is placed mid-thigh and the subject walks for 5 min. Deep venous occlusion and communicating vein incompetence is demonstrated by pain and increased prominence of superficial veins.

Jacques Calvé (1895–1954)
and Arthur Thornton Legg (1874–1939)
French and American orthopaedic surgeons respectively. Calvé, Perthes and Legg independently described the condition of osteochondritis of the hip between 1910 and 1913 and the condition is also known as Calvé–Legg–Perthes disease.

JLA Peutz (1886–1957)　　　　　**Peutz–Jeghers syndrome**
and Harold Jeghers (b. 1904)
Dutch and American physicians, respectively, who described an inherited syndrome characterised by gastrointestinal polyposis (usually hamartomatous polyps of the small bowel) and melanin pigmentation of the skin and mucous membranes. The syndrome is transmitted as an autosomal dominant.

Johann Conrad Peyer (1653–1712)　　　　　**Peyer patches**
Swiss anatomist who, in 1677, described nodules of lymphoid tissue in the small intestine.

Henry Stanley Plummer (1874–1936)　**Plummer–Vinson syndrome;**
and Porter Paisley Vinson (1890–1959)　**also called Paterson–**
　　　　　　　　　Brown–Kelly syndrome
Plummer and Vinson were American physicians at the Mayo Clinic who, in 1912, described the syndrome of dysphagia, glossitis and iron-deficiency anaemia.

Donald Ross Paterson (1863–1939)
and Adam Brown-Kelly (1865–1941)
British otolaryngologists who independently described sideropenic dysphagia in 1919.

Johannes Evangelista Purkinje　　　**Purkinje network, fibres**
(1787–1869)
Czech physiologist who, in 1839, described the subendarcardial network of cells and fibres constituting the terminal ramifications of the conducting system of the heart.

Maurice Raynaud (1834–1881)   **Raynaud disease/syndrome**

French physician who, in 1862, described the vascular disorder, now known by his name, as his graduation thesis.

Friedrich Daniel von Recklinghausen   **Von Recklinghausen disease**
(1833–1910)   **of nerve — neurofibromatosis;**
of bone — osteitis fibrosa cystica
due to hyperparathyroidism

German Professor of Pathology who wrote classic articles on neurofibromatosis in 1887 and on osteitis fibrosa cystica (hyperparathyroidism) in 1891.

Ralph Douglas Kenneth Reye (1912–1977)   **Reye syndrome**

Australian pathologist, Head of Pathology at the Royal Alexandra Hospital for Children in Sydney. He described a syndrome, in 1963, of encephalopathy and fatty degeneration of liver and other viscera in children, usually following viral infections (chicken pox, influenza) or aspirin administration.

Rhesus   **Rhesus factor**

Species of monkey sharing red cell antigens with humans.

Howard Taylor Ricketts (1871–1910)   **Rickettsia — genus of**
bacteria causing typhus
and Q fever

American pathologist who discovered the causative organisms of Rocky Mountain spotted fever and later Mexican typhus. He contracted and died from typhus during his investigations. Rickettsial organisms mostly live intracellularly in biting arthropods, causing disease when transmitted to man by the bite of the tick, louse or mite.

Sidney Ringer (1835–1910)   **Ringer solution,**
Ringer–Locke solution

British paediatrician who developed a balanced electrolyte solution isosmotic with body fluids for keeping isolated organs functional for long periods.

Frank Spiller Locke (1871–1949)

English physiologist who, in 1894, introduced an electrolyte solution with similar objectives.

Daniel Elmer Salmon (1850–1914)   *Salmonella* — **genus of Gram**
negative rod-shaped bacteria
that includes the bacterium
causing typhoid

American veterinary pathologist who discovered that dead bacteria could confer immunity against live organisms, which became the basis for the typhoid and poliomyelitis vaccines.

Sella turcica

Pituitary fossa of the sphenoid, resembling a Turkish saddle with high supports front and back.

Hugo Joseph Schiff (1834–1915)   **periodic acid-Schiff (PAS)**
reaction

German chemist. Glycogen, glycoproteins and related polysaccharides stain red in tissue sections after treatment with periodic acid and Schiff reagent.

Kiyoshi Shiga (1870–1957)   *Shigella* — **genus of Gram-negative bacillus**
Japanese bacteriologist who discovered the Shiga dysentery bacillus in 1897.

Henrik Samuel Conrad Sjögren (b. 1899)   **Sjögren syndrome**
Swedish ophthalmologist who described, in 1933, the syndrome of keratoconjunctivitis sicca, xerostomia, and lymphocytic infiltration of salivary and lacrimal glands, often associated with rheumatoid arthritis.

Robert William Smith (1807–1873)   **Smith fracture**
Professor of Surgery in Dublin after Abraham Colles. Described a fracture of the radius with forward displacement of the lower fragment. Also described cancer in burn scars and coined the term 'Marjolin ulcer'.

Sir George Frederick Still (1868–1941)   **Still disease**
Physician to the Hospital for Sick Children, London, who described the clinical features of juvenile arthritis in 1896 in his MD thesis.

William Sturge (1850–1919)   **Sturge–Weber syndrome:**
and Frederick Weber (1863–1962)   **encephalofacial angiomatosis**
English physicians who described a congenital syndrome consisting of a (usually unilateral) port-wine stain (naevus flammeus) over the trigeminal nerve distribution with an accompanying similar vascular disorder of the underlying meninges and cerebral cortex.

Jacobus Sylvius (1478–1555)   **Aqueduct of Sylvius**
French anatomist, teacher of Vesalius. He described the cerebral aqueduct connecting the third and fourth cerebral ventricles.

Friedrich Trendelenburg (1844–1924)   **Trendelenburg sign,**
position, operation, test
German surgeon who is commemorated by his sign for sapheno–femoral venous incompetence, the head-down position for pelvic surgery, the open operation for pulmonary embolectomy, and the test for pelvic stability. Signs of sapheno–femoral incompetence were actually described earlier by Benjamin Brodie.

George Grey Turner (1877–1951)   **Grey Turner sign**
English Professor of Surgery who described the sign of local loin and flank discolouration after an attack of pancreatitis.

Henry Hubert Turner (1892–1970)   **Turner syndrome**
American endocrinologist who in 1938, described a genetically determined condition with one X and no Y chromosome, outwardly female phenotype and incomplete and infertile gonads.

Antonio Maria Valsalva (1666–1723)   **Valsalva manoeuvre**
Italian anatomist who was taught by Malpighi and later became Professor of Anatomy at Bologna and taught Morgagni there. In a treatise on the ear in 1704, he described the manoeuvre of forced expiration against closed mouth and nose, testing the patency of the Eustachian tubes.

Abraham Vater (1684–1751)   **Duodenal papilla and**
ampulla of Vater
German anatomist.

Rudolf Ludwig Karl Virchow (1821–1902) Virchow triad
The leading German physician of the 19th century. He described his triad of the pathogenesis of thrombosis (vessel wall injury, stasis, changes in blood constituents) in a classic book on cellular pathology in 1858.

Richard von Volkmann (1830–1899) Volkmann contracture
German Professor of Surgery. He described the contracture in 1881 and was a major influence in introducing Listerian principles of antisepsis in Europe.

Alfred Scott Warthin (1866–1931) Warthin tumour — adenolymphoma
Professor of Pathology at Ann Arbor, Michigan. In addition to his work on salivary glands and the lymphatic system, he published a classic work on fat embolism in 1913.

William Henry Welch *Clostridium welchii*: Gram-positive
(1850–1934) sporing bacillus causative of gas gangrene
American pathologist who discovered the bacillus causing gas gangrene in 1892, he was Professor of Pathology at Johns Hopkins in Baltimore from 1884. With William Osler (Professor of Medicine), William Stewart Halsted (Surgery) and Howard Kelly (Obstetrics and Gynaecology), he developed a clinical school of outstanding (perhaps unequalled) merit.

Karl Wernicke (1848–1904) Wernicke aphasia — receptive or sensory aphasia; Wernicke encephalopathy
German neuropsychiatrist and Professor of Neurology at Breslau. In 1861, he described the area in the temporal gyrus responsible for receptive aphasia. He also described, in 1881, the eponymous encephalopathy; comprising a confused state with cerebellar signs and peripheral neuritis and due to thiamine deficiency associated with alcoholism or malnutrition.

Thomas Wharton (1614–1673) Wharton duct
English physician who described the submandibular duct in 1656.

Allen Whipple (1881–1963) Whipple operation, Whipple triad
American surgeon, Professor of Surgery at Columbia, New York. His contributions to disorders of the pancreas included description of the operation of pancreaticoduodenectomy and a description of the Whipple triad, diagnostic of a pancreatic insulinoma (low fasting blood sugar, initiation of an attack by fasting and recovery after giving glucose).

George Hoyt Whipple (1878–1976) Whipple disease — intestinal lipodystrophy
American pathologist, Dean of the School of Medicine at Rochester (New York), who conceived the idea of using a liver diet to treat pernicious anaemia and received the Nobel Prize for Medicine in 1934. Intestinal lipodystrophy, described in 1907, is a rare disease, probably infective, affecting primarily the small intestine with accumulation of lipid deposits in lymphatic tissues with subsequent systemic involvement. Macrophages in the lamina propria of the small intestine give a positive reaction to a PAS test.

Max Wilms (1867–1918) Wilms tumour — nephroblastoma
German surgeon who, in 1898, described the embryonal tumour of the kidney named after him.

Samuel Alexander Kinnier Wilson (1877–1937)

Wilson disease — hepatolenticular degeneration — cerebellar signs and cirrhosis with copper deposition

British neurologist who published his monograph on the disease bearing his name in 1912.

Louis Wolff (1898–1972), Sir John Parkinson (1885–1976) Paul Dudley White (1886–1973)

Wolff–Parkinson–White syndrome

American, English and American cardiologists, respectively. Together they described the syndrome of supraventricular tachycardia, showing a short P–R interval and widened QRS complex on electrocardiography, in 1930.

Robert Milton Zollinger (1903–1992) and Edwin Ellison (1918–1970)

Zollinger–Ellison syndrome

American surgeons from Columbus, Ohio. In 1955 they described the syndrome linking intractable peptic ulcers with tumours of the pancreas which secrete a gastrin-like substance.

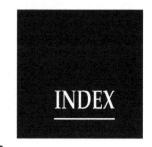

INDEX

The numbers refer to the question numbers in Section 1.

The commentaries in Section 2 are numbered in the same sequence as the questions.

(P), picture.

Printed in the United States
By Bookmasters